KETO AFTER 50

2 BOOKS IN 1

The New Ketogenic Diet Guide for Seniors. Over 500 Simple Keto Recipes and 30-Day Meal Plan - Balance Hormones, Reset Your Metabolism, Stay Healthy, and Boost your Energy.

By
KAREN TURNER

DISCLAIMER

The information in this e-book is provided for informational purposes only, and it aims to provide accurate and reliable information regarding the subject matter and topic covered.

The author and publisher do not bear any responsibility towards any person or entity with respect to any repair, damage, or financial loss resulting from or alleged resulting directly or indirectly from this electronic book.

The post is sold with the idea that the publisher is not required to provide accounting services, officially permitted or otherwise eligible. If counseling is necessary, legal, or professional, the individual practicing in the profession should be directed.

No reproduction, copying, or transmission of any part of this document electronically or in print is permitted. This publication is prohibited from registration, and this document is not permitted to store unless you obtain written permission from the publisher. All rights are saved.

The author owns all copyrights that the publisher does not own. Trademarks used are not approved, and the publication of the trademark does not contain permission or endorsement from the trademark owner.

TABLE OF CONTENT

- DISCLAIMER 2
- INTRODUCTION 10
- WHAT IS THE KETO DIET? 11
- KETO FOR WOMEN AND MAN OVER 50 ... 19
- RECOMMENDED KETO FOODS 22
- KETO RECIPES FOR WOMEN/MAN OVER 50 .. 24
- BREAKFAST 24
  - 01. Tortilla Breakfast Casserole 24
  - 02. Pecan-Banana Pops 25
  - 03. Greek Breakfast Wraps 26
  - 04. Curried Chicken Breast Wraps 27
  - 05. Baked Salmon Fillets with 28
  - 06. Cinnamon and Spice Overnight Oats 29
  - 07. Mexican Casserole 30
  - 08. Microwaved Fish and Asparagus with Tarragon Mustard Sauce 31
  - 09. Hearty Hot Cereal with Berries 32
- LUNCH AND DINNER 34
  - 10. Protein Power Sweet Potatoes 34
  - 11. Penne Pasta with Vegetables 35
  - 12. Spinach and Swiss Cheese Omelet 36
  - 13. Broiled Halibut with Garlic Spinach 37
  - 14. Quinoa with Curried Black 38
  - 15. Quinoa Pilaf 40
- GRAINS AND BEANS 42
  - 16. Mushroom Bean Spread 42
  - 17. Black Bean Burger 43
  - 18. BBQ Black Bean & Jalepeño Burger 44
  - 19. Green Pea Risotto 46
  - 20. Dilly White Beans 47
  - 21. Peppered Pinto Beans 49
- BREAD 51
  - 22. Cinnamon Bread 51
  - 23. Cheesy Flax & Chia 52
  - 24. Paleo Keto Shortbread Cookies 53
  - 25. Chocolate Gas Ingredients (Optional): 54
  - 26. Savane Bread with Coconut and Rosemary 55
  - 27. Cauliflower Coconut Bread 56
  - 28. Avocado Chocolate Bread 57
- BEVERAGES AND SMOOTHIES 59
  - 29. Garden Green Smoothie Bag 59
  - 30. Keto Vanilla Milk Shake 59
  - 31. Walnut Milk 60
  - 32. Alkaline Detox Tea 61
  - 33. Green Fruit Juice 62
  - 34. Flat Flush Juice 62
- VEGETABLES AND SALADS 64
  - 35. Salad with Plum Vinaigrette 64
  - 36. Shrimp and Cranberry Salad 65
  - 37. Tuna and Bean Salad Pockets 66
  - 38. Grilled Chicken Salad with Poppy 67
  - 39. Cucumber-Mullet-Avocado Salad 68
  - 40. Steamed Cauliflower 69
  - 41. Pomegranate, Arugula Salad 70
  - 42. Smoky Coleslaw 71
  - 43. Garlic and Herb Zoodles 72
- SNACKS 74
  - 44. Amazing chocolate cheesecake 74
  - 45. Walnut Chocolate Bites 76
  - 46. Cinnamon and caramel pudding 77
  - 47. Cheesecake Mousse 78
  - 48. Chocolate and Mint Cupcakes 79
  - 49. Pumpkin Pie Without Crust 80
  - 50. Coconut Blondies 81
  - 51. Italian Crackers 82
  - 52. Easy Granola Bars 84
  - 53. Quinoa Crunch Blueberry Muffins 85
  - 54. Keto Barueri Cocoa 87
  - 55. Baked Granola 88
- SOUP 90
  - 56. Coconut Curry Lentil Soup 90
  - 57. Easy Chicken Pasta Soup 91
  - 58. Quick Miso Soup with 92
  - 59. Hearty Shrimp and Kale Soup 93
  - 60. Black Bean Soup 94
  - 61. Curried Cauliflower Soup 96
- SIDE DISHES 98
  - 62. Toasted Pepper Jack Sandwiches 98

63. Taco Pita Pizzas..................................98
64. Italian Chicken Sandwich....................99
65. Hamburgers with Sesame Buns 101
66. Low Carb Sandwiches.......................103

SAUCES, DIPS AND DRESSINGS.................106
67. Roasted Bell Pepper Hummus 106
68. Blood Orange Vinaigrette...................107

FISH, BEEF, PORK, AND CHICKEN................109
69. Salmon and Tomato Egg Sandwiches 109
70. Pork Loin Chops with Mango Salsa 109
71. Roast Chicken with Balsamic Vinegar 111
72. Orange-Five-Spice Roasted Chicken ..112
73. Orange-Tangerine Up-the- Butt 113
74. Lemon-Sesame Chicken 114
75. Chinese Sticky Wings.........................116
76. Wicked Wings 117
77. Chicken Breast with Roasted 118
Vegetarian..120
78. Olive Tapenade on Raw Vegetable.....120
79. Pumpkin Pie Bites 121
80. Chocolate Covered Macaroons...........122
81. Low coconut macadamia bars.............123
82. Oatmeals Bars 125
83. Mini Choco Coco Cups 126

CONCLUSION..128

DISCLAIMER..131

INTRODUCTION...132

THE BASICS OF KETOSIS............................133

HEALTH BENEFITS OF KETO DIET FOR WOMEN OVER 50 138

KETO COMPARED TO OTHER DIETS 142

CAUTION FOR KETO 145

MAKING PROPER MEAL PLANS 148

WHAT TO EAT ON THE KETO DIET? 150

30 DAY KETO MEAL PLAN 156

KETO DELICIOUS RECIPES..............................157

BREAKFAST..157
84. Pizza Dip..157
85. Morning Pie..157
86. Blender Pancakes..............................158
87. Sausage Patties 159
88. Keto Breakfast Mix.............................159
89. Chicken Omelet..................................160
90. Pepperoni Pizza Omelet.....................161
91. Kale Fritters 161
92. Italian Spaghetti Casserole 162
93. Chorizo and Mozzarella Omelet..........163
94. Ricotta Cloud Pancakes with Whipped Cream..164
95. Mushroom & Cheese Lettuce Wraps..165
96. Bacon & Cheese Pesto Mug Cakes.......165
97. Cream Cheese Soufflé.......................166
98. Morning Casserole.............................167

LAUNCH & DINNER 169
99. Zesty Chili Lime Tuna Salad 169
100. Brussels Sprouts and Bacon 169
101. Super Simple Chicken Cauliflower.....170
102. Prep-Ahead Low-Carb Casserole......171
103. BBQ Pulled Beef Sando 171
104. Stuffed peppers................................172
105. Glazed salmon 173
106. Coconut shrimp................................173
107. Shrimp salad 174
108. Little Portobello pizza.......................175
109. Duck and Eggplant Casserole 176
110. Spicy Breakfast Sausage 176
111. Classic Chicken Salad.......................177
112. Creamed Sausage with Spaghetti 177
113. Chicken Fajitas with Peppers............178
114. Crispy Chicken Drumsticks...............179
115. Chicken Fillet with Brussels Sprouts 179
116. Chicken Breasts with Mustard...........180
117. Chinese-Style Cabbage with Turkey 181
118. Easy Turkey Meatballs......................181
119. Chicken with Mediterranean Sauce.182
120. Easy Roasted Turkey Drumsticks 183
121. Herbed Chicken Breasts...................183
122. Cheese and Prosciutto Chicken 184
123. Boozy Glazed Chicken 185
124. Festive Turkey Rouladen 185
125. Pan-Fried Chorizo Sausage 186
126. Chinese Bok Choy and Turkey Soup 187
127. Italian-Style Turkey Wings.................187

- 128. Easy Chicken Tacos ... 188
- DESSERT ... 189
  - 129. Greek-Style Cheesecake ... 189
  - 130. Caramel Chocolate Pudding ... 189
  - 131. Old-Fashioned Penuche Bars ... 190
  - 132. Easiest Keto Cheesecake Ever ... 190
  - 133. Chocolate Pudding ... 191
  - 134. Cranberry Cream Surprise ... 191
  - 135. Coconut Dream ... 192
  - 136 Keto Sorbet ... 192
  - 137. White Chocolate Berry Cheesecake ... 193
  - 138. Coconut Pillow ... 193
  - 139. Coffee Surprise ... 194
  - 140. Chocolate Cheesecake ... 194
  - 141. Almond Crusty ... 195
  - 142. Cheesecake Cups ... 195
  - 143. Strawberry Shake ... 195
- SOUP ... 197
  - 144. Cream of Red Bell Pepper Soup ... 197
  - 145. Stuffed Pepper Soup ... 197
  - 146. Shiitake Mushroom and Asparagus Soup ... 198
  - 147. Green Chile Chicken Soup ... 199
  - 148. Egg Drop Soup ... 200
  - 149. Vegetable Cream Soup ... 200
  - 150. Beef and Mushroom Soup ... 201
  - 151. Columbian Creamy Avocado Soup ... 202
  - 152. Chicken Avocado Soup ... 202
  - 153. Hot Avocado Curry with Shrimp ... 203
  - 154. Lamb and Herb Bone Broth ... 204
- SNACKS ... 205
  - 155. Stuffed Mini Peppers ... 205
  - 156. Homemade Wings in Spicy ... 205
  - 157. Oven-Baked Cheesy Zucchini ... 206
  - 158. Holiday Prawn Sticks ... 206
  - 159. Deviled Eggs with Peppers ... 207
  - 160. Ranch Chicken Wings ... 208
  - 161. Colby Cheese-Stuffed Meatballs ... 208
  - 162. Cheese and Artichoke Dip ... 209
  - 163. Italian Cheese Crisps ... 210
  - 164. Paprika Cheese Dipping Sauce ... 210
- VEGETARIAN KETO RECIPES ... 211
  - 165. Generous Green Bean Fries ... 211
  - 166. Traditional Roasted Asparagus ... 211
  - 167. King-Style Roasted Bell Pepper ... 212
  - 168. Tastes Like Heaven Garlic and ... 213
  - 169. Rockstar Creamy Mashed ... 213
  - 170. Appetizing Kale Chips ... 214
- KEEPING TRACK OF YOUR KETO DIET ... 215
- NEGATIVE MOMENTS AND OVERCOMING ... 218
- TIPS AND TRICKS FOR KETO WEIGHT LOSS ... 221
- CONCLUSION ... 225

BONUS EXTRA RECIPES

- BREAKFASTS ... 228
  - 171. Breakfast Egg Rolls ... 228
  - 172. Keto Air Fryer Fish Sticks ... 228
  - 173. Low Carb Mozzarella Sticks ... 229
  - 174. Homemade Sausage Rolls ... 230
  - 175. Air Fryer Tofu Scramble ... 231
  - 176. Air Fryer Hard Boiled Eggs ... 232
  - 177. Fried Cheesecake Bites ... 232
  - 178. Air Fryer Fried Parmesan Zucchini ... 233
  - 179. Keto Creamed Spinach ... 234
- Lunches ... 235
  - 180. Air Fried Cauliflower Recipe ... 235
  - 181. Keto Air Fryer Double ... 235
  - 182. Air Fryer Pork Chops & Broccoli ... 236
  - 183. Air Fryer Tuna Patties ... 236
  - 184. Air Fryer Carne Asada ... 237
  - 185. Healthy Eggplant Parmesan ... 238
  - 186. Air Fryer Radish Hash Browns ... 239
  - 187. Air Fryer Chicken Quesadilla ... 239
  - 188. Tomato Basil Scallops ... 240
  - 189. Air Fryer Keto Low Garb ... 241
- Appetizers and Side Dishes ... 242
  - 190. Air Fryer Zucchini Fries ... 242
  - 191. Roasted Turnips ... 242
  - 192. Keto Air-Fried Pickles ... 243

- 193. Air-Fried Onion Rings 243
- 194. Air Fryer Avocado Fries 244
- 195. Air-Fried Okra 245
- 196. Baked Chicken Nuggets 245
- 197. Air Fryer Egg Cups 247
- 198. Air Fryer Frittata 247
- 199. Air Fried Blooming Onion 248

Fish and Seafood 249
- 200. Perfect Air Fried Salmon 249
- 201. Air Fryer Salmon Cakes 249
- 202. Air Fryer Coconut Shrimp 250
- 203. Air Fryer Crispy Fish 251
- 204. Air Fryer Parchment Fish 251
- 205. Lemon Garlic Shrimp 252
- 206. Coconut Curry Salmon Cakes 253
- 207. Air Fryer Parmesan Shrimp 254
- 208. Keto Air Fryer Shrimp Scampi 255
- 209. Tomato Mayonnaise Shrimp 256

Poultry Food 257
- 210. Air Fryer Chicken Wings Sauce 257
- 211. Keto Thai Chili Chicken Wings 257
- 212. Keto Adobo Air Fried Chicken 259
- 213. Jalapeno Popper Stuffed Chicken 259
- 214. Herb-Marinated Chicken Thighs 260
- 215. Air Fryer Chicken Nuggets 261
- 216. Bacon Wrapped Chicken Bites 262
- 217. Air Fryer Chicken Parmesan 262
- 218. Air Fryer Keto Chicken Meatballs 263
- 219. Keto Southern Fried Chicken 264
- 220. Chicken Strips Recipe 265
- 221. Chick-Fil-A Copycat Recipe 265
- 222. Crumbed Chicken Tenderloins 266

Meat Recipes 267
- 223. Air Fryer Steak with Garlic Butter 267
- 224. Air Fryer Meatloaf 267
- 225. Air Fryer Ribeye with Coffee 268
- 226. Air Fryer Crispy Pork Belly 269
- 227. Keto Beef Satay 270
- 228. Air Fryer Bacon 271
- 229. Keto Air Fryer Meatloaf Sliders 271
- 230. Air Fried Spicy Bacon Bites 272
- 231. Keto Lasagna 272

Vegetables 274
- 232. Three Cheese Stuffed Mushrooms ... 274
- 233. Air Fryer roasted Asian broccoli 274
- 234. Cauliflower Buffalo Wings 275
- 235. Air Fryer Herbed Brussels Sprouts .. 276
- 236. Cilantro Ranch Sweet 276
- 237. Air-Fried Asparagus 277
- 238. Cauliflower Tater Tots 278
- 239. Air Fryer Pumpkin French Fries 278
- 240. Air Fryer Keto Falafel 279
- 241. Keto Air Fryer Roaste 280

Desserts 282
- 242. Chocolate Lava Cake 282
- 243. Keto Chocolate Cake 282
- 244. Air Fried Sweet Potato Dessert 283
- 245. Easy Coconut Pie 284
- 246. Air Fried Cheesecake Bites 285
- 247. Chocolate Brownies 285
- 248. Apple Cider Vinegar Donuts 286
- 249. Air-Fried Spiced Apples 287
- 250. Air Fryer Brazilian Pineapple 287
- 251. Coconut-Encrusted Cinnamon 288

VEGETABLE RECIPES OF KETO 290

Breakfast 290
- 252. Cauliflower Waffles 290
- 253. Tofu Quiche Cups 291
- 254. Cinnamon & Pecan Porridge 291
- 255. Superfood Breakfast Bowl 292
- 256. Strawberry Chia Pudding 292
- 257. Blueberry Coconut Porridge 293
- 258. Raspberry Pancakes 294
- 259. Raspberry Chia Pudding 294
- 260. Chia Berry Yogurt Parfaits 295
- 261. Warm Quinoa Breakfast Bowl 295
- 262. Banana Bread Rice Pudding 296
- 263. Apple and Cinnamon Oatmeal 296
- 264. Cinnamon Muffins 297
- 265. Chocolate Strawberry Milkshake 297

Main Dishes 298
- 266. Creamy Brussels Sprouts Bowls 298
- 267. Green Beans and Radishes Bake 298
- 268. Green Goddess Buddha Bowl 299

269. Zucchini Sage Pasta 299
270. Broccoli Stir-Fry 300
271. Kale and Cashew Stir-Fry 300
272. Tofu Green Bean Casserole 301
273. Creamy Stuffed Peppers 302
274. Zucchini Pizza Boats 303
275. Vegan Coconut Curry 303
276. Chiles Rellenos 304
277. Broccoli and Cauliflower Rice 305
278. Cauliflower Fried Rice 305
279. Mexican Zucchini Hash 306
280. Eggplant Lasagna 306
281. Spaghetti Squash Bake 307
282. Cheesy Spinach Bake 308
283. Fakeachini Alfredo 309
284. Cheesy Cauliflower Mac 'N' Cheese . 309
285. Margherita Pizza 310

Appetizers and Starters 312
286. Keto Vegan Lasagna Rolls 312
287. Stuffed Avocados 313
288. Keto Vegan Cashew Cheese 313
289. Baba Ghanoush 314
290. Avocado Fries 315
291. Keto Vegan "Cheese" Sticks 315
292. Keto Vegan Crack Bars 316
293. Vegetable Dip 317
294. Mongolian Stir Fry 317
295. Mushroom "Bacon" 318

Soups and Stews 319
296. Creamy Onion Soup 319
297. Lettuce and Cauliflower Soup 319
298. Spring Vegetable Soup 320
299. Creamy Garlicky Tofu Soup 321
300. Kale Ginger Soup with Avocados 321
301. Creamy Tomato & Turnip Soup 322
302. Italian Cheese Soup 323
303. Chilled Lemongrass 324
304. Mixed Mushroom Soup 324
305. Coconut Pumpkin Soup 325
306. Mushroom Bourguignon 325

Side Dishes 327
307. Basil Zucchinis and Eggplants 327

308. Chard and Peppers Mix 327
309. Balsamic Kale 328
310. Mustard Cabbage Salad 328
311. Cabbage and Green Beans 328
312. Green Beans, Avocado 329
313. Creamy Cajun Zucchinis 329
314. Herbed Zucchinis and Olives 330

Salads 331
315. Cherry Tomato Salad with Soy 331
316. Roasted Bell Pepper Salad 331
317. Tofu-Dulse-Walnut Salad 332
318. Almond-GojiBerry Cauliflower 332
319. Warm Mushroom and Orange 333
320. Broccoli, Kelp, and Feta Salad 334
321. Roasted Asparagus with Feta 334
322. Fresh Veggie Salad 335
323. Strawberry Salad 335
324. Tex Mex Black Bean and Avocado 336
325. Lentil Fattoush Salad 336
326. Sweet Potato Salad 337

Snacks 339
327. Chipotle Tacos 339
328. Tasty Spinach Dip 339
329. Candied Almonds 340
330. Eggplant Tapenade 340
331. Almond and Beans Fondue 341
332. Beans in Rich Tomato Sauce 341
333. Tasty Onion Dip 342
334. Special Beans Dip 342
335. Sweet and Spicy Nuts 343
336. Delicious Corn Dip 344
Roasted Almonds 344
338. Cheese Biscuits 345
339. Baked Veggie Balls 345
340. Celery Crackers 346

Desserts 348
Coconut Fat Bombs 348
342. Coconut Cupcakes 348
343. Pumpkin Truffles 349
344. Raspberry Truffles 350
345. Pistachio Gelato 350
346. Berry Bites 351

347. Espresso Cups 351	Vegetarian 375
348. Himalayan Raspberry Fat Bombs 352	386. Quick and Easy Caesar Salad 376
349. Stewed Rhubarb 352	387. Creamy Roasted Pepper Soup 376
350. Peach Cobbler 353	388. Spiralized Asian Zucchini Salad 377
351. Apple Mix 353	389. Forever Together Courgette Salad ... 378
352. Poached Plums 354	390. Roasted Cauliflower Soup 378
353. Rice Pudding 354	391. Fine Pad Thai of Very Low Carb 379
354. Cinnamon Rice 354	392. Vegetarian White Pizza 380
355. Easy Buns 355	393. Mini Shephard's Pie 380
356. Zucchini Bread 355	394. Mushroom Pasta 381
357. Pear Pudding 356	395. Basil Risotto 381
358. Cauliflower Pudding 356	396. Cheese and Asparagus Pasta 382
359. Exuberant Pumpkin Fudge 357	397. Carrot and Sweet Potato Medley 382
360. Bananas and Agave Sauce 358	398. Pesto Farfalle 383
LOW-CARB FRUITS AND BERRIES 359	399. Mexican Rice Casserole 383
BREAKFAST 359	400. Warm Collard Salad 383
361. Astonishing Hemp Seed Yogurt 359	401. Fried Broccoli Salad with Tempeh ... 384
362. Sensual Portobello Mushrooms 359	402. Tangy Nutty Brussel Sprout Salad ... 385
363. Surprisingly Keto Tomato Tart 360	ENTREES 386
364. Kalamata Olive Tapenade 361	403. Tomato Cream Soup with Basil 386
365. Silly Scallion Pancakes 361	404. Coconut Green Soup 386
366. The Keto Crack Slaw 362	405. Hearty Vegetable Soup 387
367. Feisty Grilled Artichokes 363	406. Cream Soup with Avocado 387
368. The Thundering Cinnamon 363	407. Mediterranean Artichoke Salad 388
369. Enchilada Macaroni 364	408. Fresh Avocado-Cucumber Soup 388
370. Squash Salad for the Green Lovers! 364	409. Almond Parsnip Soup 389
371. Pumpkin Pecan Oatmeal 365	410. Sauteed Spinach with Spicy Tofu 389
372. Healthy Steel Cut Oats 366	411. Cauliflower & Celery Bisque 390
373. Delicious Scramble 368	412. Crunchy Rosemary Almonds 391
374. Blueberries Oatmeal 368	413. Simple Cauliflower Popcorn 391
375. Almond Butter Oatmeal 369	414. Easy Brussels sprouts Chips 392
376. Banana Oatmeal 369	415. Crispy Apple Chips 392
377. Delicious Frittata 370	416. Crisp Radish Chips 392
378. Apple Granola 370	417. Fried Parsnip Chips 393
379. Carrot and Zucchini Oatmeal 371	418. Spicy Roasted Nuts 393
380. Cranberry Breakfast Quinoa 371	High Protein Plant-Based Recipes 395
381. Delicious Quinoa and Oats 372	419. Tofu Scramble with Spinach 395
382. Breakfast Chia Pudding 372	420. Apple Pancakes 395
MAINS 374	421. Chickpea Omelet 396
383. Stinky Roasted Garlic 374	422. Black Bean and Hummus 397
384. The Crazy Tofu Bok Choy Salad 374	423. Tempeh "Chicken" Salad 398
385. A Spicy Red Coconut Curry for Keto	424. Black Bean and Sweet Potato Chili .. 398

- 425. Lentil Soup 399
- 426. Indian Yellow Split Pea Dal 400
- 427. Mexican Casserole with Black Beans 400
- 428. Sweet-And-Sour Tempeh 401
- 429. Meatloaf Loaf 402

SOUPS AND SALADS 404
- 430. White Bean Salad 404
- 431. Gourmet Vegetarian Tabbouleh Salad with Edamame and Tofu Cheese 404
- Quinoa Salad with Fresh Mint and 405
- 433. Chickpea Spinach Salad 406
- 434. Lentil Quinoa Salad with Spinach 406
- 435. Pasta Salad with Peanut 407
- 436. Red Lentil & Olive Salad with Tofu & Mint Yogurt Dressing 408
- 437. Kale Caesar Salad 409
- 438. High Protein Kidney Bean Salad 409
- 439. Sweet Potato Salad 410
- 440. Greek-Style Salad 411
- 441. Warm Savoy Cabbage Slaw 412
- 442. Taco Salad Boats 412
- 443. Cauliflower Salad with Pecans 413
- 444. Crunchy Broccoli Salad 414
- 445. Kale Salad with Crispy Tofu Cubes .. 414
- 446. Cucumber and Zucchini 415
- 447. Crazy Asian Zucchini Salad: 416
- 448. Iconic Creamy Kale Salad: 416
- 449. Tasty Corn & Avocado Salad 417
- 450. Salad: 417
- 451. Coolest Arugula & Blueberry Salad: 417
- 452. Fantastic lean Avocado 418
- 453. Curious Courgette Salad 418
- 454. Keto Red Curry 419
- 455. Kale Soup 420
- 456. Creamy Jalapeno Soup 420
- 457. Chinese Chili Soup 421
- 458. Mushroom Soup 421
- 459. Vietnamese-Style Vegetable Soup 422
- 460. Green Chili Soup 422
- 461. Vegetarian Red Chili 423
- 462. Vegetarian Green Chili 423
- 463. Tortilla Soup 424
- 464. Keto Vegetable Soup 425
- 465. Keto Cabbage Soup 425

Sauces and Dips 427
- 466. Vegetarian Black Soup 427
- 467. Vegetarian Curried Corn Soup 428
- 468. Vegetarian Thai Coconut 429
- 469. Vegetarian Minestrone Soup 429
- 470. Fat-Free Cabbage Soup Recipe 430
- 471. Easy Vegetarian Pumpkin Soup 431
- 472. Gazpacho Soup 432

Desserts and Snacks 434
- 473. Crockpot Lasagna with Spinach 434
- 474. Black Bean Veggie Burger 434
- 475. Blueberry Tofu Smoothie 435
- 476. Fluffy 1-Bowl Sugar Cookies 436
- 477. Banana Cream Pie 438
- 478. Gluten-Free Black Beans Brownies .440
- 479. Tahini Chocolate Banana Soft Serve 440
- 480. Raw Oreos 441
- 481. Peanut Butter Cup Cookies 442
- 482. Gluten-Free Cinnamon Rolls 442

INTRODUCTION

Keto After 50 is an absolute must-have for all older women who need a thorough understanding of the Ketogenic Diet and the surprising benefits of being a woman on this diet.

I have written the guide with precision and detail, which the very nature of the diet dictates, reflecting the awareness, skills and extensive experience of both women.

The Keto Diet has become quite a popular topic in the fitness community. It has been observed to aid within the lack of weight and to lower the inflammation within the gut. New studies have shown high-quality effects for both males and females, adhering to a keto style weight-reduction plan.

The ketogenic food regimen colloquially referred to as the keto food regimen, is a popular food plan containing excessive quantities of fats, good enough protein and low carbohydrate. It is also called a Low Carb-High Fat (LCHF) diet and a low carbohydrate eating regimen.

Gone is the parable that this diet is unappetizing, unpalatable, dull and unappealing! Beautifully illustrated recipes for several different delicious dishes, beverages, snacks, and desserts are testimony to this.

The keto food plan has gained in popularity in the latest years and has turn out to be a dietary plan desired by individuals of all ages. That said, this dietary roadmap may precipitate particularly vital health blessings to folks over age 50.

The Ketogenic diet is considered one of the best diets you may comply with for weight loss and to enhance your ordinary health. Numerous studies aid the eating regimen showing giant results specifically while coupled with exercises

Let's get started!

WHAT IS THE KETO DIET?

First, a keto, or ketogenic diet, is designed to maintain your body in more of a ketosis state. Ketosis is not abnormal. It is a nation where your frame is low on carbohydrate gas. When this occurs, it begins to burn fat, instead of the carbs. The technique produces ketones. The average character does now not stay in a ketogenic nation except at some point of heavy exercise, which includes CrossFit, or all through pregnancy.

A ketogenic diet promotes very low carbohydrates and higher fat intake. The frame will in turn, use fats to produce strength. This weight loss plan has additionally been proven to lower autoimmune diseases, endocrine diseases, and additionally, has cancer combating properties.

Tracking and Macros

An ideal Keto diet should consist of:

- 70-80% Fat
- 20-25% Protein
- 5-10% Carbs

You should not be consuming more than 20g of carbs according to today to keep the typical Ketogenic food plan. I individually ate less than 10g according to today for a greater drastic revel in, but I finished my initial desires after which some. I lost 28 lbs. In a little below 3 weeks.

Understanding Ketosis and Ketones

Ketogenic diets are essentially designed to result in a kingdom of ketosis in the frame. When the quantity of glucose in the body turns into too low, the body switches to fats as an opportunity supply of electricity.

The frame has two primary gas resources which are:

- glucose
- unfastened fatty acids (FFA) and, to a lesser extent, ketones made from FFA

Fat deposits are saved in the form of triglycerides. They are normally broken down into long-chain fatty acids and glycerol. Stripping off the glycerol from the triglyceride molecule allows for the release of the three loose fatty acid (FFA) molecules into the bloodstream to be used as power.

The glycerol molecule goes into the liver, wherein three molecules of it combine to form one glucose molecule. Therefore, as your frame burns fats, it also produces glucose as a via-product. This glucose may be used to gasoline components of the brain in addition to other parts of the body that cannot run on FFA.

However, while glucose can travel through the bloodstream on its own, cholesterol and triglycerides want a carrier to transport around inside the bloodstream. Cholesterol and triglycerides are packaged in a carrier referred to as low-density lipoprotein, or LDL. Thus, the larger the LDL particle, the more triglycerides it contains.

The overall technique of burning fat deposits for electricity produces carbon dioxide, water, and compounds called ketones.

Ketones are produced by using the liver from unfastened fatty acids. There are composed of 2 companies of atoms linked collectively using a practical carbonyl group.

The frame cannot shop ketones and therefore, they should be both used or excreted. The frame excretes them either through the breath as acetone or through the urine as acetoacetate.

Ketones may be used by frame cells as a supply of electricity. Also, the mind can make use of ketones in generating about 70-75% of its strength requirement.

Like alcohol, ketones take precedence as a gas source over carbohydrates. This implies that when they're high inside the bloodstream, they need to be burned first before glucose can be used as gasoline.

What Causes Ketosis

When you begin eating fewer quantities of carbohydrates, your body receives a smaller supply of glucose to use as a power in comparison to before.

The decrease in the number of consumed carbohydrates and the subsequent discount in the amount of available glucose slowly forces the body to move into the country of ketosis. Thus, the body is going into a state of ketosis when there isn't always enough quantity of glucose available to the frame cells.

Ketosis may be a problem with diabetics. This can arise if not the use of enough insulin.

Starvation Induced Ketosis

Fasting and hunger states typically contain decreased or no intake of food that the body can digest and convert into glucose. While hunger is involuntary, fasting is a greater conscious desire you're making to deliberately no longer eat.

However, the frame enters into a "hunger mode" whenever you're sleeping while you pass a meal or while you deliberately move on a fast. The lack of food consumption outcomes in a discount on blood glucose levels. As a result, the frame starts offevolved to interrupt down its glycogen (saved glucose) shops for power.

The glycogen is transformed back into glucose and used as energy by using the frame. In this kingdom, the body additionally begins to burn its saved fats. Thus, the manufacturing of ketone bodies (ketogenesis) is induced through a lack of available glucose.

Any time the number of ketones in the blood outnumbers the molecules of glucose, the body cells will start using the ketones as their supply of electricity.

Uses and Benefits of the Ketogenic Diet

The application and implementation of the ketogenic eating regimen have multiplied considerably. Keto diets are often indicated as part of the remedy plan in some of the scientific conditions.

Epilepsy

This is largely the main reason for the improvement of the ketogenic food plan. For some cause, the price of epileptic seizures reduces while sufferers are positioned on a keto food plan.

Pediatric epileptic instances are the maximum awareness of the keto diet. Some children have experienced seizure removal after some years of the usage of a keto weight loss plan.

Children with epilepsy are generally expected to fast for some days earlier than starting the ketogenic weight-reduction plan as part of their treatment.

Cancer

Research shows that the therapeutic efficacy of the ketogenic diets against tumor increase may be enhanced while mixed with positive pills and procedures under a "press-pulse" paradigm.

It is also promising to notice that ketogenic diets pressure the cancer cellular into remission. This manner that keto diets "starve cancer" to reduce the symptoms.

Alzheimer Disease

There are numerous indications that the memory functions of patients with Alzheimer's disease improve after utilizing a ketogenic weight loss plan.

Ketones are an excellent supply of alternative power for the brain mainly while it has become resistant to insulin. Ketones also provide substrates (cholesterol) that assist in repairing damaged neurons and membranes. These all help to enhance reminiscence and cognition in people living with Alzheimer's.

Diabetes

It is commonly agreed that carbohydrates are the principal wrongdoer in diabetes. Therefore, by reducing the amount of ingested carbohydrate through the usage of a ketogenic weight loss program, there are multiplied probabilities for stepped forward blood sugar control.

Also, combining a keto food plan with other diabetes treatment plans can appreciably enhance their overall effectiveness.

Gluten Allergy

Many people with gluten hypersensitive reactions are undiagnosed with this condition. However, following a ketogenic food plan showed improvement in related symptoms like digestive discomforts and bloating.

Most carbohydrate-wealthy meals are high in gluten. Thus, by using using a keto eating regimen, lots of gluten intake is reduced to a minimum because of the elimination of a huge variety of carbohydrates.

Weight Loss

This is arguably the most common "intentional" use of the ketogenic weight loss plan today. It has discovered a niche for itself in the mainstream dieting trend. Keto diets have ended up part of many weight-reduction plan regimen because of its nicely stated facet impact of aiding weight loss.

Though to begin with maligned by many, the developing number of favorable weight reduction results has helped the ketogenic to higher embraced as a prime weight loss program.

Besides the above medical blessings, ketogenic diets also offer some general health benefits which consist of the following.

Improved Insulin Sensitivity

This is manifestly the first goal of a ketogenic diet. It facilitates stabilizing your insulin tiers thereby improving fat burning.

Muscle Preservation

Since protein is oxidized, it helps to maintain lean muscle. Losing lean muscle mass reasons an individual's metabolism to gradual down as muscle tissues are commonly very metabolic. Using a keto eating regimen truly helps to hold your muscle groups while your frame burns fats.

Controlled pH and respiration function

A keto weight-reduction plan enables to lower lactate thereby enhancing each pH and breathing function. A nation of ketosis, therefore, allows holding your blood pH at a healthy level.

Improved Immune System

Using a ketogenic food plan helps to combat off aging antioxidants while also decreasing irritation of the intestine, thereby making your immune gadget stronger.

Reduced Cholesterol Levels

Consuming fewer carbohydrates at the same time as you're at the keto diet will assist in lessening blood cholesterol levels. This is due to the increased kingdom of lipolysis. This leads to a discount on LDL cholesterol levels and a growth in HDL levels of cholesterol.

Reduced Appetite and Cravings

Adopting a ketogenic weight loss program lets you reduce both your appetite and cravings for calorie wealthy foods. As you begin eating wholesome, satisfying, and beneficial excessive-fat foods, your hunger feelings will naturally start decreasing.

Side Effects of the Ketogenic Diet

Changing to the ketogenic weight loss program isn't always that clean to evolve to mainly at the initial onset. However, remember that those facet consequences are transient. Some of them can final for a few days while others can final for months.

Therefore, you need to provide your self-time, both physically and mentally, to make the switch successfully.

While making the switch to a ketogenic weight loss plan, there are two physical changes that you may also experience. These are the keto flu and keto breath.

Keto Flu

This is one component that anyone starting a ketogenic weight-reduction plan have to brace up for. It is a situation in which you experience some of the different side consequences that come along with using a ketogenic eating regimen.

Keto flu is frequently characterized using light-headedness or mind fogginess, headaches, nausea, stomachaches, and muscle soreness. You might also revel in heightened emotions of lethargy, irritability and trouble concentrating.

Interestingly, those are all common signs and symptoms of the flu, as a result, the name. These signs and symptoms are temporary and not anybody they torment the usage of a ketogenic.

These signs and symptoms are regularly caused by the sugar withdrawal occasioned through the drastically decreased carbohydrate intake. Also, an imbalance in your frame electrolytes consisting of calcium, magnesium, potassium, and sodium can affect how your body reacts to the effect of a ketogenic food plan.

Keto Breath

There are two possible reasons put forth why human beings on ketogenic diets revel in this ordinary breath issue.

The frame does not save ketones and accordingly they have to be excreted from the body. Ketones may be excreted through the urine as acetoacetate.

They also can be excreted through the breath in the shape of acetone. So, the extra ketones you produce, the more acetone you skip out through your breath. Unfortunately, this could purpose unpleasant-smelling breath when the use of a ketogenic food regimen.

On the alternative hand, increased protein ingestion also can cause keto breath. This is because the manner the frame digest fats and proteins is pretty different. The digestion of proteins normally produces ammonia, which the frame excretes through the urine.

However, the accelerated consumption of proteins may also bring about the indigestible amounts closing in your gut system and undergoes fermentation. This produces ammonia, which is sooner or later released through your breath.

Keto breath can last for approximately a week to just under a month. It mostly depends on how nicely your frame adapts to ketosis.

Micronutrient Deficiencies

This may result from the strict regulations on carbohydrate intake. A lot of carbohydrate-wealthy foods are equally rich in vitamins and minerals.

The severe restriction on carbohydrate intake may additionally, therefore, cause deficiencies in some crucial nutrients. Therefore, we need to now not handiest be targeted at the micronutrient counting in phrases of fats, proteins, and carbohydrates; however, should also do not forget the vitamin and mineral micronutrient contents as well.

This is regularly why dietary supplements are mostly endorsed when the usage of a ketogenic food regimen. Supplementation will help to reinforce any micronutrient imbalance that might occur while using a ketogenic weight-reduction plan.

Keto Mistakes to Avoid

When you're in ketosis, your frame burns fats and uses it for energy in a green manner. This system makes the keto diet an ideal choice for folks that are looking for an easy way of dropping weight. However, in case you are following this diet and aren't losing weight, chances are which you are not in ketosis. Given underneath are some mistakes to avoid when at the ketogenic weight loss plan.

Not Reaching Ketosis

Typically, most keto dieters don't lose weight due to the fact they don't achieve ketosis. And the motive that they don't attain ketosis is that they don't reduce their carb intake. According to experts, your carb intake ought to be only 5 to 10% of your caloric intake.

Most keto diets require dieters to reduce as a minimum of 20 grams of carbs according to day. And it's why they'll not be able to burn fat. You can purchase a home testing kit and use the test strips to discover if your urine includes ketones. If the check result is positive, you're in ketosis.

Consuming a Lot of Protein

Most low-carb diets do allow some amount of protein. If you believe you studied a keto weight loss program refers to an excessive protein, low-carb food regimen, you need to assume again. The component is that this form of weight-reduction plan won't help you reach ketosis as your frame can not ruin down the excessive quantity of protein to get amino acids, after which convert the amino acids into sugar.

When on a keto eating regimen, you get your calories from fats. And fat must be as a minimum 55% of your caloric intake.

Eating a Lot of Acceptable Carbs

You may have some varieties of carbs when on the keto weight loss program, including dairy and nuts. Typically, these ingredients are rich in fat and nutrients. Therefore, they may be a perfect addition to your eating regimen. But the problem is that they have carbs in them.

Therefore, it is not a good concept to have quite a few of those meals. Ignoring this advice will save you you from maintaining ketosis.

Eating Maltitol

Usually, sugar alcohols are fine for keto dieters. They offer sweetness but don't increase the wide variety of carbs in your body. But it's essential to hold in mind that some types of alcohols do incorporate carbs.

For instance, maltitol is a type that isn't always allowed on this low-carb weight loss plan. Technically, it is low GI sugar; however, it has an impact on your blood sugar levels. Therefore, it may prevent you from attaining ketosis.

Taking Too Many Calories

If you eat extra energy than you burn, you may not be able to shed those higher pounds. In fact, in case you consume a whole lot of calories, you may advantage of fats even when you have completed ketosis.

Foods that comprise many fats have more energy compared to foods that are rich in proteins and carbs. Therefore, you must screen the power you eat on an everyday basis. If you persist with a balanced weight loss program, you could gain your goals.

So, these are a few errors you could need to keep away from to ensure the keto eating regimen works for you.

KETO FOR WOMEN AND MAN OVER 50

The benefits of being a woman on this eating regimen are pretty good. In addition to weight loss and muscle advantage, a keto food plan has a high-quality manner of assisting the endocrine system. We all realize the impact hormones have on the woman athlete.

Fluctuating hormones can motive pain, fatigue, and even depression. The link between hormones and cancer can not be denied. A keto eating regimen has proven to higher adjust the endocrine system. By doing this, it decreases the occurrence of a few cancers, thyroid disease, and diabetes.

Keto Diet Benefits for Women/Man Over 50

Keto weight loss plan adherents, particularly those elderly 50 and older, are stated to enjoy numerous capability health blessings including:

Increased physical and mental energy

As humans grow older, electricity levels might drop for quite a few biological and environmental reasons. Keto food plan adherents frequently witness a lift in strength and vitality. One reason stated occurrence takes place is that the frame is burning excess fat, which in turn receives synthesized into electricity. Furthermore, systemic synthesis of ketones tends to increase brain energy and stimulate cognitive features like awareness and memory.

Improved sleep

Individuals generally tend to sleep less as they age. Keto dieters regularly gain extra from exercising packages and grow to be tired more comfortable. Said occurrence should precipitate longer and more fruitful durations of rest.

Metabolism

Aging individuals regularly revel in a slower metabolism than they did at some stage in their more youthful days. Long-time keto dieters enjoy a greater regulation of blood sugar, which can grow their metabolic rates.

Weight loss

Faster and greater green metabolism of fats enables the body to cast off accumulated frame fats, that can precipitate the shedding of extra pounds. Additionally, adherents also are believed to revel in a discounted appetite that can lead to a dwindled caloric intake.

Keeping the burden off is crucial specifically as adults age when they may need fewer calories daily in comparison to when residing in there 20s or 30s even. Yet it's miles still important to get nutrient-wealthy food from this diet for older adults.

Since it is not unusual for growing old adults to lose muscle and energy, and excessive protein-specific ketogenic weight loss plan may be advocated using a nutritionist.

Protection against specific illnesses

Keto dieters over age 50 ought to reduce their hazard of developing ailments along with diabetes, intellectual issues like Alzheimer's, diverse cardiovascular maladies, diverse styles of cancer, Parkinson's Disease, Non-Alcoholic Fatty Liver Disease (NAFLD) and a couple of scleroses.

Aging

Aging is taken into consideration by way of a few because of the essential hazard component for human illnesses or disease. So, lowering growing older is the logical step to limit these threat factors of disease.

Good information extending from the technical description of the ketosis method offered earlier, indicates the increased strength of teens as a result and due to the usage of fat as a gas source, the body can undergo a process where it may misinterpret signs so that the mTOR signal is suppressed and a lack of glucose is obvious whereby it's far reported getting older can be slowed.

Generally for years, more than one research has cited that caloric restriction can aid in slowing growing old or even increase lifespan. With the ketogenic weight loss program it's far possible without reducing calories to have an impact on anti-aging. An intermittent fasting technique used with the keto weight loss plan can also have an impact on vascular growing older.

When a person fasts intermittently or when at the keto food plan, BHB or Beta-Hydroxybutyrate is produced that is believed to set off anti-getting old effects.

To be fair, as reported in the US National Library of Medicine National Institutes of Health article "Effects of Ketogenic Diets on Cardiovascular Risk Factors" in May 2017; the ketogenic diets, which are very low in carbohydrates and generally excessive in fat and proteins are used successfully in weight loss for the duration of the remedy of weight problems and cardiovascular diseases.

However, an essential note in the article changed into that "Results concerning the effect of such diets on cardiovascular threat elements are controversial" and "Moreover, these diets are not completely safe and can be related to a few detrimental events."

Safe to say, extra is needed than virtually researching this food plan, blessings, wonderful effects, and facet effects mainly in growing older adults by way of the net and periodicals alone. One specifically has to consult her or his medical professional about unique concerns.

General Nutritional Needs for Women/Man Over 50

"You are what you eat" how normally have we heard that? Well, I virtually agree with it, through eating healthily and for substance, there's no need to observe diets. As you reach 50 and beyond, think of aging as ripening. In other words, don't get obsessive about being stick-thin.

After all not everyone is supposed to be skinny and anyway, if you're too thin after 50 you tend to look older. Instead purpose to be wholesome and fit and discover what your healthful weight ought to be; chances are you already recognize. Beware of crash diets, and "fat-free" ingredients, they are packed complete of sugar, so do not be deceived via it all!

Healthy eating for women over 50 is all about re-learning a tasty and healthy way of eating. Eat seasonal, local produce whenever possible.

You will discover that as you age sure meals that you used to consume when you have been more youthful will give you indigestion, inclusive of "fish & chips" so alternative it with baked fish and a wholesome salad.

The secret is to get to recognize your frame and paintings with it no longer in opposition to it. Don't combat the inevitable, just assist its adjustments with not unusual sense.

Gentler Approach to Keto for Women/Man Over 50

Slowly and carefully. A ketogenic weight loss plan must not be started at a complete 100 percent. You need to decrease the amount of carbs you consume slowly. Cutting the carbs too quickly can have a poor effect. It can pressure the frame and confuse it, for that reason inflicting a wild imbalance.

Also, if pregnant or nursing, you have to use a keto weight-reduction plan no longer. During this period, eat a well-rounded weight loss plan of fruits, vegetables, dairy, and grains.

My nice advice, get your body as strong as possible, and then slowly include a ketogenic eating regimen.

RECOMMENDED KETO FOODS

Because rapid food restaurants and processed meals surround us, it can be a venture to avoid carb-rich ingredients, but proper making plans can help.

Plan menus and snacks at the least a week ahead of time, so you aren't stuck with the best high carb meal choices. Research keto recipes online; there are pretty a few great ones to pick from. Immerse yourself within the keto lifestyle, discover your favorite recipes, and stick with them.

Keto weight loss plan adherents are endorsed to consume ingredients like meat, fatty fishes, dairy products which include cheeses, milk, butter and cream, eggs, produce merchandise possessing low carbohydrate concentrations, condiments like salt, pepper and a bunch of different spices, diverse wishes and seeds and oils like olive and coconut. On the alternative hand, positive meals must be averted or strictly limited. Said items encompass beans and legumes, many fruits, edibles with excessive sugar contents, alcohol and grain merchandise.

Exercise for Over 50 in Support of Keto

Here are 10 Weight Loss Exercises for Women over 50:

1. **Walking** - Walking is taken into consideration to be one in every of the most effective physical activities for weight loss. 30 minutes walk every morning can assist you to return to shape.

2. **Jogging** - It allows you to burn those greater calories than you take in ordinary in the shape of food. Initially, you may discover it hard and may face ache on your thighs, but recollect one thing; if there may be no ache - there can be no gain.

3. **Yoga** - Famous everywhere in the world, yoga has helped millions of people to come lower back to their different sizes. The handiest kind among all other sporting events for a girl over 50, can be achieved at home sitting in your bed.

4. **Aerobic exercises** - Doing aerobics for half-hour thrice a week will increase your heart price and breathing charge. You may have a consultation of 10 minutes 3 instances at a time.

5. **Flexibility exercises** - Stretching slowly and breathing in deeply is an excellent exercise for ladies over 50 to free weight.

6. **Running** It is an excellent weight loss remedy and it burns several calories.

7. **Light household work-** Dusting, cleaning and many others is another terrific form of exercise for girls over 50.

8. **Climbing stairs-** It builds up stamina and is also very convenient.

9. **Stretching exercise** -Arm stretching and back stretching allows in burning fat.

10. **Join a gym** - Get the help of the instructor in the Gym to free weight. Your instructor will assist you to exercise to unfastened weight and get into shape.

KETO RECIPES FOR WOMEN/MAN OVER 50

Try these easy keto recipes to lose weight on a ketogenic diet, from nutritionists and bloggers. These recipes are all high in fat, low in carbs, and taste delicious, of course.

BREAKFAST

01. Tortilla Breakfast Casserole

Yield

12 servings

Nutrition

Per Serving: 447 calories, 32.6 g fat, 14.6 g carbohydrates, 25.5 g protein

Ingredients

- 1 Pound Bacon, Cooked and Crumbled
- 1 Pound Pork Sausage. Cooked and Crumbled
- 1 Pound Package Diced Ham
- 10 8 inch Tortillas, Cut in half 8 Large Eggs
- 1 1/2 Cups Milk
- 1/2 Teaspoon Salt
- 1/2 Teaspoon Pepper
- 1/2 Teaspoon Garlic Powder
- 1/2 teaspoon Hot Sauce
- 2 Cups Shredded Cheddar Cheese
- 1 Cup Mozzarella or Monterrey Jack Cheese

Instructions

1. A 9x13-inch baking dish with 2 teaspoons of butter or sprinkle with nonstick spray oil.

2. Bake 1/3 layer of tortillas in the bottom of the pot and cover with baked bacon and 1/3 layer of cheese.

3. Place another third of the tortillas in the pan and cover with the cooked and chopped sausages and place another third of the cheese in layers.

4. Repeat with the last tortilla, ham and cheese 1/3.

5. In a large bowl, combine eggs, milk, salt, pepper, garlic powder, and hot sauce.

6. Pour the egg mixture evenly over the pot.

7. If desired, cover overnight and refrigerate or bake immediately.

8. When you are ready to bake, preheat the oven to 350 degrees.

9. Bake covered with foil for 45 minutes. Find and cook for another 20 minutes until the cheese is completely melted and cooked in a pan.

02. Pecan-Banana Pops

A healthy breakfast doesn't necessarily have to be hot; in fact, this one is frozen. Make a bunch of these pops ahead of time and keep them in the freezer. They make an excellent after-school treat as well. Kids love them!

Servings

Yields 4 pops.

Nutrition

Amount Per Serving

Fat 14g, Carbohydrates 7g, and Protein 19g

Ingredients

- 4 large just-ripe bananas

- 2 tablespoons raw honey
- 4 Popsicle sticks
- 3A cup chopped pecans
- ½ cup almond butter

Instructions

1. Peel and cut one end from each banana, and insert a Popsicle stick into the cut end.
2. In a small bowl, stir together the almond butter and honey, and heat in the microwave for 10 to 15 seconds, or just until the mixture is slightly thinned. Pour onto a sheet of wax paper or aluminum foil and spread with a spatula.
3. On another piece of wax paper or foil, spread the chopped pecans — Line a small baking sheet or large plate with the third piece of wax paper or foil.
4. Roll each banana first in the honey mixture until well coated, then in the nuts until completely covered, pressing down gently, so the nuts adhere.
5. Place each finished banana onto the baking sheet. When all of the bananas have been coated, place the sheet in the freezer for at least 2 hours. For long-term storage, transfer the frozen bananas into a resealable plastic bag.

03. Greek Breakfast Wraps

This recipe is just as satisfying as that fast-food breakfast sandwich, but this wrap has far less fat and fewer calories. It's an excellent breakfast to do and reheat any time you want.

Servings

2 servings

Nutrition

Fat 10.4 g, Carbohydrate, 4.5g, Protein 10.6 g

Ingredients

- 1 teaspoon olive oil

- ½ cup fresh baby spinach leaves
- 1 tablespoon fresh basil
- 4 egg whites, beaten
- ½ teaspoon salt
- ¼ teaspoon freshly ground black pepper
- ¼ cup crumbled low-fat feta cheese
- 2 (8-inch) whole-wheat tortillas

Instructions

1. In a small skillet, heat the olive oil over medium heat. Add the spinach and basil to the pan and saute for about 2 minutes, or just until the spinach is wilted.
2. Add the egg whites to the pan, season with the salt and pepper, and saute, often stirring, for about 2 minutes more, or until the egg whites are firm.
3. Remove from the heat and sprinkle with the feta cheese.
4. Heat the tortillas in the microwave for 20 to 30 seconds or just until softened and warm. Divide the eggs between the tortillas and wrap up burrito-style.

04. Curried Chicken Breast Wraps

These quick and filling wraps deliver a lot of flavor for very few calories. Make the filling ahead of time to have on hand for work lunches and busy days.

Servings

Yields 2 servings

Nutrition

5 g total fat, 18 g carbohydrates, 28 g protein

Ingredients

- 6 ounces cooked chicken breast, cubed

- 1 small Gala or Granny Smith apple, cored and chopped
- 2 tablespoons plain low-fat yogurt
- 1 cup spring lettuce mix or baby lettuce
- 1 teaspoon Dijon mustard
- ½ teaspoon mild curry powder
- 2 (8-inch) whole-wheat tortillas

Instructions

1. In a small bowl, combine the chicken, yogurt, Dijon mustard, and curry powder; stir well to combine. Add the apple and stir until blended.
2. Divide the lettuce between the tortillas and top each with half of the chicken mixture. Roll up burrito-style and serve.

05. Baked Salmon Fillets with Tomato and Mushrooms

Salmon is an excellent source of healthy fats, especially omega-3 fatty acids. When baked with a mixture of tangy tomatoes and wild mushrooms, it's as delicious as it is healthy.

Servings

Yields 2 servings

Nutrition

Fat 12.2g, Carbohydrate 21g, Protein 25.1g

Ingredients

- 2 (4-ounce) skin-on salmon fillets
- 2 teaspoons olive oil, divided
- ½ teaspoon salt
- ¼ teaspoon freshly ground black pepper
- ½ teaspoon chopped fresh dill

- ½ cup diced fresh tomato
- ½ cup sliced fresh mushrooms

Instructions

1. Preheat the oven to 375 degrees F and line a baking sheet with aluminum foil.
2. You are using your fingers or a pastry brush, coat both sides of the fillets with ½ teaspoon of the olive oil each. Place the salmon skin-side down on the pan. Sprinkle salt and pepper equally all round.
3. In a small plate, mix the remaining 1 teaspoon olive oil, the tomato, mushrooms, and dill; stir well to combine. Spoon the mixture over the fillets.
4. Fold the sides and ends of the foil up to seal the fish, place the pan on the middle oven rack, and bake for about 20 minutes, or until the salmon flakes easily.

06. Cinnamon and Spice Overnight Oats

Yield

1 person

Nutrition

Carbohydrates: 15g | Protein: 26g | Fat: 34g

Ingredients

- 75g rolled oats
- 100ml milk
- 75g yogurt
- 1 tsp honey
- 1/2 tsp vanilla extract
- 1/8th tsp Schwartz ground cinnamon
- 20g raisins

Instructions

1. Add all ingredients to a bowl and mix well. Cover overnight or at least one hour and refrigerate.

2. Exit the refrigerator or heat it in the microwave immediately or slowly.

07. Mexican Casserole

Yield

6 servings

Nutrition

43.7 g fat; 32.8 g carbohydrates; 31.7 g protein

Ingredients

- 1-pound lean ground beef
- 2 cups salsa
- 1 (16 ounces) can chili beans, drained
- 3 cups tortilla chips, crushed
- 2 cups sour cream
- 1 (2 ounces) can slice black olives, drained
- 1/2 cup chopped green onion
- 1/2 cup chopped fresh tomato
- 2 cups shredded Cheddar cheese

Instructions

1. Preheat oven to 350 degrees Fahrenheit (175 degrees Celsius).

2. In a large fish over medium heat, cook the meat so that it is no longer pink. Add the sauce, reduce the heat and simmer for 20 minutes or until the liquid is absorbed. Add beans and heat.

3. Sprinkle a 9x13 baking dish with oil spray. Pour the chopped tortillas into the pan and then place the meat mixture on it. Pour sour cream over meat and sprinkle with olives, green onions, and tomatoes. Top with cheddar cheese.

4. Bake in preheated oven for 30 minutes or until hot and bubbly.

08. Microwaved Fish and Asparagus with Tarragon Mustard Sauce

Yield

2 servings

Nutrition

4g carbs, 33 g protein, 17g fat

Ingredients

- 12 ounces (340 g) fish fillets— whiting, tilapia, sole, flounder, or any kind of white fish
- 10 asparagus spears
- 2 tablespoons (30 g) sour cream
- 1 tablespoon (15 g) mayonnaise
- ¼ teaspoon dried tarragon
- ½ teaspoon Dijon or spicy brown mustard

Instructions

1. Draw the bottom of the asparagus spears and cut them naturally. Put the asparagus on a large glass plate, add 1 teaspoon (15 ml) of water and cover with a plate. Microwave for 3 minutes.

2. While the asparagus is in the microwave, mix sour, mayonnaise, tarragon and mustard together.

3. Remove the asparagus from the microwave oven, remove it from the pie plate and

set aside. Drain the water from the runway. Put the fish fillet in it

4. Peel the pie plate and spread 2 tablespoons (30 ml) cream mixture on them and cover the pie again and place the fish in the microwave for 3 to 4 minutes. Open the oven, remove the plate from the top of the pie plate and place the asparagus on top of the fish. Cover the pie plate again and cook for another 1-2 minutes.

5. Remove the pie plate from the microwave oven and remove the plate. Put the fish and asparagus on a serving platter. Chop any boiled sauce on a plate over fish and asparagus. Melt each with reserved sauce and serve.

09. Hearty Hot Cereal with Berries

Whole grains are not only great for your heart; they're also great for your waist.

The high fiber content makes them filling and provides slow, steady energy for your day. The addition of berries and nuts in this recipe makes it especially hearty.

Servings

Yields 4 servings.

Nutrition

Amount Per Serving

Fat 15g, Carbohydrates 17g, and Protein 19g

Ingredients

- 4 cups of water
- 2 tablespoons honey
- ½ teaspoon salt
- ½ cup fresh blueberries
- 2 cups whole rolled oats
- ½ cup fresh raspberries
- ½ cup chopped walnuts

- cup low-fat milk

- teaspoons flaxseed

Instructions

1. In a medium saucepan, bring the water to a boil over high heat and add the salt.

2. Stir in the oats, walnuts, and flaxseed, then reduce the heat to low and cover — Cook for 16 to 20 minutes, or until the oatmeal reaches the desired consistency.

Divide the oatmeal between 4 deep bowls and top each with 2 tablespoons of both blueberries and raspberries. Add ½ cup milk to each bowl and serve.

LUNCH AND DINNER

10. Protein Power Sweet Potatoes

This recipe is straightforward and quick, but it packs almost ten grams of protein per serving, which makes it a perfect fasting-day meal for keeping you full and helping you stay energized and focused.

Servings

Yields 2 servings

Nutrition

Amount Per Serving

Fat 11g, Carbohydrates 15g, and Protein 18g

Ingredients

- 2 medium sweet potatoes
- 6 ounces plain Greek yogurt
- ½ teaspoon salt
- 1/3 cup dried cranberries
- ¼ teaspoon freshly ground black pepper

Instructions

1. Heat The oven to 400 degrees F and pierce the sweet potatoes several times. Place them on a cooking plate and cook for 40 to 45 minutes, or until you can easily pierce them with a fork.
2. Cut the potatoes in half and wrap the meat in a medium bowl and keep the skin healthy.
3. Add the salt, pepper, yogurt, and cranberries to the bowl and mix well with a fork.
4. Spoon the mixture back into the potato skins and serve warm.

11. Penne Pasta with Vegetables

Even on fasting days, you can enjoy a light pasta meal.

This one is chock-full of vitamin C and iron from the spinach and tomatoes and delivers lots of flavor and satisfaction.

Servings

Yields 2 servings.

Nutrition

Amount Per Serving

Fat 12g, Carbohydrates 9g, and Protein 19g

Ingredients

- 1 teaspoon salt, divided
- ¾ cup uncooked penne pasta
- 1 tablespoon olive oil
- 1 tablespoon chopped garlic
- 1 teaspoon chopped fresh oregano
- l cup sliced fresh mushrooms
- to cherry tomatoes, halved
- l cup fresh spinach leaves
- ½ teaspoon freshly ground black pepper
- 1 tablespoon shredded Parmesan cheese

Instructions

1. In a large saucepan, bring 1-quart water to a boil. Add 1/2 teaspoon of the salt and the penne, and cook according to package directions, or until al dente (about 9 minutes). Drain but do not rinse the penne, reserving about VA cup pasta water.

2. Meanwhile, in a large skillet, heat the olive oil over medium-high heat. Add the garlic, oregano, and mushrooms, and saute for 4 to 5 minutes, or until the mushrooms are golden.

3. Add the tomatoes and spinach, season with the remaining ½ teaspoon salt and the black pepper, and saute for 3 to 4 minutes, or until the spinach is wilted.

4. Add the drained pasta to the skillet, along with with 2 to 3 tablespoons of the pasta water. Cook, constantly stirring, for 2 to 3 minutes, or until the pasta is glistening and the water has cooked off.

5. Divide the pasta between two shallow bowls and sprinkle with the Parmesan cheese. Serve hot or at room temperature.

12. Spinach and Swiss Cheese Omelet

Omelets don't need to be reserved for breakfast or brunch. An egg can be a great dinner solution on busy nights and also makes a satisfying lunch entree on weekends.

Servings

Yields 2 servings

Nutrition

Amount Per Serving

Fat 8g, Carbohydrates 12g, and Protein 18g

Ingredients

- 1 teaspoon olive oil
- 6 large egg whites, beaten
- 1 cup fresh baby spinach leaves
- 2 (1-ounce) slices reduced-fat Swiss cheese
- ½ teaspoon salt

- ¼ teaspoon freshly ground black pepper

Instructions

1. In a small skillet, heat the olive oil over medium-high heat. Add the spinach, salt, and pepper, and saute for 3 minutes, stirring often.

2. Use a spatula to spread the spinach reasonably evenly over the bottom of the pan, and pour the egg whites over the top, tilting the pan to coat the spinach thoroughly.

3. Cook for 3 to 4 minutes, occasionally pulling the edges of the eggs toward the center as you tilt the skillet to allow uncooked egg to spread to the sides of the pan.

4. When the centers of the eggs are mostly (but not wholly) dry, use a spatula to flip the eggs. Place the Swiss cheese slices on one half of the omelet, and then flip the other half over the top to form a half-moon. Cook for 1 minute, or until the cheese is melted and warm.

5. To serve, cut the omelet in half and serve hot.

13. Broiled Halibut with Garlic Spinach

Halibut is a deliciously moist fish that is loaded with heart-healthy omega-3 fatty acids. If you substitute frozen halibut, be sure to thaw it thoroughly and pat it very dry before cooking.

Servings

Yields 2 servings

Nutrition

Amount Per Serving

Fat 22g, Carbohydrates 17g, and Protein 19g

Ingredients

- 2 (4-ounce) halibut fillets, 1 inch thick
- ½ lemon (about 1 teaspoon juice)

- 1 teaspoon salt, divided
- ¼ teaspoon freshly ground black pepper
- ½ teaspoon cayenne pepper
- 1 teaspoon olive oil
- 2 cloves garlic
- ½ cup chopped red onion
- 2 cups fresh baby spinach leaves

Instructions

1. Preheat the broiler and place an oven rack 4 to 5 inches below the heat source. Line a baking sheet with aluminum foil.
2. Squeeze the lemon half over the fish fillets, then season each side with ½ teaspoon of the salt, pepper, and cayenne. Place the fish on the pan and broil for 7 to 8 minutes. Turn over the fish and cook for 6 to 7 minutes more, or until flaky.
3. Meanwhile, heat the olive oil in a small skillet over medium heat. Add the garlic and onion, and saute for 2 minutes. Add the spinach and remaining ½ teaspoon salt, and saute for 2 minutes more. Remove from the heat and cover to keep warm.
4. To serve, divide the spinach between two plates and top each portion with a fish fillet. Serve hot.

14. Quinoa with Curried Black Beans and Sweet Potatoes

The beans, quinoa, and sweet potatoes combine to deliver a healthy and filling portion of the meatless protein that is very satisfying. You can prepare the quinoa in the microwave if you prefer; follow package directions to yield one cup.

Servings

Yields 2 servings

Nutrition

Amount Per Serving

Fat 22g, Carbohydrates 17g, and Protein 19g

Ingredients

- ½ cup quinoa
- ½ teaspoon dried rosemary
- 1 cup water
- 1 cup canned black beans, drained
- ½ cup peeled and diced sweet
- 1 teaspoon mild curry powder potato (about 1 small)
- 2 tablespoons chopped fresh parsley
- ½ teaspoon olive oil

Instructions

1. Rinse the quinoa under cold running water in a fine mesh sieve. Drain very well over paper towels and then pat dry.
2. In a small saucepan, toast the quinoa for 2 minutes over medium heat, shaking frequently. Add the water, increase the heat to high, and bring the water to a boil. Cover, reduce the heat to low, and cook for 15 minutes, or until
3. the quinoa is plump and the germ forms little spirals on each grain. Remove from the heat and cover to keep warm.
4. In a small bowl, toss the sweet potato with the olive oil and rosemary.
5. Transfer to a medium skillet over medium-high heat. Saute, frequently stirring, for 6 to 7 minutes, or until well caramelized. Stir in the black beans and curry powder, reduce the heat to medium, and cook, frequently stirring, until the beans are heated through.
6. To serve, place ½ cup cooked quinoa on each plate and top with half of the bean

mixture. Garnish with the parsley.

15. Quinoa Pilaf

Yield

4 Servings

Nutrition

Amount Per Serving

Fat 22g, Carbohydrates 17g, and Protein 19g

Ingredients

- 2 tablespoons extra virgin olive oil
- 1/2 medium yellow onion, finely chopped
- 1/4 bell pepper, finely chopped
- 1 garlic clove, minced
- 2 tablespoons pine nuts
- 1 cup uncooked quinoa
- 2 cups of water
- Pinch freshly ground black pepper
- 2 tablespoons chopped fresh mint
- 2 tablespoons chopped fresh basil or Thai basil*
- 1 tablespoon chopped fresh chives (or green onions including the greens)
- 1 small cucumber, peeled, seeds removed, chopped
- Salt and pepper

Instructions

1. Rinse the box with instructions: check your quinoa box, if you recommend washing

it, place the quinoa in a large sieve and rinse it to remove water. (Some brands do not require washing).

2. Onions, peppers, garlic, pine nuts: Heat 1 tbsp. Put the olive oil over medium-high heat in a pot of 1/1 to 2 quarts. Add and cook onions, rusty peppers, garlic and pine nuts, occasionally stirring until the onions are translucent but not browned.

3. Add quinoa: add and cook uncooked quinoa, occasionally stirring for a few minutes. You can toast a little quinoa for some bread.

4. Add water, salt, stir: Add 2 glasses of water and a teaspoon of salt. Bring to a boil and reduce heat so that cheese and water shine while the pot is partially covered (enough for steam).

5. Cook for 20 minutes or until quinoa is thin and water is absorbed. Remove from heat and serve in a large bowl. Fill with a fork.

6. Add olive oil, mint, basil, onion, cucumber: add over low heat, add another tablespoon of olive oil. In chopped mint, mix basil, onion and cucumber. Add salt and pepper to taste.

7. Chill or cook at room temperature.

GRAINS AND BEANS

16. Mushroom Bean Spread

Yield: 2 packed cups (560 g), or 8 servings

Nutrition content per serving: Carbohydrates: 3g | Protein: 4g | Fat: 5g

Ingredients

- 2 packs (0.88 ounces, or 25 g, each) dried mushroom mix of choice
- 2 cups (470 ml) vegetable broth, boiling
- 1 tablespoon (15 ml) toasted sesame oil 4 cloves garlic, grated or pressed
- 2 tablespoons (8 g) sun-dried tomato halves
- 1 teaspoon dried oregano
- 1 teaspoon red pepper flakes
- 1 (246 g) cooked chickpeas or (266 g) cannellini beans
- ¼ cup (64 g) tahini
- 1 tablespoon (15 ml) olive oil
- 2 tablespoons (30 ml) liquid from jar of capers
- 2 tablespoons (30 ml) fresh lemon juice
- 2 teaspoons onion powder
- 2 tablespoons (18 g) capers, drained and minced
- Salt and pepper

Instructions

1. Wash dried mushrooms quickly and place them in a medium bowl. Add the broth above and soak for 20 minutes. Slowly remove the liquid from the fungus without discarding it. It is used during the processing of the battery, and the rest can be

refrigerated for up to a week in an air container to replace vegetable juice in any recipe.

2. Heat the oil in a large skillet over medium-high heat. Add garlic, sun-dried tomatoes, mushrooms, oranges and chili peppers. Reduce heat to medium-low and cook until lightly brown and fragrant, stirring occasionally, about 6 minutes.

3. Put cooked mushrooms, canola or peanuts, tahini, olive oil, capers, lemon juice and onion powder in a food processor. Cut the process a bit. Add and press the caps several times to spread them everywhere.

4. If necessary, spread one tablespoon of mushrooms, each tablespoon (15 ml), if necessary. Try the condiments.

5. Place in an airtight container for at least 3 hours or overnight and refrigerate until the flavors have melted. Store leftovers in the refrigerator for up to 4 days. If it is too thick for your taste after the refrigerator, add the added mushroom liquid.

17. Black Bean Burger

Yield

6-7 burgers

Nutrition

Carbohydrates: 4g, Total Fat: 11g, Protein: 8g

Ingredients

- 2 (14 ounces) cans black beans, drained, rinsed, and patted dry
- 1 Tablespoon extra-virgin olive oil
- 3/4 cup finely chopped bell pepper (1/2 of a pepper)
- 1 cup finely chopped yellow onion (1/2 of a large onion)
- 3 garlic cloves, minced (about 1 Tablespoon)

- 1 and 1/2 teaspoons ground cumin
- 1 teaspoon chili powder
- 1/2 teaspoon garlic powder
- 1/4 teaspoon smoked paprika
- 1/2 cup bread crumbs or oat flour
- 2 large eggs
- 2 Tablespoons ketchup, mayo, or BBQ sauce
- pinch salt + pepper

Instructions

1. Preheat oven to 325 degrees F (163 degrees C). Sprinkle the beans evenly on a baking sheet and cook for 15 minutes to dry slightly.

2. Also, sauté the olive oil, chopped pepper, onion, and garlic over medium heat until the peppers and onions are softened, about 5-6 minutes. Crush a little moisture. Put in a large bowl or leftover food. Stir or press everything, then add the black beans — mix jam with a fork or powder and place more significant pieces of seeds.

3. Mix about 1/3 cup in each slice.

4. For baking: Place the cooked dough on a wooden board and bake at 375 degrees F (191 degrees C) for 10 minutes on each side for 20 minutes. To Grill: Place the dough pieces on greased aluminum foil and grill on each side for 8 minutes. Heat temperature is a personal priority, as all gas stoves are different. In general, black bean burgers should be cooked at an average temperature of approximately 350 degrees Fahrenheit (177 degrees Celsius) - 400 degrees Fahrenheit (204 degrees Celsius).

5. Serve with your favorite tapas.

18. BBQ Black Bean & Jalepeño Burger

YIELD: 6 Burgers

Nutrition

Carbohydrates: 15g | Protein: 27g | Fat: 16g

Ingredients

- 2 x 400g tins black beans, drained and rinsed
- 4 spring onions
- 12-14 slices jalapeno (from a jar)
- 175 g breadcrumbs (crumbs from 4 slices of bread)
- Juice and zest of 1 lime
- 2 tsp ready chopped garlic Protein content per serving garlic puree (or 2 cloves fresh garlic, peeled and chopped)
- Handful fresh coriander, finely chopped
- 2 tbsp. soy sauce
- 2 tbsp. tahini
- Salt & black pepper

Instructions

- Put the black beans in a food processor and press several times until it is crushed but not completely purified. (Alternatively, crush them with potato sand). Pour into a large bowl.
- Chop the scallions and finely chop the slices. Add both to the bowl, followed by breadcrumbs, lemon zest and juice, garlic, coriander, soy sauce and Tahini. Season with salt and pepper.
- Mix the ingredients to combine well, then divide them into approximately 5-6 pieces (or for smaller burgers 7-8). Use your hamburger machine or shape hamburgers by hand, then place them on a cooked tray covered with baking paper

and refrigerate for as long as necessary.

- **To grill:** rinse each side with a little oil and cook for 5 minutes in the oven

- **For cooking**: Brush each side with oil and bake at 190 degrees Celsius at 375 degrees Fahrenheit for 5 minutes for 20 minutes.

- **To fry**: fry in oil for 5 minutes on each side.

- Serve with chopped avocado, tomato slices, lettuce, purple onion, gherkins, or a slice of cheese and dairy-free tomato sauce.

19. Green Pea Risotto

Yield

4 servings

Nutrition

Carbohydrates: 8g | Protein: 21g | Fat: 22g

Ingredients

- 1tbsp olive oil
- 2 French shallots, chopped
- 1 clove garlic, crushed
- 400g risotto rice
- 150ml white wine
- 750ml veg stock
- 300g frozen peas, thawed
- 200g watercress
- 1 bunch mint leaves
- zest and juice of half a lemon

- Reduced-fat crème Fraiche, to serve

Instructions

- Heat the olive oil in a pan over medium heat over medium heat and cook the rest for a few minutes until it softens, then add the garlic and cook for 2 minutes, then add the rice.

- Increase the heat and add wine to the pot. Cook 1-2 minutes and add 4 broths. Gradually add the broth and add progressively until all the liquid is absorbed and the rice is tender.

- Meanwhile, beat the peas, juices, mint and lemons in a food processor. Add the green puree to the cooked risotto, add the seasoning and cook for 1 minute.

- If desired, divide the risotto between 4 bowls and above with frame cream and some additional peas to decorate.

20. Dilly White Beans

Yield

4 servings

Nutrition

Fat: 15g Carbohydrates: 12g Protein: 9g

Ingredients

- 1½ cups ricotta
- 1½ tsp. kosher salt, divided, plus more
- 1 lemon
- 2 Tbsp. white wine vinegar
- 2 tsp. Dijon mustard
- 1 tsp. freshly ground black pepper

- ½ cup extra-virgin olive oil, divided
- 4 scallions
- 8 oz. sugar snap peas
- ½ cup dill sprigs
- 1 14.5-oz can cannellini, navy, or gigante beans
- 4 1"-thick slices crusty bread
- 1 garlic clove

Instructions

1. Using a spatula, mix 1 cup of ricotta and one tablespoon. Put the salt in a medium bowl to separate the cheese and make the ricotta soften and spread. Do not be afraid of aggression. Grate half the lemon in a small saucepan and stir to combine.

2. Divide the lemon in half and pour the water into a large bowl. Beat in 2 tablespoons. White wine vinegar, 2 tablespoons. Dijon mustard, 1 tbsp. Salt and tablespoons Sucking constantly, slowly pour in 2 cups of olive oil until the dressing is slightly thick and no longer greasy. You want to add the oil gradually so that your mixture is creamy and emulsified.

3. Cut the sliced onions and cut them in four directions. Add the dressing to the bowl and stir to combine.

4. The ends of 8 oz. If you are serving the peas, harden and discard the strands along their seams (if the knife appears to be threatening, you can use your fingers). Cut the chopped peas into diagonal slices (about the size of their beans) and add them to the bowl.

5. Chop the meatballs well and add them to the pan.

6. Chop gingerbread, seaweed or beans in a fine mesh sieve, then cover the pot. Mix to cover well. Adjust the seasoning and adjust the seasoning, adding more salt if necessary.

7. Cut the crusted bread in half (this will only make it easier to eat). Heat 2 tablespoons. Olive oil in a large medium skillet until lightly browned, about 1 minute. Reduce heat 4 Slices of bread in a single layer until golden brown and crispy at the bottom, 5 to 7 minutes (seems to be patient for a while). Transfer the fried side of the bread to a plate to make it crispy. Repeat with the remaining 2 tablespoons. Oil and 4 pieces of bread. (Why simply fry one side of the bread? The side of the filling should be strong enough to support the cheese and the end without coming out), but the other side can be soft and easy to eat. The best of both worlds. .)

8. Rub the fried portion of each bread with 1 clove of garlic. Season with a little more salt.

9. Divide the ricotta mixture between toasts. Spoon the peas and beans over it. Do not leave wings: divide the leftovers between toasts.

10. Serve and enjoy!

21. Peppered Pinto Beans

Yield

10 servings

Nutrition

Fat: 5g Carbohydrates: 6g Protein: 9g

Ingredients

- 1 tbsp. plain flour
- 30g butter
- 300ml beef stock
- 50ml cider vinegar
- 1 tbsp. Worcestershire sauce

- 2 tbsp. honey
- 2 tsp dark muscovado sugar
- 2 bay leaves
- 1 tsp black peppercorns, crushed
- 3 x 400g cans pinto beans

Instructions

1. Heat the flour and butter in a large pan and mix to form a roux.
2. Repeat cooking until cookies brown.
3. Add broth, vinegar, sauces, honey, sugar, bay leaf and pepper, then season with salt.
4. Boil, bubble for 2-3 minutes, then add beans and cook 10 minutes.
5. It can be prepared 1-2 days in advance; Refrigerate and serve again before serving.

BREAD

22. Cinnamon Bread

(with or without dairy products)

Some people are reluctant to make their bread, because they consider it a complicated process, not in this case! This is a quick and easy recipe. And the bread is perfect in texture and flavor.

Servings

10

Nutrition

- Fat 11.3g
- Carb 2.5g
- Protein 3.8g

Ingredients

1. 1/2 cup coconut flour
2. 1/2 tablespoon of baking powder
3. 1/2 tablespoon of baking powder
4. 1 tablespoon cinnamon
5. 1/4 tablespoon of Stevia Select Stevia or the sweetener of your choice (as desired)
6. 3 eggs
7. 1/3 cup pure cream or Greek yogurt **
8. 3 tablespoons salted butter **
9. 2 teaspoons of water

** For dairy products, use coconut milk and coconut oil and add 1/8 tablespoon. Salt

Instructions

1. Heat the oven to 350 degrees F. Grease and cover the bottom of the tray with parchment paper. Mix the dry ingredients with the whisk until well mixed. Add the remaining ingredients and mix well. Try the sweetness and adjust it if necessary. Let stand for 3 minutes and then stir again.

2. Put the tray in the pan with bread. Bake for 25 to 30 minutes or until the rod inserted in the center comes out clean. Let cool on the stand. Store in the refrigerator.

23. Cheesy Flax & Chia Seed Cracker Bread

Servings

28-30 crackers

Nutrition

- Fat 8.3g
- Carb 1.5g
- Protein 2.8g

Ingredients

- 1 1/2 c ground flax seeds (I used my Magic Bullet)
- 2 teaspoons chia seeds (we recommend skipping)
- 2 eggs, beaten
- Cheddar chopped 1/2 c
- 1/2 teaspoon of garlic powder
- 1/2 teaspoon salt
- 1/2 teaspoon pepper

Instructions

1. Combine all ingredients in a medium bowl and shake with your hands until a thick dough forms.

2. Spray a sheet of foil or plastic foil with non-stick spray. Form the dough into a diary with your hands and place it on the wrapper. Turn it until it is about a foot or so long and about one and a half inches in diameter. You can keep it round or tap into a square shape. Put it in the freezer for about 5 minutes, until it freezes.

3. In the meantime, preheat the oven to 350 degrees. Remove the dough from the freezer and slice into thick slices about 1/4 to 1/2 inch.

4. Place on a greased baking sheet and bake for 12-15 minutes until browned. Remove from the oven and cool. Taste.

5. Don't throw them away yet. Put something delicious in the first place and see if you can stand it. Report back. This message will self-destruct in five ... four ... ... three ... one. Just kidding. Still here. Now it's starting to crack ......

24. Paleo Keto Shortbread Cookies

Serve your Keto pie cakes with a cold glass of non-dairy milk ice cream, a warm cup of original anti-balloon coffee or a relaxing spiced milk chai for a perfect afternoon treatment.

Portions

It is perfect for 24 servings.

Nutrition

It contains 29.5 g of fat, 14 g of protein and 17.6 g of net carbohydrates per serving. Although the preparation lasts 40 minutes, the cooking time is 20 minutes.

Ingredients Shortbread:

- 1 1/3 cup (145 g) almond flour
- 1/4 teaspoon sea salt
- 1/3 cup plus 1 teaspoon (80 g) of butter or grass-fed ice

- 4 tablespoons (40 g) of erythritol monk fruit mix, such as Lakanto
- 1/2 teaspoon vanilla extract
- 1 tablespoon (8 g) coconut flour
- 1 tablespoon (8 g) of collagen peptides
- 1 crushed short vanilla collagen protein bar

25. Chocolate Gas Ingredients (Optional):
- ounces (134 g) of quality dark chocolate (at least 85% cocoa), chopped
- 3 tablespoons avocado oil
- 2 tablespoons low-fat cocoa

Instructions:
1. In a food processor, mix all the ingredients with a short peel, except the collagen bar, until combined.
2. Carefully remove and spread the dough with a pin until it is approximately 3.5 mm thick.
3. Cut the cakes with the round chalk cutter and freeze them for 30 minutes.
4. Preheat the oven to 350 degrees and prepare a perforated tray with parchment or silicone coating.
5. Remove the cakes from the freezer, place them on the baking sheet and bake for about 8 minutes or until golden brown. The baking time will vary depending on the oven, the baking tray and the baking thickness.
6. Allow the shortbread to cool completely before adding icing.
7. While the cakes are cooling, prepare the glaze: Using a double boiler on the plate, lightly melt the chocolate and oil until well combined. Mix in cocoa foods.
8. Use chocolate chip cookies and sprinkle with collagen crumbs.

26. Savane Bread with Coconut and Rosemary

You often don't associate coconut with salt flavors, but it works well here. The texture is slightly drier than some Ketogenic bread recipes, making it an excellent option to serve with paleo soups or pate. Coconut flour gives this bread a lighter texture, which means you can use this recipe to try different flavor options.

Servings

3

Nutrition

Fat 11.3 g, Carb 2.5 g, Protein 3.8 g

Ingredients

- 4 eggs
- 1/4 cup olive oil
- 1/4 cup coconut milk
- 1 teaspoon freshly ground rosemary
- 1 teaspoon baking soda
- 1 teaspoon coarse salt
- 1/3 cup flax seeds
- 3/4 of coconut flour cane

Instructions

1. Preheat oven to 180C (350F).
2. In a bowl, mix the eggs, olive oil, coconut milk, and rosemary with a hand mixer until smooth.
3. Add flax seeds, soda, and sea salt and mix well.
4. Add coconut flour and mix well. So far, the mixture is quite dry.
5. Scrape the dough with a spatula in a baking dish and form a beautiful loaf of bread

with your hands. (You can also place the dough in a small basket and spread it with a spatula).

6. Bake for 45 minutes or until an inserted stick comes out clean.

27. Cauliflower Coconut Bread

This recipe is perfect for cauliflower lovers! It is based on a French cauliflower cake recipe and is an ideal companion for serving soups and stews. Coconut flour gives this bread a lighter texture and is also rich in fiber and nutrients that support bone health and blood sugar problems. If you have any remains, refrigerate them and then reheat them in the oven. A lot of Ketogenic bread tastes so good when served hot!

Servings

8

Nutrition

- Fat 10.2 g
- Carb 5.8 g
- Protein 6.2 g

Ingredients

- 1 cauliflower with a small head, cleaned and minced in small flowers
- 1/4 cup extra virgin olive oil
- 1/4 cup unsweetened almond milk, coconut milk or whole milk
- 6 eggs
- 3/4 cane coconut flour
- 1/2 teaspoon baking
- 1/2 teaspoon sea salt
- 1 teaspoon of garlic powder

Preparation

1. Preheat oven for frying.

2. Place the chopped cauliflower on a baking sheet lined with aluminum foil, sprinkle with olive oil, salt and pepper (in addition, not included in the ingredients list) and fry until the fork is tender and fried. Meanwhile, combine the remaining ingredients in a large mixing bowl.

3. Lower the oven to 350. Bend the roasted cauliflower in the dough. Put the mixture in a well-greased pan of bread.

4. Bake 25-30 minutes until browned.

5. Cut and serve. Refrigerate the leftovers and reheat in the toaster oven.

28. Avocado Chocolate Bread

This bread is IF friendly and is so delicious that you probably want to have it for dessert! Avocado, almond flour, and cocoa powder: the perfect combination for tasty bread.

Servings

8

Nutrition

- Fat 26g
- Carb 13g
- Protein 10g

Ingredients

- 2 ripe avocados, mash
- 3 tablespoons (45 ml) coconut oil
- 3 whispered eggs
- 2 cups (240 g) almond flour

- 1/2 cup (48 g) cocoa powder
- 1 teaspoon (4 g) of baking soda
- 1/2 teaspoon (1 g) baking powder
- 1 teaspoon (5 ml) vanilla extract
- Stevia, to taste
- Salt spray

Instructions

1. Preheat the oven to 175 F (350 F).
2. Mix everything.
3. Place in a pan with bread.
4. Bake 40 to 45 minutes until you can deep a toothpick, and it comes out without any stain.

BEVERAGES AND SMOOTHIES

29. Garden Green Smoothie Bag

Yield

1 Serving

Nutrition

Calories: 49, Carbohydrate: 9 g, Fat: 0.5 g, Protein: 3 g

Ingredients

- 1/4 cup chopped celery (1 small stalk)
- 1/4 cup chopped fennel (1/4 large head)
- 1/4 cup chopped romaine or green leaf lettuce
- 1/4 cup frozen peas
- 2 Tbs. non-dairy milk or water
- 1 Tbs. fresh parsley leaves
- 1 Tbs. chopped fennel fronds
- 1 Tbs. lemon juice
- 4 ice cubes

Instructions

Place all ingredients in a blender and blend until smooth. Season with salt and pepper, if desired.

30. Keto Vanilla Milk Shake

Smooth and fluffy vanilla milkshake! Add almond butter to this vanilla milkshake Keto.

Use almond milk as a low carb alternative to whole milk.

Servings

It is perfect for 2 servings.

Nutrition

It contains 41 g of fat, 8 g of protein and 3 g of net carbohydrates per serving. The preparation lasts 5 minutes and

ingredients

- 1 cup unsweetened almond milk
- 1/4 cup thick cream *
- 1 cup crushed ice
- 2 teaspoons almond butter
- 1/2 spoon. Vanilla extract
- Stevia sweetener according to taste (6-7 drops)
- Mineral salt tip
- Optional: sliced almonds, flax seeds, hazelnuts, cinnamon

Instructions

1. Put all the ingredients in the blender and mix until all the ice is crushed and the milkshake is thick

31. Walnut Milk

Yield

12 1/4 cup servings

Nutrition

Fat 6g, Carbohydrates 1g, Protein 1g

Ingredients

- 1 cup walnuts
- 3.5 cups of filtered water

- 1/4 tsp cinnamon

Instructions

2. There are two ways to prepare this recipe. If you are in a hurry, boil the nuts for 10 minutes to soften them; otherwise, moisten them for at least 8 hours at night.

3. Wash soaked (or boiled) nuts. Place the soaked nuts in the blender, add the filtered water + cinnamon, and mix over high heat for 1 minute until uniform.

4. Strain through a bag of nut milk (there must be at least pulp with nuts) + Store in a glass container in the refrigerator for 3-4 days.

32. Alkaline Detox Tea

Yield

2 servings

Nutrition

Fat 5g, Carbohydrates 0.8g, Protein 1g

Ingredients

- 500ml filtered water
- 1/4 tsp powdered cardamom
- 1/4 tsp powdered cinnamon
- 1/2 tsp powdered ginger
- 1/2 tsp powdered turmeric
- 1/2 lemon

Instructions

1. There are two ways to prepare this recipe. If you are in a hurry, boil the nuts for 10 minutes to soften them; otherwise, moisten them for at least 8 hours at night.

2. Wash soaked (or boiled) nuts. Place the soaked nuts in the blender, add the filtered water + cinnamon, and mix over high heat for 1 minute until uniform.

3. Strain through a bag of nut milk (there must be at least pulp with nuts) + Store in a glass container in the refrigerator for 3-4 days.

33. Green Fruit Juice

Yield

4 cups

Nutrition

Carbohydrates: 7.7g | Protein: 5.6g | Fat: 10g

Ingredients

- 1 bunch curly kale roughly chopped
- 1 large lemon peeled and quartered
- 1-inch ginger peeled
- 1 large cucumber cut into long strips
- 2 large granny smith apples cored and sliced
- 4 whole celery stalks

Instructions

1. Wash and prepare the vegetables.
2. Juices listed, respectively.
3. Optional: push through a sieve (if you don't like dough)
4. Drink fast, and enjoy it! * *

34. Flat Flush Juice

Yield

3 servings

Nutrition

Fat 3g, Carbohydrates 1g, Protein 1g

Ingredients

- 1 pink grapefruit peeled
- 1 tangelo peeled
- 2 leaves chard
- 1 lemon peeled
- 1 small bunch mint

Instructions

Wash all produce thoroughly and chop into sizes that will fit into your juicer. Juice all ingredients and serve over ice.

VEGETABLES AND SALADS

35. Salad with Plum Vinaigrette

The truth is, my favorite way to eat most stone fruits—from peaches to plums to cherries—is understandable. I often find that they don't need much embellishment to taste fantastic. After all, the last thing I want to do is obscure the fresh summer flavor that I've waited nine long months to experience again.

Servings

This recipe makes 4 servings.

Nutrition

32 g protein, 20 g carbs, 23 g fat

Ingredients

- 1 head butter lettuce
- 1/2 small red onion
- 2 medium carrots
- 1 small beet
- 1 cucumber, chopped
- 1/2 cup button mushrooms
- 1 avocado, cubed Vinaigrette Ingredients:
- 1/2 cup olive oil
- 1 tbsp. ume plum vinegar
- 1 lemon, juiced
- 1 tsp ginger powder

Directions

1. Make the salad: Combine the lettuce, onion, carrots, beet, cucumber, and

mushrooms in a large bowl.

2. Make the vinaigrette: Combine the olive oil, vinegar, lemon juice,2. and ginger powder in a small bowl and whisk together.

3. Top the salad with fresh avocado and vinaigrette. Divide the salad3. into 4 equal servings.

36. Shrimp and Cranberry Salad

Dried cranberries add a tart touch of flavor to this fresh shrimp salad. Using steamed shrimp from your seafood counter makes this a very fast lunch to prepare.

Servings

Yields 4 servings.

Ingredients

- 1 dozen large (26-30 count) cooked
- ½ cup sliced red onion shrimp, peeled and deveined
- ¼ cup lime juice
- ¼ teaspoon ground cumin
- ¼ teaspoon paprika
- 2 cups chopped romaine lettuce
- ½ yellow bell pepper, chopped
- ½ orange bell pepper, chopped
- ½ cup dried cranberries
- ½ cup of your favorite homemade or store-bought balsamic vinaigrette

Instructions

1. In a small bowl, toss the shrimp with the lime juice, cumin, and paprika, and let them sit for 30 minutes in the refrigerator. Drain.

2. In a large bowl, combine the lettuce, onion, bell peppers, and cranberries until evenly combined.

3. Add the marinated shrimp and balsamic vinaigrette and toss again. Divide between 4 salad plates and serve.

Nutrients

1. Calories 165g
2. Fat 15g
3. 3g protein
4. Carbs 7g

37. Tuna and Bean Salad Pockets

This light but filling recipe is a great one for workday lunches. It packs well and the flavor gets better the longer it has a chance to sit, so prepare the salad the night before and pop it into a pita pocket and then into your lunch bag in the morning.

Servings

Yields 4 servings.

Ingredients

- 4 whole-wheat pita pockets 1 (6-ounce) can tuna packed in water, drained
- ½ (15-ounce) can pinto beans, rinsed and drained
- ¼ cup diced white onion
- 2 tablespoons light mayonnaise
- teaspoon spicy brown mustard
- ½ teaspoon celery seed
- ½ teaspoon freshly ground black pepper
- 1 cup chopped romaine lettuce

Instructions

1. If the pitas are unsliced, slice them so that there is a pocket-like opening, being careful not to cut through the sides or bottoms.

2. In a small mixing bowl, combine the tuna, pinto beans, onion, mayonnaise, mustard, celery seed, and pepper; mix well.

3. Divide the lettuce between the pita pockets, then fill each one with one-quarter of the tuna salad.

Nutrients

- Fat 18g
- 6g protein
- Carbs 9g

38. Grilled Chicken Salad with Poppy Seed Dressing

Salads are easy to put together, and when made with lots of fresh, high-fiber vegetables, they provide lots of food for very few calories. This salad not only tastes great but also fills you up nicely, too.

Servings

Yields 2 servings.

Nutrition

Amount Per Serving

Fat 32g, Carbohydrates 17g, and Protein 42g

Ingredients

- 2 tablespoons light olive oil
- 1 tablespoon apple cider vinegar
- 1 teaspoon Dijon mustard
- 1 tablespoon poppy seeds

- ½ cup chopped cooked chicken breast
- 1 cup chopped romaine lettuce
- 1 medium unpeeled cucumber, sliced
- 1 medium red bell pepper, chopped
- 1 small red onion, chopped

Instructions

1. In a medium mixing bowl, whisk together the olive oil, cider vinegar, Dijon mustard, and poppy seeds for about 1 minute, or until well blended and smooth.
2. Add the chicken, lettuce, cucumber, bell pepper, and onion, and toss well until evenly coated.
3. Divide between two salad plates and serve immediately.

39. Cucumber-Mullet-Avocado Salad

Cucumber salad avocado with lime, and feta this fits with delight! Here this tasty salad, with so many of my favorite flavors, these have what with low carbohydrate level, IF, low glucose level, gluten-free, vegetarian diet South Beach.

Servings

1 serving

Ingredient

- 1 cucumber, chopped
- 1/4 red onion, thinly sliced
- 1 sausage olive oil
- 1/2 avocado
- Freshly chopped bran and parsley
- Apple cider vinegar

- Salt for taste

Direction

1. Mix the cucumber, onion, parsley and mint in a bowl.
2. In a small bowl, whisk the apple cider vinegar, olive oil, and sea salt.
3. Drop the dressing with vegetables and enjoy!

Nutrients

- Calories 778
- Fat 61g
- 22g protein
- Carbs 52g

40. Steamed Cauliflower

Yield

1 cup

Nutrition

Carbohydrates: 4g, protein: 2g, Fat: 5g

Ingredients

- 1 head cauliflower, cut into florets
- 4 teaspoons extra-virgin olive oil
- ¾ teaspoon coarse kosher salt
- ¼ teaspoon freshly ground pepper
- 4 teaspoons chopped fresh herbs

Instructions

1. Boil an inch or two of water in a large pot heated by an electric steamer.
2. Add the cauliflower to the steam basket, cover the pan, and cook until the cauliflower is tender, 4 to 5 minutes.
3. Remove the steaming basket from the pot and pour the water.
4. Empty the cauliflower from the steaming basket in the bowl. Sprinkle with oil and sprinkle with salt and pepper.
5. Rinse Add the vegetable and vegetable cover. Serve immediately.

41. Pomegranate, Arugula Salad

Instead of relying on fat for aroma, this fresh garnish uses a variety of flavors and textures to impress guests: crispy, Romanian spicy; crunchy and crunchy pomegranate seeds; And delicious, slightly sweet fish. It is also nutritious, with nuts that contribute to monounsaturated fats (the good type) and pomegranates that offer a good dose of fiber, vitamin C and antioxidants.

Portions

This recipe makes 4 servings.

Ingredients

- 4 cups arugula
- 1 small fennel bulb, thinly sliced
- 1 cup pomegranate seeds
- 1/4 cup blood orange eggplant

Instructions

1. Combine relatives, slices of fennel and pomegranate seeds in a large bowl.
2. Chop the salad with orange eggplant (see recipe below) and divide it into 4 equal portions. Enjoy!

Nutrition

1. 145.8 kcal

2. 4g protein

3. 14.8 g of carbohydrates

4. 10 g of fat

42. Smoky Coleslaw

Yield

5 servings

Nutrition

Carbohydrates: 4g | Protein: 1g | Fat: 7g

Ingredients

- 6 cups shredded cabbage
- 1 cup shredded carrots
- 1/2 cup sliced celery
- 1/2 cup sliced toasted almonds
- 1/2 cup mayonnaise
- 1 tablespoon apple cider vinegar
- 1 teaspoon spicy brown mustard
- 2 teaspoons brown sugar
- 1/2 teaspoon smoked paprika
- 1/2 teaspoon chipotle powder
- 1 teaspoon kosher or sea salt
- Fresh cracked black pepper, to taste

Instructions

3. Preheat the oven to 425 degrees Fahrenheit. Line a baking sheet with removable paper.

4. Combine butter, miso paste, maple syrup, soy sauce, rice wine vinegar, sesame seeds, and chopped red pepper in a small saucepan over medium heat: Cook, blisters, until melted and syrupy, about 5 minutes.

5. Pour the carrots, parsley, and fennel in a large bowl and sprinkle with salt and pepper. Transfer to a baking sheet and spread in a single layer. Bake for 35-40 minutes until the vegetables are tender and caramelized.

43. Garlic and Herb Zoodles

Yield

4 servings

Nutrition

Protein 10.7 g, Carbohydrate 11.2 g, Fat 14.3 g

Ingredients

- 3 long, thin zucchini
- freshly grated parmesan cheese
- significant pinch steak seasoning (store-bought or see notes for recipe)
- 1 stick salted butter (1/2 cup,) softened to room temperature
- 2 Tablespoons chopped fresh parsley
- 1 Tablespoon finely minced fresh rosemary
- 1 Tablespoon finely minced fresh thyme
- 1 garlic clove, pressed or minced
- squeeze fresh lemon juice

Instructions

1. Spiral the zucchini with the thickest strand of the noodle leaf to create zodiacs and then add them to a can on top of a bowl. Gently salt and then stir with your fingers to cover and refrigerate for 30 minutes to an hour to drain the excess liquid. Remove the zoodles from the refrigerator and dry them with paper towels or paper towels.

2. Meanwhile, add the garlic and herb butter ingredients in a small bowl and then stir to combine and set aside. It can be done a few days before or even several weeks because the butter freezes well.

3. After drying and pressing the trays, heat a 12-inch roll over medium heat. Add 2 tablespoons of garlic butter and melt, add the zest and the sauce to a boil for 2-3 minutes and add more butter. Turn off the heat if desired and then grate in Parmesan cheese to add flavor.

SNACKS

44. Amazing chocolate cheesecake

In addition to being the richest, densest, and lowest carb recipe on the planet, this triple creamy, decadent chocolate cheese will make all your dreams come true. You don't need sugar or gluten with this fantastic recipe.

Servings

It is perfect for 12 meals.

Nutrition

It contains 32.98 g of fat, 7.75 g of protein, and 5.22 g of net carbohydrates per serving. Although the preparation lasts 15 minutes, the cooking time is 2 hours.

Ingredients

— 1/4 1 1/4 cup almond flour

- 1/4 cup cocoa powder
- 1/4 cup Swerve sweetener
- 3 tablespoons melted vegan butter
- 6 ounces' dark chocolate without chopped sugar
- 1 tablespoon of vegan butter
- 24 ounces softened cream cheese
- 1/2 cup Swerve sweetener
- Sweetener with 1/1 cup of powder
- 1 tablespoon vanilla extract
- 3 large eggs at room temperature
- 1/4 cup cocoa powder
- 1/3 cup thick cream at room temperature

- 2 teaspoons melted butter to brush the sides of the pan
- 3/4 fresh cane
- Swerve Sweetener 1/3 cup
- 3 oz. chopped chocolate
- 1/2 teaspoon vanilla extract

Instructions
1. Preheat oven to 325F. In a medium bowl, mix the almond flour, cocoa powder, and sweetener. Stir the melted butter until well combined.
2. Press the mixture well into the bottom of a 9-inch bow-shaped container. Bake 10 to 12 minutes, then remove and reduce oven temperature to 300F.
3. In a small saucepan over medium heat, melt the dark chocolate with butter, mix until smooth. Set aside to cool.
4. In a large bowl, beat cream cheese until smooth. Beat the sweeteners and vanilla extract, then beat the eggs one by one, scraping the sides and sides of the bowl as necessary.
5. Add cocoa powder and thick cream until well combined, then mix the melted chocolate until the mixture is completely smooth.
6. Brush the parts of the pan with melted butter, being careful not to disturb the crust. Pour the filling into the pan and shake gently from side to side so that it comes out evenly.
7. Bake 55 to 60 minutes or until the filling is ready, but only a little in the center.
8. Remove and let cool for 15 minutes, then wrap a sharp knife around the inside of the pan to loosen. Let cool completely. After cooling, remove the sides, cover well in a plastic wrap and refrigerate for at least 3 hours.
9. In a medium saucepan over medium heat, combine the cream and the sweetener. Bring to a simmer, then remove from heat and add chopped chocolate and vanilla.

Let stand for 5 minutes and then beat until smooth.

10. Pour over the top of cold cheese, letting it drain slightly on the sides. Cool until ready.

45. Walnut Chocolate Bites

Yield

16 servings

Nutrition

Fat: 4g, Carbohydrates: 5 G, Protein: 2 G

Ingredients

- 1 ½ cup Old Fashioned oats
- 3 tablespoons dark cocoa
- ½ teaspoon cinnamon
- Generous pinch salt
- 1 cup pitted soft dates, 4 ounces
- 3 tablespoons almond butter
- 3 tablespoons dark pure maple syrup
- 3 tablespoons chopped walnuts, toasted
- 3 tablespoons mini chocolate chips

Instructions

1. Put the oatmeal in a food processor and process until it is frozen. Transfer to a medium bowl. Add cocoa, cinnamon and salt and mix to combine.
2. Apply the dates in the food processing and press several times to break them down. Add and process almond butter and maple syrup, crush the sides if necessary to

make a thick paste.

3. Add the dough to the bowl and pot and stir with a tablespoon of silicone to begin to resemble crushed cookie dough, about 2 minutes. Continue the work of the dough, clean with your hands if necessary to convert the oatmeal mixture into a coherent dough. Add nuts and chocolate chips. Kneel well. Turn the form into 14 balls. If used, rinse with chocolate. Refrigerate the refrigerator to adjust the chocolate.

46. Cinnamon and caramel pudding

Sweet, fluffy, and delicious: this cinnamon and caramel pudding is everything you want it to be. Perfect for leftover bread crumbs or a grilled dinner, this easy pudding recipe uses muffins and a caramel rum sauce to melt it.

Servings

It is perfect for 6 servings.

Nutrition

It contains 18 g of fat, 2 g of protein, and 8 g of net carbohydrates per serving. Although the preparation lasts 10 minutes, the cooking time is 1 hour.

Ingredients

- 3 eggs 3/4 cup thick cream
- 1/2 splendid cane
- 1/4 cup unsweetened caramel topping
- 1 cup almond flour
- 1/4 teaspoon of baking powder
- 1 cup of cottage cheese, a shell full of fat
- 1/4 teaspoon cinnamon

Instructions

1. Beat all the ingredients with the mixer until they are as foamy and soft as possible;

there will still be a lot of cottage cheese.

2. Pour into an 8x8 "glass baking dish with butter and sprinkle extra cinnamon.

3. Bake at 350 ° F for about 1 hour or until the countertop is golden brown.

47. Cheesecake Mousse

Cheesecake Mousse is a light and airy Keto recipe that is quick and easy to prepare. This low carb dessert is excellent with chocolate or fruit sauce.

Servings

It is perfect for 6 servings.

Nutrition

It contains 27.8 g of fat, 3.7 g of protein, and 16.5 g of net carbohydrates per serving. The preparation lasts 5 minutes.

Ingredients

- 8 ounces softened cream cheese
- 1/3 cup low carbohydrate sweetener or erythritol powder
- 1/8 teaspoon concentrated stevia powder
- 1 1/2 teaspoons vanilla extract
- 1/4 teaspoon lemon extract
- 1 cup thick whipped cream or regular thick cream

Instructions

1. Beat the cream cheese until smooth.
2. Mix the extract of erythritol, stevia, vanilla, and lemon until well combined.
3. In a separate bowl, beat the thick cream with the mixer until stiff peaks form.
4. Fold half the whisk in the cream cheese mixture until it is well incorporated. Fold the other half of the whip.

5. Beat with an electric mixer until it is soft and fluffy.

6. In the refrigerator for at least two hours. Pipe or spoon in individual dishes. Melt with fresh fruit or unsweetened chocolate if desired.

48. Chocolate and Mint Cupcakes

Mint and chocolate glaze are beautiful. You will love to pee and eat it! This dessert is Keto, Paleo, GAPS, and low carb, with only small variations for each diet. Chocolate cupcakes are moist and tasty! The glaze has two flavors: both are delicate, fun and chocolate, to create such a beautiful swirl!

Servings

It is perfect for 8 servings.

Nutrition

It contains 11.4 g of fat, 4.4 g of protein, and 4.6 g of net carbohydrates per serving.

Ingredients

Chocolate cupcakes (dairy-free)

- 3/4 cup hot coconut butter

- Sweet 2/3 cup of practical sweetener Monk fruit sweetener (see the link below in the Recipe Notes or low carb sweetener) works for Keto, honey for GAPS / Paleo, coconut sugar/maple syrup and Paleo

- 1/2 cup hot melted coconut oil or other liquid fats: hot melted butter/ice, warm melted butter, avocado oil

- Trade 1/2 cup of fair trade cocoa powder, see the recipe notes to see the link to good cocoa

- Temperature 2 eggs at room temperature (not cold); You can do this by putting cold eggs in a glass of hot tap water for 30 minutes

- 1/4 cup coconut flour

- 1/4 cup whole coconut milk (not frozen)

- 1 teaspoon jelly
- Optional 1 teaspoon of optional peppermint oil (you can make simple chocolate cupcakes if you wish).
- 1/2 teaspoon of baking soda
- 1/4 teaspoon sea salt

49. Pumpkin Pie Without Crust

Sweet pumpkin kiss, juicy coconut and lemon, all wrapped in a creamy filling.

This is a wonderful low in carbohydrates, at its best!

Servings

It is perfect for 10 servings.

Nutrition

It contains 10 g of fat, 2 g of protein, and 2 g of net carbohydrates per serving. While the preparation lasts 10 minutes, the cooking time is 40 minutes.

Ingredients

- 2 tablespoons of butter, to grease the baking dish
- 4 tablespoons grated coconut without sugar
- 15 oz. pumpkin
- 2/3 heavy fresh cane
- 1-ounce butter
- -% teaspoon salt
- 2 teaspoons pumpkin pie
- 2 teaspoons coconut flour (optional)
- -% lemon, just dowry

- 1 teaspoon of baking powder
- 3 eggs
- 1/4 cups of thick cream, to serve

Instructions

1. Cut the squash into cubes and place it in a pan. Add wheat, butter and salt and boil over medium heat.
2. Lower the heat, boil until the pumpkin is soft. It will take at least 15 ¬20 minutes. Stir occasionally.
3. When the squash is soft, add the remaining ingredients, except the eggs and mix until a smooth puree is obtained with a hand blender, an immersion blender or a food processor.
4. Beat the eggs in a separate bowl with a hand mixer for 2-3 minutes. Add the purified pumpkin and mix well.
5. Heat the oven to 200 ° C to 400 ° F. Grease a 9 "baking dish with butter and apply the coconut flakes evenly.
6. Pour the oven into the oven and bake for about 20 minutes or until halfway through.

50. Coconut Blondies

A wonderful batch of coconut flour blondies, which now made me notice that this is a recipe to come back and play with the aromas. It is a light recipe for blond coconut.

Portions

It is perfect for 9 servings.

Nutrition

It contains 17 g of fat, 4 g of protein and 6 g of net carbohydrates per serving. Although the preparation lasts 5 minutes, the cooking time is 20 minutes.

Ingredients

- 1/2 cup (113 g) untreated butter
- 1/2 cup (105 g) of erythritol or sugar substitute
- 4 eggs
- 1/2 cup (56 g) coconut flour
- 1/4 cup (56 g) coconut milk
- 1/2 cup (30 g) unsweetened coconut
- 1 tablespoon vanilla extract
- 1/4 teaspoon baking powder
- 1/4 teaspoon salt

Instructions

1. Preheat oven to 180C / 350F degrees
2. Grease and line an 8-inch baking sheet with parchment paper.
3. In a bowl, mix the butter and erythritol until smooth.
4. Add the eggs, stirring in the oven once.
5. Then add the vanilla extract and coconut milk and beat until smooth.
6. Then add coconut flour, dried coconut, baking powder and salt. Mix until smooth.
7. If the mixture is too thick, add more coconut milk (coconut flour may vary between brands).
8. Bake on the baking sheet and bake for 25-30 minutes until firm and golden brown.
9. Let cool in the pan for at least 30 minutes.
10. Cut into squares and enjoy!

51. Italian Crackers

These tasty cookies are an excellent way to recover part of the crisis. With the option of adding several flavors, you can make this recipe for any taste, or you can choose Ingredients for a particular occasion. You can increase the number of ingredients by making these cookies as a buffet meal.

Servings

6

Nutrition

- Fat 11.3 g
- Carb 2.5 g
- Protein 3.8 g

Ingredients

- 1/2 (143 g) Almond flour
- 2 teaspoons (30 ml) olive oil
- 3/4 teaspoon (5 g) of salt
- 1/4 tablespoon (0.5 g) basil
- 1/2 teaspoon (1 g) thyme
- 1/4 teaspoon (0.5 g) oregano
- 1/2 tablespoon (1 g) onion powder
- Garlic powder 1/4 teaspoon (0.5 g)

Instructions

1. Preheat oven to 177 °C (350 °F).
2. Mix all the ingredients well to form a dough.
3. Form the dough into a long rectangular log (use a sheet or film to wrap the money) and then cut it into thin slices (approximately 0.5 cm) thick. Gently place each slice on a baking sheet lined with parchment paper. It does about. 20-30 cookies,

depending on size.

4. Bake 10 to 12 minutes.

52. Easy Granola Bars

This recipe is much better for you than any business granola bars, which are frequently weighed down with high-fructose corn syrup and less solid grains. These bars heat up in a jiffy and will keep in a hermetically sealed compartment for as long as a multi week—that is, if they keep going that long.

Servings

Yields 1 dozen bars.

Nutrition

Amount Per Serving

Fat 14g, Carbohydrates 8g, and Protein 17g

Ingredients

- teaspoon coconut oil
- 1 cup pecan pieces
- 1 cup raw pumpkin seeds
- l cup chopped walnuts
- l cup dried cranberries
- l cup dried apricots, chopped
- l cup unsweetened coconut flakes
- ½ cup coconut oil, melted
- ½ cup almond butter
- ½ cup raw honey
- ½ teaspoon pure vanilla extract

- ½ teaspoon salt
- 1 teaspoon ground cinnamon

Instructions

1. Preheat the oven to 325 degrees F. Grease a 9-by-13-inch baking pan with the 1 teaspoon of coconut oil and set aside.
2. In a large bowl, combine the pecans, pumpkin seeds, walnuts, cranberries, apricots, and coconut flakes, and toss to mix well.
3. In a small saucepan over low heat, combine the melted coconut oil, almond butter, honey, vanilla, salt, and cinnamon, and heat just until the honey is melted.
4. Transfer the nut mixture to the baking pan, pressing down to spread it evenly. Pour the honey mixture evenly over the top.
5. Bake for 35 to 40 minutes, or until golden. Let the mixture cool to room temperature before cutting into equal bars. Store in an airtight container for up to 1 week.

53. Quinoa Crunch Blueberry Muffins

Yield: 12 muffins

Nutrition content per muffin: Carbohydrates: 4g | Protein: 5g | Fat: 6g

Ingredients

For the topping:

- ¼ cup (28 g) slivered almonds, chopped
- 2 tablespoons (22 g) dry quinoa
- 1 tablespoon (15 g) packed brown sugar
- 1 tablespoon (7 g) quinoa flour
- 1 tablespoon (15 ml) neutral-flavored oil

For the muffins:

- Protein content per serving cup (70 g) raw cashews
- 1¼ cups (295 ml) unsweetened plain vegan milk
- 2 tablespoons (14 g) ground flaxseed
- 2 teaspoons pure vanilla extract
- 3 tablespoons (45 ml) neutral- flavored oil
- ⅔ cup (94 g) all-purpose flour
- 1 (56 g) quinoa flour
- ¼ cup (30 g) almond meal
- ⅔ cup (170 g) packed brown sugar
- 1 tablespoon (8 g) cornstarch
- 2 teaspoons baking powder
- 1 teaspoon ground cinnamon
- Protein content per serving teaspoon fine sea salt
- ¼ cup (33 g) chopped dried apricots
- ⅔ cup (109 g) fresh blueberries

Instructions

1. Preheat the oven to 375°F (190°C, or gas mark 5). Line a 12-cup muffin pan with paper liners.
2. **To make the topping:** Using a fork, stir together the almonds, quinoa, brown sugar, and quinoa flour in a small bowl. Add the oil and stir to combine. It will be a little crumbly.
3. **To make the muffins:** Blend the cashews, milk, ground flaxseed, and vanilla in a small, high-powered blender until smooth. Add the oil and blend until combined,

but do not emulsify.

4. Whisk together the flours, brown sugar, cornstarch, baking powder, cinnamon, and salt in a medium-size bowl. Stir in the apricots and blueberries. Pour the liquid ingredients into the dry ingredients and stir to combine. Do not over stir, but there should be no floury spots. Spoon about ¼ cup (72 g) of batter into each cup. Divide the topping evenly on the muffins, using about 2 teaspoons on each. Bake for 28 to 32 minutes until golden brown. Cool on a wire rack.

54. Keto Barueri Cocoa

Do you want a Keto chocolate bar that reminds you of Bounty Bars? The chocolate and coconut combination always drove me crazy, so it was only a matter of time until I made a Keto version of a chocolate and coconut bar.

Portions

It is perfect for 12 servings.

Nutrition

It contains 22 g of fat, 11 g of protein and 4 g of net carbohydrates per serving. Although the preparation lasts 5 minutes, the cooking time is 20 minutes.

Ingredients

- Coconut layer:
- 2 cups shredded coconut
- 1/3 c of coconut oil, melted
- 1/4 cup granulated concealer as the So Nourished sweetener
- Chocolate cover layer:
- 3 squares of Baker's unsweetened chocolate (3 ounces of chocolate)
- 1 tablespoon coconut oil
- 1-2 tablespoons nutritive sweetener

Instructions

Coconut layer from below

1. Insert the coconut, coconut oil and sweetener into a food processor with the S blade. Process until the ingredients form a dough that comes out of the sides, scraping the sides as necessary.

2. Press the coconut mixture into the bottom of a silicone pan or in 12 ways. Place the pan in the freezer while preparing the cover.

Chocolate coating

1. Heat coconut oil and chocolate to 50% microwave power until melted. Add the sweetener if you use unsweetened chocolate.

2. Spread evenly over the frozen coconut layer. Place in the refrigerator for 30 minutes.

3. Remove the freezer. Rotate the silicone molds inward to release the frozen content. They are stored very well in a freezer in the freezer.

55. Baked Granola

Yield

5 cups

Nutrition

Carbohydrates: 5g | Protein: 12g | Fat: 16g

Ingredients

- 1/2 cup canola oil or other neutral oil, such as coconut or olive oil
- 1/2 cup honey or maple syrup
- 1/2 teaspoon ground cinnamon
- 1/2 teaspoon salt

- 3 cups old-fashioned rolled oats
- 1 cup sliced almonds
- 1 cup raisins or other dried, chopped fruit

Instructions

1. Heat the oven to 300 degrees F and glue a baking sheet with parchment paper. Fix a shelf in the middle of the oven and heat it to 300 degrees Fahrenheit. Sprinkle a baking sheet with anchovy paper. Reserve

2. Multiply the oil, honey, cinnamon, and salt. Put the oil, honey, cinnamon and salt in a large bowl and mix to combine.

3. Add oats and almonds and stir until foamy. Continue and measure barley and almonds directly in the oil mixture; do not worry if you add a little more barley or almonds; the granule is very generous. Stir to cover well.

4. Spread the oatmeal on the ready baking sheet. Transfer the mixture to a prepared baking sheet and spread it on a uniform layer. If the granule lacks a hook, use a spatula to press it into the pot.

5. Bake for 20 minutes, stirring halfway. Bake, stir for about half a minute, about 20 minutes. The granule is prepared when the toasts are golden and almond; It still feels like it's coming out of the oven, but it's drying out.

6. Remove from the oven, add fruit, fry and crisp. Place the baking sheet on a wire and sprinkle the raisins or nuts. If you want to bulk granulate, press and pat the granule before cooling, which helps you stay together. Cool completely before storing it.

7. Store in reserved containers. Transfer the cooled granule to an airtight container for long-term storage at room temperature.

SOUP

56. Coconut Curry Lentil Soup

Yield

4 servings

Nutrition

Amount Per Serving

Fat 24g, Carbohydrates 13g, and Protein 18g

Ingredients

- 2 tablespoons virgin coconut oil or extra-virgin olive oil
- 1 medium onion, finely chopped
- 2 garlic cloves, finely chopped
- 1 2½-inch piece ginger, peeled, finely grated
- 1 tablespoon medium curry powder (such as S&B)
- ¼ teaspoon crushed red pepper flakes
- ¾ cup red lentils
- 1 14.5-ounce can crushed tomatoes
- ½ cup finely chopped cilantro, plus leaves with tender stems for serving
- Kosher salt, freshly ground pepper
- 1 13.5-ounce can unsweetened coconut milk, shaken well
- Lime wedges (for serving)

Instructions

1. Heat oil in a medium skillet over medium heat. Cook the onions, continually stirring, until golden brown, about 8-10 minutes.

2. Add and cook the garlic, ginger, curry powder, and red chili powder, stir to remain fragrant for about 2 minutes. Add lentils and cook for 1 minute, stirring.

3. Add tomato, coriander cup, generous salt and 2 cups water. Add the season with pepper and a cup of coconut milk to store and add the remaining coconut milk to the pot.

4. Bring the mixture to a boil. Reduce heat and simmer, occasionally stirring, until lentils soften 20-20 minutes. Eat more soup and pepper if necessary.

5. Divide the soup between the cucumber bowls. The strain is preserved with coconut milk and covered with more cantaloupe. Serve with slices of lime.

57. Easy Chicken Pasta Soup

Heat the pasta daily or two early, and after depleting, place it in a resealable pack in the ice chest until prepared to utilize. This bit of prep work makes this soup a lunch that takes only ten minutes to make.

Servings

Yields 4 servings.

Nutrition

Amount Per Serving

Fat 32g, Carbohydrates 18g, and Protein 42g

Ingredients

- 3 cups chicken stock
- 1 cup of frozen green beans
- 1 cup frozen sliced carrots
- 1 (6-ounce) can flaked chicken, drained
- 1 teaspoon chopped fresh tarragon
- 1 teaspoon fresh thyme leaves

- ½ teaspoon salt
- ½ teaspoon freshly ground black pepper
- 1 cup cooked mini-shell pasta
- ½ cup shredded Parmesan cheese

Instructions

1. In a large saucepan, bring the chicken stock to a boil over high heat. Add the green beans and carrots and reduce the heat to medium. Cover and let simmer for 5 minutes.
2. Add the chicken, tarragon, thyme, salt, and pepper, and simmer for 4 minutes more. Remove the pan from the heat and stir in the cooked pasta.
3. To serve, divide between 4 bowls and top with the Parmesan.

58. Quick Miso Soup with Bok Choy and Shrimp

If you appreciate Asian flavors, you'll love this basic, snappy soup. It meets up in only a couple of moments, making it an incredible formula for your busiest evenings. It warms well, so it's likewise the correct decision for a workday lunch.

Servings

Yields 2 servings

Nutrition

Amount Per Serving

Fat 2g, Carbohydrates 5g, and Protein 16g

Ingredients

- 2 cups of water
- ¼ cup white miso paste
- 8 large (34-40 count) raw shrimp, peeled and halved

- 1 cup cubed firm tofu
- 2 green onions, chopped
- 1 cup chopped bok choy

Instructions

1. In a medium saucepan, bring the water to a boil over high heat. Add the shrimp and boil for 1 minute.
2. Reduce the heat to low and stir in the bok choy. Simmer for 2 minutes, then stir in the miso and tofu. Simmer for 1 minute more.
3. To serve, divide between two soup bowls and sprinkle with the green onions.

59. Hearty Shrimp and Kale Soup

This delicious soup packs a lot of cell reinforcements from the carrots and kale, in addition to a sound measure of protein from the shrimp and beans. It's scrumptious, straightforward, and fulfilling.

Servings

Yields 2 servings.

Nutrition

Amount Per Serving

Fat 18g, Carbohydrates 17g, and Protein 21g

Ingredients

- teaspoon olive oil
- cloves garlic
- 1/4 cup chopped onion
- cups chopped fresh kale
- 1 cup thinly sliced fresh carrots

- 1/2 teaspoon salt
- 1/2 teaspoon freshly ground black pepper
- 1/2 cups vegetable stock
- 8 mediums (36-40 count) raw shrimp, peeled and halved
- l cup canned great northern beans, drained
- 1/2 cup chopped fresh parsley

Instructions

1. In a medium saucepan, heat the olive oil over medium heat. Add the garlic, onion, kale, and carrots, and saute for 5 minutes, stirring often.
2. Season the vegetables with the salt and pepper, then add the vegetable stock. Simmer, uncovered, for 30 minutes, or until the carrots are fork-tender.
3. Increase the heat to high and bring the soup to a boil. Add the shrimp and cook for 2 minutes, or until the shrimp are pink and somewhat firm. Reduce the heat to low.
4. Use a fork to mash about one-quarter of the beans. Stir all the beans into the soup and add the parsley. Simmer for 2 minutes, or until heated through.
5. Ladle into soup bowls and serve hot.

60. Black Bean Soup

Yield

6 servings

Nutrition

Calories 342, Carbohydrate 36g, Fat 6.1g, Protein 18.7g

Ingredients

- 2 tablespoons extra-virgin olive oil

- 2 medium yellow onions, chopped
- 3 celery ribs, finely chopped
- 1 large carrot, peeled and sliced into thin rounds
- 6 garlic cloves, pressed or minced
- 4 ½ teaspoons ground cumin
- ½ teaspoon red pepper flakes (use ¼ spoon if you're sensitive to spice)
- 4 cans (15 ounces each) black beans, rinsed and drained
- 4 cups (32 ounces) low-sodium vegetable broth
- ¼ cup chopped fresh cilantro (optional)
- 1 to 2 teaspoons sherry vinegar, to taste, or 2 tablespoons fresh lime juice
- Sea salt and freshly ground black pepper, to taste

Instructions

1. Heat olive oil in a large Dutch oven or pot of soup over medium heat to dry. Add onions, celery and carrots and a pinch of salt. Cooking, continually stirring, until the vegetables soften, about 10 to 15 minutes.

2. Add garlic, cumin, and red pepper shells and cook for 30 seconds until fragrant. Pour in beans and broth and cook over medium heat. Cook, if necessary, to keep the sprinkler soft, reduce heat until the liquid is aromatic and the beans are tender about 30 minutes.

3. Transfer about 4 cups of soup to the mixer, close the lid tightly and mix until smooth (never pour the mixer over the filling line and never be careful with steam coming out of the mixer). Too hot) Or use a blender to mix some soup.

4. Return the noodle soup to the pot, add the melon juice, vinegar/lemon juice and salt and pepper to taste. Serve.

61. Curried Cauliflower Soup

Rich, vegetarian cauliflower soup made with coconut milk and spiced with Thai curry glue. This solid, encouraging soup formula is ideal for cold days.

Servings

This recipe makes 3 servings.

Ingredients

- 2 tbsp. olive oil
- 1 onion, chopped
- 1 large head of cauliflower, cut into florets
- 2 cups chicken bone broth 1 cup filtered water
- 1/4 cup full-fat coconut milk
- 3/4 cup almond milk
- 1/2 tsp coriander
- 1/2 tsp turmeric
- 1 1/2 tsp cumin
- 2 tbsp. fresh parsley, chopped
- 1 tbsp. honey, for drizzling (on each serving) salt and pepper, to taste

Directions

1. Preheat the oven to 375 degrees F. Spread out the onion and cauliflower in a single layer on a baking sheet. Drizzle with olive oil and sprinkle with salt and pepper. Roast for 15-20 minutes until golden. Stir once or twice over the 15-20 minutes.

2. Place the cauliflower and onions in a large pot and add the bone2. Broth and cup of water. Stir in the coriander, turmeric, cumin, and a pinch of salt. Bring to a boil and let boil for 5 minutes. Remove from heat.

3. I am using an immersion blender, food processor, or regular blender,3. puree the

ingredients until smooth. Stir in the coconut milk and almond milk and warm the soup to serve.

4. Divide the soup into 3 equal servings. Garnish with fresh parsley.

Nutrition
- g protein
- 11 g carbs
- 14.7 g fat

SIDE DISHES

62. Toasted Pepper Jack Sandwiches

Toasting, as opposed to flame broiling, your cheddar sandwich includes huge amounts of fulfilling crunch while discarding additional fat. These toasted cheddar sandwiches pack a great deal of fiery flavor into each nibble.

Servings

Yields 2 servings.

Nutrition

Amount Per Serving

Fat 22g, Carbohydrates 17g, and Protein 19g

Ingredients

- 2 slices reduced-calorie pepper jack cheese
- ½ cup fresh arugula leaves
- 4 thin slices fresh tomato
- 4 slices reduced-calorie whole wheat bread

Instructions

1. Preheat the oven to 350 degrees F.
2. Place 1 slice of cheese on each of 2 slices of bread; top each with 2 slices of tomato and half of the arugula. Top with the remaining bread slices and put the sandwiches on a baking sheet in the center of the oven.
3. Toast for 4 minutes, then turn over and toast for 2 to 3 minutes more, or until the bread is golden and the cheese is melted. Cut each sandwich in half to serve.

63. Taco Pita Pizzas

Yield

4 servings

Nutrition

17g fat, 5g carbohydrate, 35g protein.

Ingredients

- 1-pound lean ground turkey
- 1/3 cup finely chopped onion
- 1 can (4 ounces) chopped green chilies, drained
- 4 whole wheat pita breads (6 inches)
- 1 cup salsa
- 1 cup shredded reduced-fat Mexican cheese blend
- 1 cup shredded lettuce
- 1 medium tomato, seeded and chopped

Instructions

1. In a large fish, cook turkey and onions over medium heat until the meat is no longer pink. Drain Add the peppers. Place the cakes on the baking sheet.
2. Spread 2 tablespoons of sauce on each pizza. Cover with turkey mixture. Sprinkle with cheese. Bake at 400 degrees for 4-10 minutes or until the cheese melts. Serve with lettuce, tomato and remaining sauce.

64. Italian Chicken Sandwich

The Italian sandwich is a modified type of the IF microwave bread but added with special Italian spices that are tasty to make it taste unique. You can prepare this bread with chicken fillings or your desired Italian fillings.

Servings

Nutrition

- Fat 65g
- Carb 4g
- Protein 33g

Ingredients

For chickens

- 1 chicken breast (200 g), cut into thin pieces
- 1 egg, whispered
- 1 teaspoon (3 g) garlic powder
- 1/4 teaspoon (.5 g) of pepper
- Sprinkle with salt and pepper.
- Avocado oil or olive oil to fry the chicken.

For Italian bread without cereals

- 1/3 cup (35 g) almond flour
- 1/2 tablespoon (1 g) of Italian spices
- 1/4 teaspoon (1 g) garlic powder
- 1/2 teaspoon (1 g) of baking powder
- 1/8 teaspoon (1 g) of salt
- 1 egg, whispered
- 2 and 1/2 tablespoons (37 ml) of ice (or butter if tolerated, coconut oil or olive oil) melted

For serving with

- Mustard salad, paleo, and Romanian mayonnaise

Instructions

1. Heat the oven to 205 C (400 F).
2. Put all the bread ingredients in a cup and mix well.
3. Insert the cup in the microwave and microwave for 90 seconds.
4. Let the bread cool for a few minutes, then remove it from the cup and cut it into 4 slices.
5. Place the slices on a baking sheet and bake in the oven for 4 minutes.
6. Cut the chicken breast into thin slices, about the size of the pan (so that the chicken pieces do not break the bread too much).
7. Prepare the coating for the chicken pieces by mixing the egg, garlic powder, pepper, salt, and pepper.
8. Put 2 tablespoons of olive oil in a pan. Soak each piece of chicken in the egg mixture and then place it in the pan. Roast over medium heat until the outside of the chicken is browned and then the chicken is fully cooked. Put the chicken pieces on a plate.
9. Put the sandwiches together, smearing some mustard and mayonnaise on 1 slice of bread, add some salad leaves, then place a slice of chicken on top. Eat like an open-faced sandwich or sit on top of another slice of cereal-free Italian bread.

65. Hamburgers with Sesame Buns

These hamburger burgers not only allow us to eat with our hands again but also allow us to throw away all our favorite treats without problems.

Servings

2

Nutrition

- Fat 70 g
- Carb 23 g
- Protein 41 g

Ingredients

For sesame rolls:

- 98 g coconut flour
- 2 tablespoons (14 g) psyllium powder peel
- 1 teaspoon (2 g) baking powder
- salt knife tip
- 3 medium eggs (132 g)
- 1 tablespoon (15 ml) melted coconut oil
- 2 teaspoons (10 ml) sesame oil, plus an extra brush
- 1 teaspoon (5 ml) white balsamic vinegar
- 1 tablespoon (14 g) sesame seeds

For the patties:

- 257 g of ground beef 9.1 oz.
- 1/2 teaspoon garlic powder
- salt and freshly ground black pepper
- 2 tablespoons (30 ml) olive oil

toppings:

- 2 leaves of butter salad
- 2-4 slices of tomatoes
- 2-4 large red onion rings

- 1/2 avocado, peeled and sliced

Instructions

To make rolls:

- Preheat oven to 180 ° C to 350 ° F.
- Combine coconut flour, psyllium husk powder, baking powder and salt in a large bowl. Put aside.
- In another bowl, beat the eggs, coconut oil, sesame oil, vinegar, and 3 oz. (88 ml) of water together.
- Add the wet mixture to the dry and double mixture to combine.
- Divide into two portions and form each part in a hamburger roll (taking into account that you will cut it in half once completed)
- Put the bread on a tray lined with parchment paper. Spread some sesame oil on the rolls and spread on the sesame seeds.
- Bake in the oven for 35-40 minutes. Remove and reserve.

To make stains:

1. Combine ground beef with garlic powder, salt and freshly ground black pepper. Divide into two portions and form each portion in a hamburger dressing.
2. Heat the olive oil in a thick nonstick skillet and fry over medium heat until cooked, occasionally turning to create a golden crust.
3. Prepare hamburgers by cutting sesame in half and adding your favorite toppings.

66. Low Carb Sandwiches

The look and texture of the kitchen are so good that nobody would suspect that they are healthy! Ideal for sandwiches, these delicious snacks can also be fried, offering you an excellent version of sandwiches. When you roll them, place the dough between the parchment sheets and it will not stick to the pin.

Servings

10

Nutrition

- Fat 25.9 g
- Carb 11 g
- Protein 13.2 g

Ingredients

- 1 low-carb flatbread recipe
- 2 tablespoons Dijon mustard
- 2 teaspoons mayonnaise
- ½ pound black forest ham
- 6 ounces thinly sliced
- 1 medium green apple, thinly sliced
- Oil or melted butter to brush off the sandwich

Instructions

1. Preheat the panini press.
2. Cut the bread into 10 sections, then cut the center of each section to get two flat and thin slices.
3. In a small bowl, mix mustard and mayonnaise.
4. Take two appropriate sections of bread and spread one side with the mustard/mayonnaise combination. Layer with slices of cheese, meat and green apple. Repeat with the remaining sections of bread.
5. Grease each sandwich with melted oil or butter.

6. Put the sandwiches in the press and roast until the bread is fried and the cheese has melted.

SAUCES, DIPS AND DRESSINGS

67. Roasted Bell Pepper Hummus

Yield

12 servings

Nutrition

Amount Per Serving

Fat 26g, Carbohydrates 14g, and Protein 15g

Ingredients

- 3/4 cup roasted red bell peppers
- 3 1/2 cups soaked and cooked chickpeas/garbanzo beans
- 1/4 cup tahini paste
- 2 tbsp. extra virgin olive oil
- 1 1/2 tbsp. fresh lemon juice
- 1 1/2 tsp crushed fresh garlic (or more to taste)
- 3/4 tsp smoked paprika (or more to taste)
- 1/4 tsp salt (or more to taste- I usually use about 1/2 tsp)
- 1/4 tsp cayenne pepper (or more to taste)
- Warm water as needed

Instructions

1. Use grilled jams or make your own.
2. If using canned peas, rinse and rinse. If you are using dry peas, after soaking them, wash and rinse them, then apply them on the stove for 60-90 minutes to soften. Drain the beans and let them cool to room temperature.

3. You can peel boiled peas to make this super creamy hummus. Gently press each pea to remove the skin, then remove the skin before processing. While this step is not completely necessary, it ensures that your humus becomes very soft and creamy.

4. Make your food processor with blade accessories. Add chili, peas, dough, olive oil, lemon juice, garlic and spices to this processor.

5. Press the material for about 60 seconds and then straighten until smooth. If the mixture looks too thick, add one tablespoon at a time and mix for consistency. Try this mixture and add more salt, lemon juice, garlic or garlic to taste. Mix again to mix additional equipment.

6. Pour into a bowl and cool completely before stirring. Hamas gets a little cooler because it gets colder. They are grilled with pita bread, pita chips, crackers, or topping.

68. Blood Orange Vinaigrette

This live and citrus dressing gets sweetness from blood oranges, the taste of lemon juice and some ginger from the ears and mustard from whole grains. Try it in a simple salad of roasted potatoes, French fries, and almonds, or stir it over fried beets and segmented blood oranges for a mild winter salad.

Portions

This recipe makes 2 servings.

Nutrition

36g Fat, 13g Carbs, 2g Protein

Ingredients

- 2 oranges, with juice
- 1/2 cup olive oil
- 2 tablespoons plum vinegar

Addresses

1. Combine all the ingredients in a small bowl and beat together

2. Noodles with pumpkin and vegetable salad

3. Have you tried making noodles with vegetables? I like to make pasta dishes with fresh and healthy vegetables. It's not that I don't like traditional noodles, I'm a fan of almost any pasta dish. However, there is something satisfying to know that the noodles are full of fresh and healthy vitamins, instead of naked carbohydrates!

FISH, BEEF, PORK, AND CHICKEN

69. Salmon and Tomato Egg Sandwiches

This breakfast sandwich is far healthier and more substantial than anything you can pick up at the drive-through; it's also a lot tastier, but it only takes a few minutes to prepare.

Servings

Yields 4 servings.

Nutrition

Amount Per Serving

Fat 22g, Carbohydrates 17g, and Protein 19g

Ingredients

- ½ cup unsalted walnuts, chopped
- 4 medium peaches, sliced
- 4 (6-ounce) containers vanilla Greek yogurt

Instructions

1. Toast the English muffins while you prepare the eggs.
2. In a medium skillet, heat the olive oil over medium-high heat. Add the salmon and tomatoes to the pan and saute, frequently stirring, for 4 minutes.
3. Pour the eggs over the top, season with the salt and pepper, and scramble, frequently stirring, for about 2 minutes, or until the eggs are set.
4. Place the English muffin halves on 4 plates and top each bottom half with one-quarter of the egg mixture. Top with arugula and the other muffin half.

70. Pork Loin Chops with Mango Salsa

This formula is overflowing with enhancing and is fulfilling enough to cause you to overlook that you're fasting. The salsa is shockingly better made a day ahead, so permit it to marinate in the cooler short-term with the pork hacks.

Servings

Yields 2 servings

Nutrition

Amount Per Serving

Fat 22g, Carbohydrates 17g, and Protein 19g

Ingredients

- 2 pork loin chops, ¾ inch thick
- ½ cup lime juice
- Juice of 1 large orange
- 1 large just-ripe mango, peeled and diced
- ½ cup diced green bell pepper
- ½ cup diced red bell pepper
- 1 small jalapeno pepper, seeded and diced
- 1 tablespoon chopped fresh cilantro
- ½ cup diced red onion
- 1 tablespoon chopped fresh parsley
- ½ teaspoon salt
- ¼ teaspoon freshly ground black pepper

Instructions

1. Place the pork chops in a freezer bag and add the lime and orange juices. Seal, shake to mix well and place in the refrigerator overnight.

2. In a small bowl, combine the mango, red onion, bell peppers, jalapeno, cilantro, and parsley. Stir to mix very well. Cover and refrigerate overnight.

3. Preheat the broiler and line a baking pan with aluminum foil.

4. Season each pork chop on both sides with the salt and pepper. Place on the pan and broil for 4 to 5 minutes on one side, then turn over and cook for 4 to 5 minutes more. Place each pork chop on a plate, spoon the salsa over the top, and serve.

71. Roast Chicken with Balsamic Vinegar

Yield

4 servings

Nutrition

Carbohydrates: 2g | Protein: 44g | Fat: 16g

Ingredients

- 1 cut up broiler-fryer Bay Leaves Salt or Vege-Sal Pepper
- 3 to 4 tablespoons (45 to 60 ml) olive oil
- 3 to 4 tablespoons (42 to 56 g) butter
- ½ cup (60 ml) dry white wine 3 tablespoons (45 ml) balsamic vinegar
- Preheat the oven to 350°F (180°C, or gas mark 4).

Instructions

1. Wrap a sheet or two of leaves under the skin of each slice of chicken and sprinkle each slice with salt and pepper and place them in the grill pan.

2. Soak the chicken with olive oil and cover with the same butter. Roast in the oven for 1 V2 hour and rotate each piece every 20 to 30 minutes. (This makes the skin gloriously crisp and pleasant.)

3. When the chicken is ready, place it on a plate and pour the fat from the pan. Put the

pan over medium heat and pour the wine and balsamic vinegar.

4. Mix this loop and dissolve the delicious sweets that are glued in the cooking pan.

5. Boil this in just a minute or two, pour into a pot or jar and serve with chicken.

6. Throw in bay leaves before serving.

72. Orange-Five-Spice Roasted Chicken

Yield

5 to 6 servings

Nutrition

32 g protein, 3g carbs, 17g fat

Ingredients

- 3 pounds (1.4 kg) chicken thighs
- ¼ cup (60 ml) soy sauce
- 2 tablespoons (30 ml) canola or peanut oil
- 1 tablespoon (15 ml) lemon juice
- 1 tablespoon (15 ml) white wine vinegar
- 1 tablespoon (1.5 g) Splenda
- 2 tablespoons (40 g) low-sugar orange marmalade
- 2 teaspoons five-spice powder

Instructions

1. Put the chicken in a large plastic bag. Mix everything. Reserve a little marinade for weight loss and pour the rest into the bag. Seal the bag and press the air as you go. Turn the bag over to cover the chicken and place it in the refrigerator. Allow for at least two hours and this is a good time.

2. Heat the oven to 375 degrees Fahrenheit (190 degrees Celsius). Remove the chicken from the refrigerator, pour the marinade and place the chicken in a pan and fry the chicken for 1 hour.

3. Reserved with Marinade 2 or 3 times, be sure to use clean containers every time you eat to avoid cross-contamination.

73. Orange-Tangerine Up-the- Butt Chicken

Yield

5 servings

Nutrition

5g carbs, 40 g protein, 16g fat

Ingredients

- 3½ to 4-pound (1.6 to 1.8 kg) whole roasting chicken
- 1 teaspoon salt or Vege-Sal
- 1 teaspoon Splenda
- 1 drop blackstrap molasses (It helps to keep your molasses in a squeeze bottle.)
- 1 teaspoon chili powder
- 3 tablespoons (60 g) low-sugar orange marmalade
- 1 12-ounce (360-ml) can tangerine Diet-Rite soda, divided (Make sure the can is clean!)
- 2 to 3 teaspoons oil
- 1 teaspoon spicy brown mustard

Instructions

1. Prepare your grill for indirect cooking - if you have a gas stove, just light it on one side. If using charcoal, place the lighter on one side of the grill and light.

2. Remove the chicken's neck and towels and wash the chicken and dry it with paper towels.

3. In a small bowl of salt or Vege-Sal, mix Splenda, molasses and red pepper powder. Pour half of the mixture (1/8 teaspoon) into a bowl and store. Rub the rest into the chicken hole.

4. Mix the orange marmalade with low sugar in the reserved spice mixture. Open the tangerine boxes and pour 3.2 cups (160 ml). Put N cup (60 ml) of the beverage in a jam/spice mixture and mix - you can drain or throw away the remaining siphon you poured. Now, using a church-style console door, pull several holes at the top of the can. Cover the box with non-stick cooking spray and place it in a deep bowl. Carefully place the chicken on the tables and place the can inside the chicken cavity. Rub the chicken with oil.

5. Okay, you're ready to cook! Make sure you put a pan. Set the chicken to rotate vertically on the beverage cans on the side of the oven, not above the fire, and gently spread the drums to create a tripod effect. Close the grill and cook the chicken at 250 degrees Fahrenheit (130 degrees Celsius) or about 75 to 90 minutes or until the juices are evident when the bone sticks. You can also use a meat thermometer. Must have 180 degrees Fahrenheit (85 degrees Celsius).

6. While the chicken is cooking, add the mustard to the jam/soda/spice mixture and mix all the ingredients. Use this mixture for the chicken dough for the last 20 minutes or fry.

7. When the chicken is finished, carefully separate it from the grill. Grill gloves are useful here or use hot pads and piles. Wrap the tins and separate them from the chicken and discard. Allow the chicken to rest for 5 minutes before sculpting. Meanwhile, heat each remaining sweetened sauce until boiling and serve as a chicken sauce.

74. Lemon-Sesame Chicken and Asparagus

Chicken and asparagus go together perfectly, and this formula consolidates them with a trace of lemon and the additional mash of sesame seeds.

Servings

Yields 2 servings

Nutrition

Amount Per Serving

Fat 27g, Carbohydrates 17g, and Protein 38g

Ingredients

- 8 ounces' skinless chicken breast tenders (or quartered chicken breast)
- ½ cup plus 1 tablespoon lemon juice, divided
- 1 teaspoon salt, divided
- ¼ teaspoon freshly ground black pepper
- 1 teaspoon chopped fresh rosemary
- 6 medium spears fresh asparagus, cut into 2-inch pieces
- ½ teaspoon olive oil
- 2 tablespoons sesame seeds

Instructions

1. Pound out the chicken tenders with a mallet or the heel of your hand until they are a uniform ½ inch thickness. Place in a freezer bag with the ½ cup lemon juice and marinate for 2 hours or overnight.
2. Preheat the broiler and line a baking pan with aluminum foil.
3. Season the chicken on both sides with ½ teaspoon of the salt and the pepper, and place on the pan. Sprinkle with the rosemary.
4. In a small bowl, toss the asparagus with the olive oil, remaining 1 tablespoon lemon

juice, and remaining ½ teaspoon salt. Arrange the asparagus around the chicken on the pan.

5. Broil the chicken for 4 to 5 minutes, then turn it over and stir the asparagus, and broil for 4 to 5 minutes more.

6. Divide the chicken and asparagus between two plates and sprinkle with the sesame seeds.

75. Chinese Sticky Wings

Yield: Approximately 28 pieces

Nutrition

Nutrition

17g fat, 6 g carbohydrates, 18g protein

Ingredients

- 3 pounds (1.4 kg) chicken wings
- ¼ cup (60 ml) dry sherry
- ¼ cup (60 ml) soy sauce
- ¼ cup (60 ml) sugar-free imitation honey
- 1 tablespoon (6 g) grated ginger root
- 1 clove garlic
- ½ teaspoon chili garlic paste

Instructions

1. If complete, cut the wings to "resistance". Put the wings in a large plastic bag that can be used.

2. Mix everything else and reserve a little marinade to loosen and pour the rest into the bag. Seal the bag and press the air as you go. Turn the bag several times to cover

the wings and chill in the refrigerator for several hours (a whole day is bright).

3. Preheat the oven to 375 degrees Fahrenheit (190 degrees Celsius or marked gas 5). Pull the bag, pour the marinade and place the wings on a shallow plate and allow them to cook for one hour in the oven, then marinate every 15 minutes. Use a clean container every time you eat.

4. Serve with lots of napkins!

76. Wicked Wings

Yield

Nutrition

18g fat, 7 g carbohydrates, 20g protein

Ingredients

- 4 pounds (1.8 kg) chicken wings
- 1 cup (100 g) grated Parmesan cheese
- 2 tablespoons (2.6 g) dried parsley
- 1 tablespoon (5.4 g) dried oregano
- 2 teaspoons paprika
- 1 teaspoon salt
- ½ teaspoon pepper
- ½ cup vegan butter

Instructions

1. Heat the oven to 350 degrees F (180 degrees Celsius or gas 4). Line a shallow pan with foil. (Do not miss this step or clean the pan a week later.)

2. Saving interesting things, cut the wings into "sticks". (Not sure what to do with wing tips? Freeze them for soup. Have a good broth.)

3. Combine parmesan and parsley, oregano, pepper, salt and pepper in a bowl.

4. Melt the butter in a shallow bowl or pan

5. Soak each roast in butter, roll in cheese and spice mixture and place in lined pan.

6. Bake for 1-hour B and then beat to avoid making a double recipe!

7. Yield: About 50 pieces

8. Each has only carbohydrates, fiber and 4 grams of protein.

77. Chicken Breast with Roasted Summer Veggies

This formula warms well, so set it up on an end of the week or at night and pack in singular holders to take for your lunch during the week. Test with other occasional vegetables to shift the flavors.

Servings

Yields 4 servings.

Nutrition

Amount Per Serving

Fat 42g, Carbohydrates 21g, and Protein 39g

Ingredients

- 4 (4'to 5-ounce) skinless chicken breasts
- 1 teaspoon plus 1 tablespoon olive oil, divided
- 1 teaspoon salt, divided
- ½ teaspoon freshly ground black pepper, divided
- ½ teaspoon ground turmeric
- 1 medium zucchini, thinly sliced
- yellow squash, thinly sliced
- l medium white onion, sliced ½ inch thick

- 1-pint cherry tomatoes 1 teaspoon dried parsley 1 teaspoon dried oregano

Instructions

1. Preheat the oven to 400 degrees F and line a baking pan with aluminum foil.

2. Rub both sides of the chicken breasts with 1 teaspoon of the olive oil and season them with ½ teaspoon of the salt, ½ teaspoon of the pepper, and the turmeric. Place the chicken on the pan.

3. In a medium bowl, combine the zucchini, squash, onion, and tomatoes. Add the parsley and oregano and then drizzle with the remaining 1 tablespoon olive oil. Toss the vegetables well until they are evenly coated, and spread around the chicken breasts on the pan.

4. Bake in the center of the oven for 15 minutes, turn over the chicken and stir the vegetables, and then bake for 10 to 12 minutes more, or until the chicken juices run clear.

5. To serve, place 1 breast on each plate and top with one-quarter of the vegetables.

Vegetarian

78. Olive Tapenade on Raw Vegetable Slices

Olive tapenade is an extraordinary spread to present with wafers for a simple gourmet tidbit or oeuvres for any gathering where you're anticipating veggie lover or vegetarian visitors (or just visitors who like great nourishment!). This basic and simple hand crafted olive tapenade formula utilizes two sorts of olives to give a satisfying shading blend to the dish.

Servings

This recipe makes 4 servings.

Ingredients

- 1 cup pitted Kalamata olives
- 2 tbsp. capers
- 3 tbsp. olive oil
- 2 cloves garlic
- 1/4 cup fresh parsley
- 1 cucumber, sliced
- 1 large carrot, sliced

Directions

1. Place the olives, capers, olive oil, garlic, and parsley in a blender or1. Food processor.
2. Blend on low speed for a few seconds, until thick paste forms.
3. Divide the tapenade and vegetable slices into 4 equal servings.
4. Spread the tapenade on top of the carrot and cucumber slices with a knife, or simply dip the slices into the tapenade.

Nutrition

- 1.25 g protein
- g carbs
- 14.5 g fat

79. Pumpkin Pie Bites

Yield

2 servings

Nutrition

Carbs: 6g | Protein: 3g | Fat: 6g

Ingredients

- 15 oz. pumpkin puree (425 g), 1 can
- 12 oz. evaporated milk (355 ml), 1 can
- ¾ cup sugar (150 g)
- 1 teaspoon cinnamon, extra for taste
- ¼ teaspoon ground cloves
- ½ teaspoon ground ginger
- ½ teaspoon salt
- 2 eggs
- 2 pie crusts, refrigerated
- Whipped cream
- Ice cream

Instructions

1. In a bowl, mix the dry ingredients well.

2. Add the egg and zucchini and mix.

3. Gradually add evaporated milk, stirring constantly.

4. Preheat oven to 350 degrees Fahrenheit (180 degrees C).

5. With the glass lid, cut 12 4-inch (10 cm) rings from the foot cover. Press on each cup of muffin oil hook.

6. Gently pierce the bottom of the housing with a fork.

7. Fill each leg with the stuffing.

8. Bake for 20 to 30 minutes, until golden brown on top.

9. Add your favorite ice cream or cream with cinnamon powder.

10. To enjoy!

80. Chocolate Covered Macaroons

These little macaroons are sweet, sticky, and delightful with every bite. Each macaroni has a beautiful aroma of coconut, almonds, and chocolate, with 90% of calories from fat. It's like a perfect little fat pump, packed in a beautiful small kitchen.

Servings

It is perfect for 8 servings.

Nutrition

It contains 7.23 g of fat, 0.86 g of protein, and 1.53 g of net carbohydrates per serving. While the preparation lasts 10 minutes, the cooking time is 20 minutes.

Ingredients

- 1 cup shredded coconut
- 1 large egg white
- ¼ cup of erythritol
- ½ Almond spoon extract

- 1 salt point
- 20 grams of unsweetened chocolate (Lily's works great)
- 2 tablespoons coconut oil

Instructions

1. Preheat the oven to 350 ° F and spread a cup of chopped walnut and coconut sweetened in a thin layer on a baking sheet lined with parchment paper.
2. After the oven is hot enough, place the coconut to fry a little. This should take about 4-5 minutes. This step is optional, but it provides an additional coconut flavor.
3. While the coconut is fried, beat the egg white until it becomes foamy and double in size.
4. Now slowly add the erythritol and the salt tip while mixing. Add almond extract to turn ordinary coconut macaroni.
5. When the coconut flakes have fried and cooled, add them, and fold everything.
6. Using a small scoop of ice cream (or your hands), wrap the macaroni balls well and place them gently on a baking sheet lined with parchment paper. Bake until golden brown, about 15 minutes.
7. While baking, melt the chocolate by melting coconut oil and unsweetened chocolate. Stir continuously to make sure the chocolate does not burn.
8. After removing the noodles from the oven, pour the chocolate over each of them. If you choose to dip the macaroni in the chocolate, be sure to let them cool completely before handling them. Enjoy!

81. Low coconut macadamia bars

Keto coconut macadamia bars could be my new favorite low carb treatment. Almond flour crust with coconut butter without powder and macadamia topping.

Portions

It is perfect for 16 servings.

Nutrition

It contains 19.3 g of fat, 3.1 g of protein and 4.3 g of net carbohydrates per serving. Although the preparation lasts 15 minutes, the cooking time is 55 minutes.

Ingredients

Cortex:

- 1 1/4 cups almond flour
- 1/3 cup Swerve sweetener
- 1/4 tablespoon salt
- 1/4 cup cold and cut into small pieces

filling:

- 1/4 cup butter
- 1/2 cup of Swerve sweetener
- 1/2 cup coconut cream (thick top of a can of coconut milk)
- 1 1/3 cup of coconut
- 3/4 cup chopped macadamia nuts
- 1 egg yolk
- 1/2 teaspoon vanilla extract

Instructions

Cortex:

- Preheat oven to 350F. Combine almond flour, sweetener and salt in a food processor. Pulse to combine. Sprinkle the butter and continue stirring until the mixture looks very fine.
- Press in the base of an 8-inch square pan and bake for 15 minutes or till lightly

browned. Set aside and let cool while preparing the filling.

filling:

1. 3/4 In a saucepan over moderate heat, melt the butter. Conquer on until smooth.
2. 3/4 Macadamia mix coconut, egg yolk and vanilla extract until well blended. Pour over the crust.
3. Bake 35 to 40 minutes, Before the edges brown. Remove from the oven and let fresh cutting into bars.
4. The center will not be fixed but will strengthen as it cools.

82. Oatmeals Bars

Yield

16 squares

Nutrition

Carbohydrates: 9g, Protein: 4g, Fat: 16g

Ingredients

- 1 cup organic melted butter
- 1/2 cup honey
- 2 eggs
- 1 teaspoon baking soda
- 1/2 teaspoon sea salt
- 1 teaspoon pure vanilla extract
- 2 cups old fashioned oats
- 2 cups whole wheat flour

Instructions

1. In a large bowl, melt the butter and sugar. Add the egg, sweet boil, salt and vanilla and mix well. Add barley and flour and mix to combine well. (Add any optional section. See notes for suggestions)

2. Spread the mixture on an 8 × 8-inch baking sheet with parchment. Bake in the oven at 350 degrees for 20-25 minutes until golden brown. To enjoy!

83. Mini Choco Coco Cups

Yield

20 Mini Cups

Nutrition

Carbohydrates: 6g, Protein: 4g, Fat: 12g

Ingredients

- 2 Egg Whites
- 2 1/2 cups Desiccated coconut unsweetened
- 6 oz. Dark chocolate
- 1/2 cup Cream heavy/whippping
- 1/4 cup Butter, melted unsalted
- 1 tablespoon Erythritol Low carb sweetener

Instructions

1. Preheat oven to 180C / 350F.
2. Add the egg and coconut in a white bowl. Mix well
3. Add the sweetened and melted butter and stir well.
4. Lightly grease a muffin pan.
5. Put a tablespoon of the coconut mixture in the muffin pan and press to cover. Add

more if necessary.

6. Bake for 8 to 10 minutes until golden brown. Fresh in tin.

7. Slowly heat the cream and add the chocolate.

8. Strain until the chocolate is completely mixed, then pour into the coconut cups.

9. Refrigerate in the refrigerator for 2 hours.

10. Eat, enjoy and enjoy!

CONCLUSION

Congratulations on making it to the end of this ***keto Cookbook for Women Over 50*** navigation guide and collection of delicious recipes.

Keto diets have genuinely come on strong in the past year and a half and for a valid reason. It's an excellent way to not handiest shed that unwanted weight quickly, however also a unique manner to get healthy and stay that way.

For people who have attempted the Keto Diet and are nonetheless on it, it's higher than only a diet. It's a manner of life, a very new lifestyle.

But like any most critical shift in our lives, it isn't always an easy one; it takes a high-quality amount of commitment and determination.

I hope you find this guide useful and helpful as I have.

Thanks, and enjoy it!

KETO DIET AFTER 50

The Complete Ketogenic Diet Guide for People Over 50 to Lose Weight, Boost Energy and Stay Healthy. Includes Easy And Tasty Recipes.

By
KAREN TURNER

DISCLAIMER

The information in this e-book is provided for informational purposes only, and it aims to provide accurate and reliable information regarding the subject matter and topic covered.

The author and publisher do not bear any responsibility towards any person or entity concerning any repair, damage, or financial loss resulting from or alleged resulting directly or indirectly from this electronic book.

The post is sold with the idea that the publisher is not required to provide accounting services, officially permitted or otherwise eligible. If counseling is necessary, legal, or professional, the individual practicing in the profession should be directed.

No reproduction, copying, or transmission of any part of this document electronically or in print is permitted. This publication is prohibited from registration, and this document is not allowed to store unless you obtain written permission from the publisher. All rights are saved.

The author owns all copyrights that the publisher does not own. Trademarks used are not approved, and the publication of the brand does not contain permission or endorsement from the trademark owner.

INTRODUCTION

I need to start by congratulating you on getting this **Keto After 50 Cookbook** guide.

You are a real champ for deciding on to take charge of your fitness by being greater precise about what you eat.

And, quite honestly, there are few dietary selections better than keto. By sticking with the keto weight loss plan, you are putting your body in the best position to address things like acne, heart diseases, cancer, or even Parkinson's disease.

Of course, it is going without saying that the ketogenic food regimen is in no way magic. It will require a few matters from you like a commitment to peer the weight-reduction plan through regardless of what. Your frame will omit the eating plan it had grown used to and protest this switch to low-carb and high-fats ingredients in several ways.

You might revel in what is referred to as keto flu, to be discussed at length on this book. It consists of insomnia, insatiability, a few discomforts to your digestive system, nausea, and fatigue. This isn't unusual, and we will speak the ways you can minimize these signs until your body receives on track with your wholesome decision.

Finally, the keto food plan and its results afterward are quite impressive. It's no surprise that you are keen to learn more about this ingesting plan, and you'll simply love the keto recipes in this book. But, you should supply a short visit to your medical doctor to know if you are accurate to go keto.

That said, let's dive a touch more in-depth into what the keto weight loss plan virtually is.

THE BASICS OF KETOSIS

The original idea at the back of the ketogenic weight loss plan (keto food plan) is that it increases the consumption of fats and reduces the consumption of carbohydrates. In this way, you positioned your frame in a country of fasting. Your body uses ketones as a supply of daily electricity as opposed to glucose. This interprets into higher fitness for you.

A basic idea of the power was given from your meal is broken down below:

- Fat makes up to 60-70% of your meal
- Protein makes as much as 15-30% of your meal
- Just 5-10% of electricity is derived from carbs

With this plan, your frame stays in a country of ketosis. By default, your body chooses to run on glucose, which is were given specifically from carbs. In situations in which you restrict your consumption of carbs, your body will switch to a country of fasting. In this country, your body turns to a secondary supply of power, which occurs to be fat. Fat within the frame receives broken down into compounds called ketones, which then acts as an alternative supply of fuel.

The Ketogenic Diet: A Compromise from Fasting

Initially, the result of the fasting approach turned into an alternative impressive. However, one glaring hassle of fasting is that it's miles simplest temporary. Although effects confirmed that fasting helped to govern those seizures, one can't make rapid forever. Many sufferers complained that when they lower back to their usual diet, the seizures returned too.

After that, some other doctors commenced developing with a modified model of fasting. This involved lowering food wealthy in carbs rather than just every food. According to Dr. Wilder of the Mayo Clinic, he found out that the seizure price of a few epileptic sufferers reduced while there was a discount of blood sugar. When foods wealthy in fats but low in carbs have been eaten, the patients experienced fewer seizures similar to when they were on entire fasting. This led to the creation of a ketogenic eating regimen, which facilitates the body to mimic the metabolic procedure that happens in a fasting country.

Types of Keto Diet

As I have said within the advent, keto diets force the frame into ketosis, central to the breakdown of fat into ketones, which then serves as a chief source of electricity for the frame.

There are several methods of bringing or forcing your frame into ketosis, and there are numerous exceptional styles of ketogenic diets. However, the end goal of all the types of keto eating regimen stays the same, even though all of them share some similarities- they may be all high in nutritional fats and occasional in the carb.

I have compiled a listing of some styles of keto diets useful to girls of over 50 years. They include:

The Standard Keto Diet (SKD)

This keto food regimen incorporates a very low carb, with a mild amount of protein and a high-fats weight loss program. It usually carries between 70 to 75 percent of fat, 20% of protein, and 5-10% of carbs.

To spoil it to grams consistent with day, regular widespread keto weight loss plan would contain:

- 20-50g of carbohydrate
- No set restrict for fat
- 40-60g of protein

The nutritional fats provide a whole lot of calories in a keto diet. Therefore, its fats inside the weight loss plan have no restriction, as the need can differ extensively for specific individuals.

Keto food regimen participants must include sufficient consumption of vegetables, mainly non-starchy ones. This kind of keto food plan has recorded fulfillment in supporting many humans to lose weight, improving heart fitness, and controlling blood sugar.

Very-Low-Carb Ketogenic Diet (VLCKD)

This is another name for a fashionable ketogenic food plan with very-low-carb content material.

Well Formulated Ketogenic Diet (WFKD)

This form of ketogenic food plan originated from Steve Phinney, a leading researcher in keto diets. It has a comparable blueprint as that of SKD. Being well formulated is that the proteins, fats, and carbs follow the ratio of SDK and, therefore, can pressure your body into ketosis.

MCT Ketogenic Diet

This variation of keto food plan still follows the SKD. However, it's miles targeted on having medium-chain triglycerides as the vital supply of the fats content of the eating regimen. MCT is present in coconut oil and maybe were given as MTC oil and emulsion liquids. In reality, it has been implemented in treating epilepsy. This is because of the theory that it offers humans room to consume extra protein and carbs even as keeping their body in ketosis. This notion originates from the reality that MCT generates excess ketones in line with grams than the long-grain triglycerides found in regular fat.

It is crucial to know that MCT can cause diarrhea and belly disenchanted if eaten in a massive amount on its one. To save you this, you need to have meals containing a balance of non-fats and MCT fats. However, it's miles unknown if MCT has more significant advantages on blood sugar or weight loss.

Calorie-Restricted Ketogenic Diet

It is quite similar to SKD. However, calorie consumption is at a hard and fast amount. Although consequences have proven that keto food plan is successful no matter eating a restricted quantity of calories or not, that is due to the fact being on keto gives satiety, which facilitates to prevent immoderate eating.

Cyclical Ketogenic Diet (CKD)

This sort of keto is a little higher accommodating to carbs. It is also known as carb-lower back loading. It occurs in a few days in which carbs are eaten. For instance, a keto food plan is taken for 5 days; then followed by using two days in which more than the usual quantity of carb is made.

This variant of keto is designed for athletes who need the better carb to rebuild the glycogen lost in exercises. If you're a lady over 50 years and you have interaction in practices regularly, then this type is probably only for you.

Targeted Ketogenic Diet (TKD)

This is also just like SKD; besides that, you could devour carbs in exercising times. It is at the borderline among SKD and cyclical ketogenic food regimen that we could you

devour carbs any day you apply. It relies upon at the idea that carbs are eaten before any athletic hobby undergoes a good deal better processing, as they're transformed by using muscles for power once they act.

High Protein Ketogenic Diet

In this weight loss program, higher protein is taken extra than in SKD. It has a ratio of 60% fat, 5% carbs, and protein content of 35%. Results from some studies endorse that a keto weight-reduction plan with a little more protein is higher robust for humans who want to lose weight. However, much like other varieties of keto food plan, there's a shortage of empirical findings in determining any health hazard with doing it for a protracted time.

Now, many humans often partner illness and pain with getting older, however growing older does no longer always suggest getting sicker. We are going to take a look at how the ketogenic weight loss program can affect your fitness with aging. Diet and way of life have lots to play on how wholesome and how long you live. We are going to observe the blessings of keto food plan for women over the age of fifty in details.

The "Classic Keto" Approach

The whole idea in the back of keto is simple: patients are stored in fasting kingdom if their carb consumption is reduced, so their frame turns to fats as the primary source of fuel, as opposed to glucose. The nutritional ratio shifts to fats, and the structure makes use of an acid called ketone bodies for power production. In conclusion, the keto food plan makes your frame assume it's in a country of starvation; therefore, your metabolism modifications to that in the fasting state.

Another physician in the Mayo clinic is credited for standardizing the keto diet. This caused the "classic keto" technique we comply with today. This is a traditional technique in which the ratio of fat to carbs and proteins is 4:1. In this approach, 90% of your calories are from fats, with protein and carbs making up 6 and 4 percent, respectively. This technique is considered the gold general. A ratio of 3:1 is also beneficial.

Below are foods taken into consideration acceptable within the ketogenic weight-reduction plan, and have remained so throughout its history.

- Non-starchy vegetables: cabbage, leafy greens, cauliflower, broccoli, onions, and peppers
- Fat dairy: milk, cheese products, and yogurt
- Protein: Fish, soybeans, shellfish, chicken, and eggs
- Seeds and nuts: pistachios, pumpkin seeds, sunflower, almonds, and walnuts
- Fats: plants and animal fat
- Non-starchy fruits: avocados, coconut, berries, rhubarb

Initially, a whole lot of emphasis changed into place at the significance of accurate measurements that allows you to achieve correct outcomes. Because of this, foods were measured on the gram basis earlier than eating.

The result of these measurements became a food regimen that might deal with epilepsy and can be taken for a longer time. Currently, the fundamentals of a keto food plan are exceptionally the same. According to nutritionists, participants need to eat one gram of protein for every kilogram of body weight. Also, 10¬15 grams of carbs ought to be taken per day while the rest of the food plan should be made of fats.

Ketogenic Food Regimen Results

After the ketogenic food plan has become famous for treating epilepsy, numerous benefits became apparent. The children handled with the food regimen had been noticed to be more fabulous alert and much less irritable. They had no issues dozing at night and had extra electricity inside the day.

However, this consuming method becomes dismissed with the advent of anticonvulsant drugs, which later have become the preferred choice of treatment. With time, the weight-reduction plan lost its popularity, and fewer dieticians knew of its proper use. This brought about the mistaken use of the food regimen, primarily to unfavorable results. This created the rumor that it's far horrific for fitness. In just a rely of time, the weight loss program lost all its popularity, and only a few had the expertise of it.

Returning to Mainstream Attention

Up until 1990, the ketogenic eating regimen remains all but forgotten. Although it turned into studied, it turned into taken into consideration a historical curiosity instead of a medical fact.

The go back of ketogenic eating regimen owes loads to the TV show, Dateline. In an episode of October 1994, there has been a case of a two-year-antique Charlie. He had severe epilepsy, and his seizures have been getting out of hand until he came throughout keto. Charlie was being handled at John Hopkins hospital, and at that time, just about ten children have been on a keto weight loss plan every year.

With time, Charlie's seizures became higher and better because of the ketogenic food regimen he had to get right of entry to. This led to a sizeable scientific hobby in keto. With this, many humans became extra and more significantly interested in the keto food regimen.

Beyond epilepsy: Modern Keto Diet

After the reintroduction of the keto weight-reduction plan, many hospitals started providing it as a useful alternative in treating epilepsy. Currently, almost each primary youngsters' hospital gives a keto weight loss plan as an available choice. It also continues to attract extra-scientific hobby, for its role in managing some neurological troubles is turning into productive.

The tale of the keto weight loss program goes beyond epilepsy. The ingesting plan isn't any longer best considered as a remedy for a rare medical problem; as a substitute, it is also now widely known for its ability to help human beings lose weight. However, it isn't clean while it has become famous for its weight-dropping position.

Akins weight loss program became widely considered inside the early and the late nineties. This weight-reduction plan has a comparable perspective of carbs. Interestingly, the renewed hobby in keto weight loss program compelled many researchers to carefully look into what it can offer to the health of many human beings, and so far, their findings have even amazed those researchers.

Today, plenty of humans take into account keto for health reasons, apart from reducing seizures. And they do so because of its many blessings, which we will discuss within the next chapter.

HEALTH BENEFITS OF KETO DIET FOR WOMEN OVER 50

Keto weight loss plan adherents, mainly those elderly 50 and older, are stated to enjoy several capability fitness advantages. Here are some of these advantages of keto weight loss plans for girls over 50.

Weight Loss

This is probably the number one purpose why many people do keto. First and foremost, the initial weight loss is because of a lack of water because of a discount in carbs intake. Also, your frame makes use of up the saved carb it has.

Even, the keto weight loss plan consequences in extra weight loss because it breaks down any to be had fat for fuel.

Cutting out carbs indeed method your body gets less sugar; refined carbs method you get a higher pleasant of strength and food. Once you get adjusted to the diet, you will find out you get a regular supply of power without the need to snack anytime soon. In order words, the keto diet additionally prevents excessive eating, as you don't get hungry very frequently.

Preventing Diseases and Treatment

Other than weight reduction and epilepsy, keto also plays sure roles in the treatment and prevention of diseases. These include:

Metabolic Syndrome

Some researchers have set up that some adults with metabolic problems who participated in keto lost extra fats and frame weight than those on a standard weight loss program rich in introduced sugar and processed food.

Type 2 Diabetes

According to a have a look at published by using the Journal of Obesity and Eating Disorders in September 2016, the keto diet can assist human beings with type 2 diabetes. Currently, evidence aid that keto can help in handling the disease. It improves the HbA1c levels inside the blood. However, you should talk to your health practitioner before going with keto. See keto weight loss program and diabetes for more information.

Bipolar Disorder

In conditions of type 2 bipolar syndrome, keto can help in stabilizing modes. A look at published in the Journal Neurocase in October 2012 suggested that it could be a new powerful form of remedy than medications.

Obesity

Keto food regimen is a tried and proven technique if you need to lose weight. Very-low-calorie keto weight-reduction plan is compelling in helping overweight people shed pounds and abdominal fat. It also preserves lean frame mass when undergoing weight loss.

Dementia and Alzheimer's Disease

Published research in the 2013 February version of Journal Neurobiology of Ageing determined out that older adults on keto diets had better functioning memory just six weeks after. The director of the Alzheimer's Prevention Clinic in Weil Cornell Medicine and New York-Presbyterian in New York City, Richard Isaacson, is in the assist of low-carb diets for patients to delay growing older in bran and the maximum familiar shape of dementia, Alzheimer's.

Parkinson's Disease

According to a Professor of Clinical Psychiatry at the University of Cincinnati College of Medicine, Ohio, Robert Krikorian, keto diets may be implemented to hold cognitive functions.

Certain Cancers

Together with radiation and chemotherapy, a keto food plan may be used in cancer therapy, even though more studies desires to be carried out on the way to go about the application of keto weight-reduction plan to most cancers treatment.

Insulin Resistance

As you develop older, your body tends to emerge as extra proof against insulin—another motive why women over 50 benefit weight are traceable to insulin-related problems like diabetes. Diabetes can bring about many troubles, which include loss of imaginative and prescient and kidney. A Keto weight loss plan is a proven remedy that manages diabetes because it increases insulin sensitivity.

Bone Health

Osteoporosis is one of the many conditions related to age. The density of your bone turns into reduced, inflicting it to come to be greater brittle and fragile. This situation is pronounced in older girls above the age of fifty years. Taking extra calcium by taking more milk products is probably helpful. However, it doesn't do enough. Ironically, the countries with the very best charge of dairy intake have the very best costs of osteoporosis. Consequently, the keto weight loss plan is using away a better treatment. It is low in toxins, interrupts absorption, and consists of many micronutrients in preference to just having calcium.

Inflammation

Due to aging, you will note increased pain from accidents and arthritis. When your frame is in ketosis, it produces a small number of substances known as cytokines- it promotes inflammation.

Nutrient Deficiencies

Older adults, mainly women, frequently have higher deficiencies in essential nutrients like:

- Iron: its lack can cause mental fatigue and fog.
- Vitamin B12: deficiency can motive neurological illnesses, including dementia.
- Fats: deficiency can lead to troubles with cognition, imaginative and prescient, pores and skin, and vitamin deficiencies.
- Vitamin D: deficiency ends in cognitive impairment in older adults. It causes an increased danger of coronary heart disease or even contributes to cancer danger. Therefore, a ketogenic weight loss plan with satisfactory assets of animal protein can complement these crucial vitamins.

Managing Blood Sugar

As we said earlier, there is a connection between mind-related problems like Alzheimer's disease, Parkinson's, and dementia and terrible blood sugar.

- Excessive consumption of carbs, especially fructose, can spread up brain-related situations (fructose is hugely reduced in the keto food plan)
- Absence of nutritional LDL cholesterol and fats, both of which are plentiful in keto food plan
- Ketosis facilitates in protecting towards oxidative stress
- Applying keto weight-reduction plan in coping with blood sugar troubles improves response to insulin and forestalls memory issues that come with age

Keto for Ageing

Keto diets offer plenty of vitamins per calorie. This is vital because you are older; you need fewer calories. However, you still need an identical amount of vitamins as you did in your younger days. You could have a stricter time residing on junk food, not like when you had been younger. This approach is essential to eat foods that guide your health and fight diseases. This can help you live an exciting lifestyle while getting old gracefully. You want to take in more magnificent optimal meals and avoid immoderate and empty calories observed in sugar-wealthy foods like grains. You want to increase the amount of nutrient-wealthy proteins and fat you consume.

Carb-rich ingredients are pushed using society and aren't beneficial to your long term health. Carb low diets containing excessive quantities of plant and animal fat are way better for increasing insulin sensitivity. It also slows down cognitive decline, making your overall health higher.

It's no longer too late to enhance your possibilities of functioning and feeling as you get older. You can start doing higher and eating higher. Keto for girls over 50 years is another danger to repair some of the damage performed in your younger days while you didn't pay attention to what you did eat.

The in advance you begin to make those changes to enhance your weight, immunity, and blood sugar, the better your chances of living better and longer.

In conclusion, all of us get older. However, we will all control our satisfaction with life as we get even older. Keto diets assist you in enhancing your health so that you can thrive instead of being in pains and illness as you get farther away from fifty.

KETO COMPARED TO OTHER DIETS

Again, the keto food plan isn't the handiest diet that exists in the global health and wellness. You are afforded a wide variety of alternatives and methodologies that you can choose to undertake for yourself. This type of range and diversity inside the enterprise of weight-reduction plan is continually going to be good. This way, people are going with the intention to discover the weight-reduction plan that first-class fits their very own private wishes and their lifestyles. And if you are one who is contemplating adopting the keto food plan for your personal life, then you're going to need to know just how it compares to different options.

And that is going to serve as the topic for this chapter. You are going to receive a glimpse into what the keto weight-reduction plan sincerely is and how it stacks up relative to the other famous diets obtainable on the market. This sort of comparative evaluation would be capable of doing things. One, it will let you gather perspective on the weight loss plan enterprise and the variety of alternatives which might be to be had with a purpose to try. And, it will offer you a more informed opinion and a more strong resolve for whatever healthy diet weight-reduction plan you do eventually pick to adopt for yourself inside the future.

Keto as the Best Diet Plan Out There

It's proper that there are undoubtedly many weight loss plan plans obtainable at the market, and it'd be too arrogant to say that the keto weight loss plan is high-quality among them all. However, it would be fair to mention that the keto eating regimen is a high-quality one for you for my part if it takes place to serve your wishes and your goals higher effectively.

The keto food plan is a low-carb diet that is designed to place the human frame into a heightened ketogenic state, which might inevitably result in higher pronounced fat burn and weight loss. It is a reasonably accessible food regimen with a variety of keto-friendly meals being readily available in marketplaces at highly low prices. It isn't an eating regimen that is reserved most effectively for the affluent and elite.

As some distance as effectiveness is concerned, there's just no denying how impactful a keto eating regimen maybe for someone who wants to lose a drastic quantity of weight in a wholesome and managed manner. The keto weight-reduction plan also enforces discipline and precision for the agent by incorporating macro counting and meal journaling to ensure accuracy and accountability in the weight-reduction project. There are no external factors that can impact how robust this weight loss plan may be for you. Everything is all within your control.

And lastly, it's a reasonably sustainable weight loss plan, for the reason that it doesn't merely compromise on taste or range. Sure, there are lots of restrictions. But ultimately, there are lots of alternatives and workarounds that can assist stave off cravings. If these kinds of standards and reasons observe to you and your personal life, then it could genuinely be safe to say that the keto food plan is a high-quality one for you.

What Sets Keto Apart from Others?

But how precisely does keto stack up against other weight loss plan plans obtainable? Well, if your purpose for dieting is weight loss, then it would be prudent to investigate different diets that are similar to the keto eating regimen's goals of inducing weight reduction and fats burn. You should advantage a higher understanding of these diets and why the keto eating regimen would, in all likelihood, nonetheless be the better one for you. The three foods which are most usually compared to the keto weight loss plan in phrases of meal composition and bodily effects are Atkins, paleo, and Whole30.

Atkins

The Atkins and keto diets are so similar in the feel that they both promote a high intake of fat, mild consumption of protein, and minimum intake of carbohydrates. Typically, while on Atkins, a person's typical diet would be composed of 60% fat, 30% protein, and 10% carbohydrates. This is still a relatively minimal carbohydrate composition even when you take into consideration the keto breakdown of 75% fat, 20% protein, and 5% carbohydrates.

The problem with Atkins isn't found in better carbohydrate consumption. It's, in most cases, located inside the elevated consumption of protein. Any extra protein that the body doesn't dissipate for muscle constructing or repair is converted into glucose. And that glucose goes to be used for energy in preference to the stored fat that you could have, at this moment making the metabolic fee of your frame slower. The keto diet nonetheless offers you the protein blessings of constructing and repairing muscles without compromising the advantages of ketosis at equal time.

Paleo

The paleo food regimen is one that is gaining full-size popularity in the cutting-edge health industry. It stems from the studied nutritional practices of the Paleolithic era, which was depending on the hunter-gatherer system of food rationing and production. It is a food regimen that focuses entirely on complete ingredients that are free from any processing. Food items which include wheat, grains, dairy, legumes, processed sugars, processed oils, corn, processed fats, etc. are prohibited. It specializes in the high intake of meats and non-starchy greens.

Like the keto weight-reduction plan, the paleo diet additionally takes place to be a low-carb diet that emphasizes a better consumption of fat and proteins. However, it doesn't indeed restrict the wide variety of carbohydrates or energy that a person might take on day by day basis. It's a weight loss plan that focuses entirely on the composition of meals without the quantity of it, and that may be problematic for several people who've very particular bodily composition dreams.

Whole30

Whole30 is a stricter model of the paleo weight-reduction plan. It is a diet plan that is primarily dependent on a thirty-day application of strict eating under paleo principles. It removes the consumption of processed foods, starchy vegetables and carbohydrates, sweeteners, dairy products, legumes, and higher. Once the thirty-day period is over, you're then recommended to reintroduce certain food groups step by step in your weight-reduction plan and examine what kind of impact or effect these will have on you. This is how you will be capable of discovering what type of food you've got a trendy intolerance to.

However, the Whole30 weight loss program doesn't certainly issue in macro counting and calorie counting either. That manner that humans at the Whole30 weight loss plan are nevertheless at risk of gaining weight and getting fat despite the restrictive nature of the weight loss program.

These might most uncomplicated be 3 examples of similar nutritional packages and methodologies, and there are so many other diets obtainable that the keto food regimen can simply be as compared to. However, that would probably make for another ebook. The factor that this bankruptcy is merely looking to build and emphasize is that there are usually going to be sure caveats in any kind of nutritional philosophy. There will be benefits, and there could be cons as well. The quality sort of eating regimen isn't the only that every single individual within the international is going to discover fulfillment in. Instead, it's the one that is going to allow you to attain all your very own private health dreams and dreams. And it might be very tough to deny the fact that the keto weight loss plan manages to do precisely that for such a lot of different forms of humans within the international.

CAUTION FOR KETO

Yes, Keto is beneficial, and yes, it has a whole lot of benefits, but it is no small element, and so, it should be approached with caution. Here are some tips you have to hold in thoughts earlier than embarking on Keto.

Make Use of Recipes You Can Trust

Keto involves a variety of meal planning, and this single segment is where several human beings get it wrong. Your food is now not allowed to be careless, and you must note the whole thing that is going into your mouth. If you're embarking on a Keto weight loss plan, you should use recipes you may trust. The methods should be useful, safe, and delicious. Keto must now not take out the enjoyment in your food. Luckily, you have your hands on the excellent e-book for Keto aspirants underneath 50.

You May Additionally Need a Physician

If you have got had any trouble with blood sugar, insulin degrees, or diabetes, consult your medical doctor before embarking on Keto. Do not make any dietary adjustments as massive as Keto to your diet without first informing your physician. He or she is in a significant role to manual you correctly. See your physician.

It Will Be Difficult at First

Keto isn't any walk within the park. However, human beings continue on the path of Keto no matter the initial trouble due to the fact the consequences are glaring after a quick while. When you kick-begin Keto, you may be afflicted by low blood sugar, sluggishness, and constipation. However, they'll all put on off in a few days in case you are spiritual about it.

Can Keto Have Side Effects?

Yes. Keto can have aspect consequences. Keto may have adverse side results if it's far wrongly done. Keto cuts down on carbs and replaces them with fat. However, if the replacement isn't correctly carried out, a variety of negative facet results may also occur. This is why it is incredibly vital to begin the Keto weight loss program armed with the proper information and recipes, which might be all included in this book.

If you do no longer employ exceptional meal plans and recipes, you'll lack vitamins that your body needs. With Keto, you should no longer lack proteins, and so, your food needs to be planned.

Reaching Ketosis

Reaching the state of ketosis isn't always so truthful for many people. To effectively reach ketosis, there are some steps you need to take.

- Eat the right food- Ketosis relies lots on what you consume. To reach ketosis, you need to first reduce down on the carbohydrates you take in. Secondly, you want to soak up a good deal of extra fat in your diets. However, you should simply soak up any grease, you should ensure to take in healthy fat. Taking in unhealthy fat can reason extra harm than good.

- Exercise- To efficiently reach ketosis, you have to make sure to exercise. It mustn't be intensive. However, long walks, jugs, biking, and other sports can help your frame reach ketosis.
- Try intermittent fasting- Some human beings integrate intermittent fasting with ketosis. The motive is that, as you progress, your starvation pangs are significantly decreased and you will discover intermittent fasting easy. Even while you do now not plan to, you'll locate yourself doing it. It is certainly not compulsory, but in case you are utilizing ketosis to lose weight, intermittent fasting is a great bonus.
- Take masses of culmination and greens- Fruits and greens for snacks will maintain your body healthy, assist, and revitalize your skin.
- Include coconut oil on your weight loss plan- Coconut is compulsory in case you want to reach ketosis. Coconut oil carries wholesome fat. It allows the body to attain ketosis and includes four varieties of MCTs. It is considered one of the excellent tools for inducing ketosis. If you have got in no way made use of coconut oil before, begin slowly and increase your intake gradually.

What Are Macros?

'Macros' is short for macronutrients. These macronutrients are the essential vitamins your frame needs. These vitamins are-

- Carbohydrates: In this group, we've got sugars, fibers, and starches. Carbohydrates are damaged down into glucose or blood sugar. Your body can then use it as energy or store it as glycogen on your liver or for your muscles.
- Proteins: Proteins are observed in fish, meat, eggs, and lentils inclusive of beans.
- Proteins are vital for a whole lot of functions inclusive of cellular signaling, the building of tissues, constructing of enzymes, as well as hormones. It is additionally crucial for various immune capabilities.
- Fats: Fat is located in oils, butter, nuts, meat, fatty fish, and avocado. Fat is used for numerous essential matters within the body. It helps keep body temperature and produce hormones. It also enables the frame to absorb vitamins.

The Keto diet focuses on providing ok tiers of protein and substituting carbs for healthful fat.

Although a few foods have the vitamins you need, they'll also have an excessive level of carbs. This is why it's miles important to test the nutritional composition of any food before incorporating it into your food plan

Getting Started with Keto Over 50

There are diverse forms of Keto diets. At 50 and above, you cannot merely employ the everyday Keto weight-reduction plan. This is because, at this age, every and the entircty you eat matters. You turn out to be what you eat, and so, it's miles critical which you make use of the proper variation of Keto.

You can't employ the traditional Keto weight loss program because it isn't suitable for older persons. Whatever Keto eating regimen, you'll be on must be ideal on your age and take into consideration that your frame doesn't metabolize as fast as previously. It isn't what we need to hear, but it is what we want.

What not to consume while Ketoing:

- Sugar
- Starches and food high in carbohydrates
- Too an awful lot fruit because it carries sugar while in massive quantities.
- Beer and Alcohol

Keto Diet for Below 50 VS Keto for Above 50

Those who are more youthful than 50 years of age discover that they can stick to traditional Keto diets without a problem. They have schedules, cheat days, and other gear that help them. Missing a day or does not have too severe repercussions as they can make up. However, one over 50, Ketoing has to be taken extra seriously, indeed, because it is harder to lose weight.

Due to the reality that it will become more challenging to lose weight, numerous over 50's have made Ketoing the 'rule' and no longer the exception. A careful have to look at this book will display that every one the exceptional recipes have been transformed into Keto forms. Carbs had been taken and replaced with fats and proteins are particularly favored.

When 50 or above, your Keto weight loss plan needs to be observed religiously. This was once a hassle as most of the things we loved simply involved a variety of carbs. Luckily, that is now not the case. With the right recipe e-book, you'll find it a good deal more straightforward to do without carbs.

Remember to run any dietary changes by way of your doctor.

MAKING PROPER MEAL PLANS

For those who are new to the Keto Diet, the manner to meal plan might seem both full of possibility and complete of pitfalls. The reality is that the high-quality solution is the KISS method (Keep It Simple Stupid). The key to this food regimen is to make sure which you are keeping everything inside your proper ratios. This is the virtually important part of the Keto Diet.

When you stay inside the ratios which you need to be in, what's going to happen is that you can make sure which you get the maximum out of your weight-reduction plan. That is why you want to realize your precise amounts of carbs, proteins, and high fats.

However, this is just the primary step; the following component to think about is what precisely can you eat? Well, there may be proper news, there are lots of alternatives with proteins. One factor which you have to do is make sure that you stick to only three or four distinct assets of protein. This is a way that you may make life clean on yourself. One of the resources of protein needs to be eggs. They are undoubtedly clean and versatile, and eggs also are ridiculously cheap. Another extraordinary idea is using seafood.

The smaller forms of seafood are higher; for example, sardines are an excellent supply of protein due to the fact they are excessive in Omega-3, which has a ton of blessings for the body. Some different seafood consists of salmon, shrimp, cod, or even oysters. That said, many of these specific meats can get expensive. Also, if you can get grass-fed or natural beef, that is always higher than going with the traditional types which meats which have a higher quantity of fat content.

Here are a few sources of protein again, adjust in case you are on a budget:

- Grass-fed beef
- Wild-caught seafood
- Pork; preferably pasture-raised
- Eggs - the vegetarian weight-reduction plan is the standard
- Grass-fed chicken
- Yogurt in moderation

Oils additionally have a few very magnificent homes as correctly, and what you're cooking with will genuinely affect your development at the Keto Diet. One of the terrific suggestions for adding taste is to prepare dinner your vegetables in Extra Virgin Olive Oil or bacon fat. This is an excellent manner to get the flavor. Avocado oil and the olive oil additionally works well with salad dressings. When you decide that you need to marinate food, make sure to use avocado oil. Butter of path is excellent to cook with, and uncured bacon is both a top-notch element to render fat from and also to eat.

Also, the rendered fat has a better smoke point so that you can feel assured that you won't have to address the oxidized LDL cholesterol. This is responsible for the hardening of arteries, the building of plaque, and that is what causes heart disease as correctly.

Choosing your vegetables is also very important, and the aspect which you need to do is get dark leafy greens like spinach and kale. There are others as accurately, along with bok choy. The top information is when you are using butter and bacon fats for cooking these greens, you will enjoy their flavors. These vegetables are loaded with specific nutrients that your frame needs, along with calcium and other vitamins and minerals, to be able to make up for any deficiencies that you could have had like changed into described in the preceding chapters. Plus, they have got amazingly complex flavors and can be used in so many distinct approaches.

There are lots of other veggies to use as nicely, so don't get stuck in a kale and spinach cycle because consequences in the building up of different oxalates and the end consequences are kidney stones. No one desires to address that Mushrooms also are suitable and have a low quantity of net carbs, asparagus, Brussel sprouts, zucchini, onions, and bell peppers all do the activity too. Throw in a few balsamic kinds of vinegar and you have a few super flavors. These vegetables additionally tolerate the grill truly correctly also.

The fruit is something that must be used moderately, and the key with fruit is making positive that you are all approximately the berries. Blackberries, raspberries, blueberries, and strawberries are best due to the fact they may be each high in fiber and also in antioxidants. Furthermore, win, and dark chocolate additionally has brilliant energy with the Keto Diet as well. There are lots of other things to recollect too. Make positive that the fruit is lower in sugar, due to the fact this may keep away from the increase within the insulin, and that creates problems with the Keto Diet.

Once you've got the meals that you need to eat, the following step is making positive which you are cooking it the manner which you need. There are some specific techniques which you must use. The first is that you need to make sure that you're going certainly one of three approaches. The excellent strategies are the usage of a stress cooker, the range top, or firing up the grill.

There are masses of exciting thoughts as nicely. Bone broth is something this is genuinely amusing to make throughout meal prep, and it is carried out with the pressure cooker. There is also dishes like Keto lasagna, pulled pork, keto cheesecake, ground beef dishes, tough boiled eggs, or even veggie lasagna. When you replicate on wherein you were and how a long way you have got come, you will observe which you had been eating a bunch of starches together with pasta, rice, mac and cheese, baked potatoes, etc. The strain cooker is one of the subtle ways that you can prepare meals in a wholesome manner, and it makes life a lot easier.

Once you've got meal prep completed, you will observe how it's so easy to have the meals you want when you want it. There are precise healthful breakfasts, lunches, dinners, and snacks available. If you are not a snacker, simply add to the alternative food, and this could help you live together with your Keto Diet.

WHAT TO EAT ON THE KETO DIET?

So in considering the foods which can be allowed at the keto diet and the fact that you will be giving up your sugary treats and severely limiting your carbohydrate intake, you are in all likelihood thinking that the keto food regimen is the most restrictive weight loss program ever. But it truly isn't. Even with the carb restrictions, there are many accurate tasting carbs that are allowed on the weight loss plan.

Many of the reviews on the keto food plan will insist which you ought to devour natural greens and grass-fed meat best and use butter and ghee crafted from the milk of grass-fed cows. Eggs need to come from chickens fed with natural feed, and all fish must be wild-caught. Cheese ought to also be made from the milk that has organically fed or grass-fed cows. While this is food in its purest form and it'd be fine if we could all stick with those rules, it just isn't always necessary. For one thing, this kind of food is more significantly high priced than regular meals. It can be tougher to source on the grocery store, mainly if you live in a rural place that might not have a specialty meals store. And even though large chains and massive box stores are doing their exceptional to carry a greater variety of natural meals, their selection won't always be excellent.

You will eat quite correctly and lose weight merely excellent eating the same forms of ingredients that other people consume, so long as you're following the recommendations of the keto food regimen.

That being said, what foods does one devour on the keto food plan? There are many exclusive meals which are allowed at the keto weight loss plan, so many of which you have not to be tired of your food picks.

At the beef counter, any beef, bird turkey, or beef is ultimately allowed because those meals are no carb foods, and they will fulfill your protein necessities and a number of your fat requirements. Since no one desires to sit around chewing on a stick of butter, it's miles essential to an appearance in your protein choices to additionally fulfill a number of your fat necessities in each day weight loss program. When choosing cuts of red meat, you want to live far from the lean cuts and go for the ones that have extra fat on and in them, which interprets into dietary fat, even though all meat has a few fat contents.

A very lean three-ounce sirloin tip steak has thirty 9 grams of protein and five and one 1/2 grams of fat. A three-ounce filet mignon has thirty-three grams of protein and twelve grams of dietary fats. The rib-eye steak is probably the highest fat content material steak with thirty-eight grams of fat and thirty grams of protein. Since the fats part of the eating regimen is better in total than the protein part, it's far essential to go for the extra fatty cuts of meat. Dark meat bird could have better fats content than white meat fowl. A 3-ounce fowl breast will have thirty-one grams of protein and three and one-half of grams of fats, while a thigh with the skin on weighs in at twenty-five grams of protein and fifteen and one-half of grams of fat. And they informed us the pores and skin was horrific for us!

Also, look for fatty meats in the shape of bacon and sausage. Any form of sausage will do and will assist in adding variety for your food regimen. Check the substances at the label to look for delivered carbs or sugars. For carb words, you need to search for anything that ends in saccharide—mono, poly, or di. Also, search for glycogen, dextrin, cellulose, maltose, galactose, lactose, fructose, dextrose, sucrose, and glucose. Sugar phrases are saccharose, maple sugar, invert sugar, milk sugar, lactose, malt sugar, maltose, levulose, fructose, fruit sugar, dextrose, grape sugar, beet sugar, confectioner's sugar, brown sugar, corn sugar, cane sugar, and sucrose.

That is lots of words to don't forget; however, you will soon get used to studying food labels and knowing what you ought to and have to eat now not.

Hotdogs are also a great meat desire; this is complete of fats and provides protein. Again, make sure to study the label and look for components. At the seafood counter, nearly anything goes. While some fish and seafood do have carbs, the amounts are quite small according to a 3-ounce serving:

- Squid 2.62 net carbs
- Shrimp .74 net carbs
- Scallops 2.01 net carbs
- Oysters 3.33 net carbs
- Clams 2.19 net carbs
- Mussels 3.14 net carbs
- Crab 0 net carbs

Anything else that comes from the fish display case is a no-carb food. Net carbs are the carbs you want to be counted. Net carbs are received using taking the whole carbohydrate wide variety and subtracting the fiber amount, on account that fiber is a carb; however, it can be digested and passes out of the frame without including to overall frame weight. Fish is not extremely high in fats; however, it is carb loose and is a fantastic addition to any weight loss program. There are, however, a few fish that will provide you with both fats and protein (servings are 3 ounces):

- Trout 4.9 grams fat16 grams protein
- Tuna2.five grams of fat20 grams protein
- Whitefish12 grams38 grams protein
- Salmon27 grams40 grams protein
- Herring17 grams33 grams protein
- Mackerel34 grams25 grams protein
- Kippers4.nine grams10 grams protein

Kippers and tuna are not particularly high in fats; however, they made a list for every other reason: they are superb with other foods. Kippers are much like sardines and can be eaten with full fats cheese for a fast snack. Tuna may be blended with total fats mayonnaise for a meal or a snack.

Moving over to the deli counter, you may discover a treasure of delicious keto-friendly foods. Here you can buy sliced roast pork, turkey, and fowl. You will locate pre-packaged or clean sliced pepperoni, salami, and pastrami. You also can purchase pre-made tuna salad, egg salad, and fowl salad. Just do not forget to check the label for brought ingredients that you may not need to be ingesting. You can also discover sliced cheeses and shredded cheeses, which are a fantastic compliment to any meal. However, sliced and shredded cheese will have a minimal-carb count number because they have to be made softer for slicing or shredding. Block robust cheese is the quality desire because it has no carbs.

In the dairy case, search for complete fat butter and ghee. Ghee is nothing extra than clarified butter. It is made by using simmering butter over low heat until the milk solids and water rise and can be removed. Heavy cream can be used in recipes to thicken them, or it could be whipped and used to top berries for a sweet dessert. The more extended cheese treatment plans, the lower the carb be counted might be, but all cheese is very low in carbs for a one-ounce serving:

- American cheese 1.97 grams net carbs
- Blue cheese 066 grams net carbs
- Brie cheese 013 grams net carbs
- Camembert cheese .13 grams net carbs
- Cheddar cheese .36 grams net carbs
- Colby cheese .72 grams net carbs
- Feta cheese 1.16 grams net carbs
- Gouda cheese .63 grams net carbs
- Gruyere cheese .10 grams net carbs
- Havarti cheese .79 grams net carbs
- Mexican blend cheese .64 grams net carbs
- Monterey cheese .19 grams net carbs
- Mozzarella cheese .79 grams net carbs
- Muenster cheese .31 grams net carbs
- Neufchatel cheese .83 grams net carbs
- Parmesan cheese .91 grams net carbs
- Provolone cheese .60 grams net carbs
- Ricotta cheese .86 grams net carbs
- Romano cheese 1.03 grams net carbs

- Swiss cheese 1.51 grams net carbs

Also inside the dairy case, you'll need to pick out up a few more essential things to be used to add flavor and fats to your meals (carb counts are in line with half-cup serving):

- Full fat cottage cheese 3.02 grams net carbs 10 grams fat
- Full fat cream cheese .77 grams net carbs 29 grams fat
- Full fat yogurt (plain) 6 grams net carbs .7 grams fat
- Eggs .6 grams net carbs 5 grams fat

Yogurt should be simple to be low carb; added fruit is introduced carbs. And Greek yogurt could have a better protein depend than regular yogurt will. Yogurt is not high in fat; however, it is a superb food to have on hand for a fast snack or to mix with berries for a quick addition to any meal.

The produce counter is where things begin to get tricky. Fruits and greens have carbohydrates. Certain fruits and veggies are higher than others and are allowed on the keto food plan to provide the body with some carbs and fiber while preserving a lower carb counts. These are the things you will need to buy at the produce counter (all carb counts are for a three-ounce serving):

- Spinach 1 gram
- Lettuce (all types) 2 grams
- Avocado 2 grams
- Cucumber 3 grams
- Asparagus 2 grams
- Tomato 3 grams
- Eggplant 3 grams
- Cabbage 3 grams
- Zucchini 3 grams
- Cauliflower 3 grams
- Kale 3 grams
- Broccoli 4 grams
- Green bell peppers 3 grams
- Red bell peppers 4 grams
- Yellow bell peppers 5 grams
- Brussel sprouts 5 grams
- Green beans 4 grams

These carb counts are all in net carbs. It is ideal to consume those ingredients due to the fact your body still desires a few carbs to feature, and all of these foods will offer you fiber, which is vital for right intestinal health. You can also get a few threads from the few culminations which are advocated at the keto weight loss plan. Remember that fruits have herbal sugar that's a carbohydrate. These counts are for a three-ounce serving:

- Raspberries 5 grams
- Blackberries 5 grams
- Strawberries 6 grams
- Blackberries 4 grams
- Plum 7 grams
- Lemon 6 grams
- Lime 6 grams
- Coconut (meat) 6 grams
- Cantaloupe 7 grams
- Watermelon 7 grams

The listing of allowed fruits is much shorter than the list of allowed vegetables. Another manner to have a look at is this: in case you are eating twenty grams of carbs each day, that would be a serving of cantaloupe (3 ounces), a serving of watermelon, and a serving of strawberries. Or for that equal twenty grams, you may have a meal of green beans (3 ounces), spinach, cucumber, avocado, zucchini, tomato, and broccoli. So you see it is far better to get your carb count number in vegetables and no longer fruit. However, don't cut-price the result because everyone desires something candy in their eating regimen, and berries will fill the bill.

In the rest of the store you will discover many meals which might be allowed at the keto weight-reduction plan:

- Olive oil, coconut oil, avocado oil
- Lard
- Canned fish like tuna, sardines, salmon, crab, and anchovies
- Olives*
- Sauerkraut
- Hot sauce*
- Mayonnaise, full fats*
- Mustard*
- Vinegar*
- Broth and bouillon cubes

- Herbs and spice
- Pork rinds* (first-rate for breading foods)
- Tea, coffee, and membership soda
- Mushroom
- Bottled water
- Flavored water additives and not using a sugar
- Check the label to search for delivered sugar or starch

When you're shopping, the handiest buy the foods that you will eat. It makes no sense to shop for sardines if you don't like sardines or zucchini if you don't like zucchini. At the same time, strive to maintain your thoughts open to attempting new tastes. You might discover the person you surely want broccoli when the child you became her nostril up.

You will keep away from sugar in any form. This means you'll not eat any nutrition waters, fruit juices, sports drinks, and soft drinks. Do not even move down the aisle that has candy, cookies, donuts, canned fruit, frosting, cake mixes, brownie mixes, and boxed snack cakes. Stay away far from the cereal aisle, which means no breakfast bars, bloodless cereal, or toaster treats.

You will no longer be consuming bread in any form—this approach no sandwich bread, rolls, hot canine buns, or cinnamon rolls. The keto eating regimen does not allow potatoes, rice, or pasta. Stay away from the chip aisle.

It is vitally crucial to don't forget to consume real meals. Following one of the keto food plan plans will require more significant meal planning than you might presently be used to, but it's miles well worth the effort in the end. There can be times when it's far beneficial to prepare several days' well worth of meats and maintain them inside the fridge to make quick luncheon meals. Even if you are a single person, you could cook a whole roast or an entire turkey breast and either devour on it all week or freeze half for later use.

And do not forget that following the keto weight loss program does now not mean that giving up treats or proper food. You will find that there is a limitless array of meal pointers and snacks, even dessert ideas, as a way to follow the keto requirements and hold you are feeling complete and satisfied. Don't be afraid to discover many specific food alternatives while growing your menus. You will be surprised just how desirable and how flexible the keto consuming plan surely is.

30 DAY KETO MEAL PLAN

You will find all of the recipes used for this meal plan in the recipe chapter.

Week 1

Day 1

Breakfast:

Launch:

Dinner:

Shopping List for Keto Meals

The following are the foods that are emphasized on a keto diet.

Healthy, fatty fish such as tuna, salmon, etc.

Healthy oils such as avocado oil, coconut oil, olive oil, etc.

All types of full-fat cheese and full-fat cream cheese, sour cream, creme Fraiche.

Unsweetened almond/coconut milk, or other nut milk Eggs

Butter, total fat Avocados

Walnuts, almonds, cashews, and other nuts

Chia seed and flaxseed

Olives

Bacon

Unsweetened beverages Heavy cream

Healthy low carb, non-starchy veggies such as leek, fennel, spinach, kale, broccoli, tomatoes, other greens, etc.

All types of berries but in small quantities

Herbs and most spices

KETO DELICIOUS RECIPES

BREAKFAST

84. Pizza Dip

Servings: 4

Prep + cook time: 37 minutes

Ingredients

- ¼ cup sour cream
- ½ cup mozzarella cheese
- 4 oz. cream cheese softened
- ¼ cup mayonnaise
- Salt and ground black pepper to taste
- ½ cup tomato sauce
- ¼ cup Parmesan cheese, grated
- 1 tbsp. green bell pepper, seeded and chopped
- 6 pepperoni slices, chopped
- ½ tsp Italian seasoning
- 4 black olives, pitted and chopped

Directions:

1. In a medium bowl, mix sour cream, mozzarella cheese, cream cheese, mayonnaise, salt, and pepper. Put mixture into 4 ramekins. Add in such orders: a layer of tomato sauce, layer Parmesan cheese, chopped bell peppers, diced pepperoni, Italian seasoning, chopped black olives.
2. Preheat oven to 350 F.
3. Place ramekins in the oven and cook for 20 minutes. Serve.

85. Morning Pie

Servings: 3

Prep + cook time: 33 minutes

Ingredients:

- 3 oz. Parmesan cheese, sliced into thick pieces
- 5 medium eggs, beaten
- 8 oz. full-fat cream cheese
- 4 cloves garlic, peeled and minced
- 1 tsp salt
- ½ tsp cayenne pepper
- 1 tbsp. butter
- 4 oz. cream

Directions:
1. Put Parmesan cheese in the baking form.
2. Place the baking form in the oven and cook for about 5 minutes on 360 F.
3. In a medium bowl, whisk eggs. Add cream cheese and mix well.
4. In another bowl, combine garlic with salt and cayenne pepper.
5. Add garlic to egg mixture and stir well.
6. Heat a pan, add and melt butter.
7. Pour egg mixture in the pan and cook for 3 minutes on medium-high heat, stirring constantly.
8. Place scrambled eggs on Parmesan cheese in the baking form.
9. Top with a cream and back baking form to the oven. Cook for 10 minutes on 360
10. Remove the dish from the oven and let it cool for about 10 minutes. Serve.

86. Blender Pancakes

Servings: 1

Prep + cook time: 22 minutes

Ingredients:
- 2 large eggs, beaten
- scoop vanilla protein powder
- oz. cream cheese
- 10 drops liquid stevia
- ¼ tsp salt 1/8 tsp cinnamon

Directions:
1. Place eggs, vanilla, and cream cheese in blender or food processor and pulse it well.

2. Add liquid stevia, salt, and cinnamon to the food processor and blend until smooth.
3. Preheat pan on medium heat and spread pancake batter into 4-5" diameter rounds.
4. Bake on both sides until cooked.
5. Serve with sugar-free maple syrup or butter.

87. Sausage Patties

Servings: 3

Prep + cook time: 27 minutes

Ingredients:

- 1 lb. minced pork
- Salt and ground black pepper to taste
- ½ tsp sage, dried
- ¼ tsp thyme, dried
- ¼ tsp ground ginger
- 3 tbsp. Coldwater 1 tbsp. coconut oil

Directions:

1. In a small bowl, combine salt, sage, pepper, thyme, ginger, and water.
2. In a medium bowl, combine spice mix with pork.
3. Make patties and set aside.
4. Add coconut oil to the pan and preheat it on medium-high heat.
5. Transfer patties to pan and cook for 5 minutes, then flip, and prepare them for 3 minutes more.
6. Serve.

88. Keto Breakfast Mix

Servings: 6

Prep + cook time: 42 minutes

Ingredients:

- 1 tsp turmeric
- ½ tsp oregano
- 1 tsp cilantro
- 1 tsp salt

- ½ tsp ground black pepper
- 1 tsp paprika
- 1¼ cup bacon, chopped
- 1 tbsp. Butter oz. White mushrooms, sliced 1¼ cup zucchini, diced oz. Cauliflower, divided into florets oz. asparagus, cut in half 2 cloves garlic
- 1 white onion, sliced
- 1 cup chicken broth

Directions:

1. In a small bowl, mix turmeric, oregano, cilantro, salt, pepper, and paprika.
2. Season bacon with spice mixture, stir well.
3. Heat up a pan, add and melt butter.
4. Add bacon to the pan and cook for 5 minutes on medium heat, stirring constantly.
5. Add mushrooms, zucchini and cauliflower, stir and cook for another 2 minutes.
6. Stir in asparagus, garlic, and onion and pour the chicken broth.
7. Simmer for 10 minutes until vegetables are softened.
8. Serve warm.

89. Chicken Omelet

Servings: 1

Prep + cook time: 30 minutes

Ingredients

- 2 eggs, beaten
- Salt and ground black pepper to taste
- Olive oil spray
- 1 oz. rotisserie chicken, cooked and shredded
- tomato, cored and chopped
- bacon slices, crumbled
- 1 small avocado, peeled and chopped
- 1 tbsp. mayonnaise
- 1 tsp mustard

Directions:

1. In a medium bowl, whisk together eggs, salt, and pepper.
2. Preheat the pan on medium heat, add some Cook oil, pour in egg mixture, and cook for 5 minutes.
3. Place chicken, tomato, bacon, avocado, mayonnaise and mustard on one half of omelet. Then fold the omelet.
4. Close pan with lid and cook for about 5 minutes.
5. Serve warm.

90. Pepperoni Pizza Omelet

Servings: 1

Prep + cook time: 27 minutes

Ingredients

- Cooking spray
- 3 large eggs, beaten
- 1 tbsp. heavy cream
- 4 oz. pepperoni slices
- 4 oz. mozzarella cheese, shredded
- Salt and ground black pepper to taste
- Dried basil to taste
- 2 bacon strips

Directions:

1. Preheat pan on medium heat and drizzle with cooking spray.
2. In a bowl, combine eggs with heavy cream.
3. Pour mixture in the pan and cook until almost done. Then add some pepperoni slices to one side.
4. Sprinkle cheese, black pepper, salt, and basil over pepperoni and fold omelet over.
5. Cook for 1 minute more.
6. Meanwhile, in another pan, fry bacon strips until cooked.
7. Serve omelet with cooked bacon.

91. Kale Fritters

Servings: 6

Prep + cook time: 25 minutes

Ingredients:

- 7 oz. kale, chopped (tiny pieces)
- 10 oz. zucchini washed and grated
- 1 tsp basil
- ½ tsp salt
- ¼ cup almond flour
- ½ tbsp. mustard
- 1 large egg
- 1 tbsp. coconut milk
- 1 white onion, diced
- 1 tbsp. olive oil

Directions:

1. In a medium bowl, mix kale and zucchini.
2. Add basil and salt and stir.
3. Add almond flour and mustard. Stir well.
4. In another bowl, whisk together egg, coconut milk, and onion.
5. Pour egg mixture into the zucchini mixture and knead the thick dough.
6. Preheat pan with olive oil on medium heat.
7. Shape pancakes with the help of a spoon and put them in the pan.
8. Cook pancakes for about 2 minutes per side.
9. Transfer pancakes to a paper towel to remove excess oil.
10. Serve hot.

92. Italian Spaghetti Casserole

Servings: 6

Prep + cook time: 65 minutes

Ingredients:

- 1 spaghetti squash, halved
- Salt and ground black pepper to taste
- 4 tbsp. butter
- 2 cloves garlic

- 1 cup onion
- 4 oz. tomatoes
- oz. Italian salami, chopped
- ½ cup Kalamata olives, chopped
- ½ tsp Italian seasoning
- medium eggs
- ½ cup fresh parsley, chopped

Directions:
1. Heat the oven to 400 F.
2. Put the squash on the baking sheet. Sprinkle with salt and pepper.
3. Add 1 tablespoon butter and place in oven—Cook for 45 minutes.
4. Meanwhile, peel and mince garlic; peel and chop the onion; core and chop tomatoes.
5. Preheat pan on medium heat, add and melt 3 tablespoons butter.
6. Add onion, garlic, salt, and pepper, sauté for 2 minutes, stirring occasionally.
7. Add chopped tomatoes and chopped salami. Stir and cook for 10 minutes.
8. Add chopped olives and Italian seasoning. Stir and cook for 2-3 minutes more.
9. Remove squash halves from the oven and scrape the flesh with a fork.
10. Combine spaghetti squash with salami mixture in pan.
11. Shape 4 spaces in the mixture and crack an egg in each.
12. Sprinkle with salt and pepper and place pan in the oven.
13. Cook at 400 F until eggs are done.
14. Top with parsley and serve.

93. Chorizo and Mozzarella Omelet

Servings: 1

Prep + cook time: 20 minutes

Ingredients:
- 2 eggs
- 6 basil leaves
- 2 ounces' mozzarella
- 1 tbsp. butter

- 1 tbsp. water
- 4 thin slices chorizo
- 1 tomato, sliced
- Salt and black pepper, to taste

Directions:

1. Whisk the eggs along with the water and some salt and pepper. Melt the butter in a skillet and cook the eggs for 30 seconds. Spread the chorizo slices over. Arrange the sliced tomato and mozzarella over the chorizo. Cook for about 3 minutes. Cover the skillet and continue cooking for 3 more minutes until the omelet is completely set.
2. When ready, remove the pan from heat; run a spatula around the edges of the omelet and flip it onto a warm plate, folded side down. Serve garnished with basil leaves and a green salad.

94. Ricotta Cloud Pancakes with Whipped Cream

Servings: 4

Prep + cook time: 20 minutes

Ingredients

- 1 cup almond flour
- tsp low carb baking powder
- ½ tbsp. swerve
- ⅓ tsp salt
- ¼ cup ricotta cheese
- ⅓ cup of coconut milk
- large eggs
- 1 cup heavy whipping cream

Directions:

1. In a medium bowl, whisk the almond flour, baking powder, swerve, and salt.
2. Set aside.
3. Then, crack the eggs into the blender and process on medium speed for 30 seconds. Add the ricotta cheese, continue processing it, and gradually pour the coconut milk in while you keep on blending.
4. In about 90 seconds, the mixture will be creamy and smooth.
5. Pour it into the dry ingredients and whisk to combine.

6. Set a skillet over medium heat and let it heat for a minute. Then, fetch a soup spoonful of mixture into the skillet and cook it for 1 minute.
7. Flip the pancake and cook further for 1 minute. Remove onto a plate and repeat the cooking process until the batter is exhausted.
8. Serve the pancakes with whipping cream.

95. Mushroom & Cheese Lettuce Wraps

Servings: 4

Prep + cook time: 30 minutes

Ingredients:
- 6 eggs, separated into yolks and whites
- 2 tbsp. almond milk
- 1 tbsp. olive oil
- Sea salt, to taste for the Filling: 1 tsp olive oil
- 1 cup mushrooms, chopped
- Salt and black pepper, to taste
- ½ tsp cayenne pepper
- 8 fresh lettuce leaves
- 4 slices gruyere cheese
- 2 tomatoes, sliced

Directions
1. Mix all the ingredients for the wraps thoroughly.
2. Set a frying pan over medium heat. Add in ¼ of the mixture and cook for 4 minutes on both sides.
3. Do the same thrice and set the wraps aside, they should be kept warm in a separate pan over medium-high heat, warm 1 teaspoon of olive oil. Cook the mushrooms for 5 minutes until soft; add cayenne pepper, black pepper, and salt for seasoning.
4. Set 1-2 lettuce leaves onto every wrap. Split the mushrooms among the covers. Top with tomatoes and cheese.

96. Bacon & Cheese Pesto Mug Cakes

Servings: 3

Prep + cook time: 7 minutes

Ingredients:
- ¼ cup flax meal
- egg
- tbsp. heavy cream
- 2 tbsp. pesto
- ¼ cup almond flour
- ¼ tsp baking soda
- Salt and black pepper, to taste
- Filling:
- 2 tbsp. cream cheese
- 4 slices bacon
- ½ medium avocado, sliced

Directions:

1. Mix the dry muffin ingredients in a bowl. Add egg, heavy cream, and pesto and whisk well with a fork. Season with salt and pepper. Divide the mixture between two ramekins.

2. Place in the microwave and cook for 60-90 seconds. Leave to cool slightly before filling.

3. Meanwhile, in a nonstick skillet, over medium heat, cook the bacon slices until crispy. Transfer to paper towels to soak up excess fat. Set aside. Invert the muffins onto a plate and cut in half, crosswise. Assemble the sandwiches by spreading cream cheese and topping with bacon and avocado slices.

97. Cream Cheese Soufflé

Servings: 3

- Prep + cook time: 35 minutes <u>Ingredients:</u>
- 1/3 cup spinach, chopped roughly
- 1 tsp coconut oil
- ¼ cup white onion, peeled and diced
- 1 egg, beaten
- ½ cup cream cheese
- ¼ cup coconut flour
- 1 tsp salt 1 tsp paprika

Directions:

1. Place spinach in blender or food processor and blend until texture smooth.
2. Preheat pan with coconut oil on medium heat.
3. Add onion and sauté for about 5 minutes, continually stirring until onion turn golden brown.
4. In a medium bowl, combine egg, cream cheese, and coconut flour.
5. Season mixture with salt and paprika, stir well.
6. Add the cooked onion to mixture and stir.
7. Pour soufflé in baking dish.
8. Place dish in the oven at 365 F and bake for 10 minutes
9. Remove the baking dish from the oven and
10. whisk it carefully. Serve.

98. Morning Casserole

Servings: 4

Prep + cook time: 45 minutes

Ingredients:

- 3 eggs, beaten
- 8 oz. ground chicken
- 1 tsp salt
- 1 tsp oregano
- ½ tsp dried basil
- tsp dried cilantro
- ½ tsp cayenne pepper
- green bell peppers, deseeded and chopped
- 1 and 1/3 cup cauliflower, divided into florets
- 1 tbsp. olive oil
- 6 oz. Cheddar cheese, grated

Directions:

1. In a medium bowl, combine eggs with chicken.
2. Season mixture with salt, oregano, basil, cilantro, and cayenne pepper. Stir well. In another bowl, mix bell peppers and cauliflower.

3. Grease baking dish with olive oil.
4. Add chicken mixture to a baking dish, lay cauliflower mixture on top, and sprinkle with Cheddar cheese.
5. Cover baking dish tightly with aluminum foil.
6. Place the form in oven at 360F and cook for 10 minutes. Remove foil and bake dish for another 10 minutes.
7. Remove baking dish from oven and let it cook for 5-7 minutes. Serve.

LAUNCH & DINNER

99. Zesty Chili Lime Tuna Salad

Servings: 4

Prep time: 5 minutes

Ingredients

- 1 tablespoon of lime juice
- 1/3 cup of mayonnaise
- 1/4 teaspoon of salt
- 1 tsp of Tajin chili lime seasoning
- 1/8 teaspoon of pepper
- 1 medium stalk celery (finely chopped)
- 2 cups of romaine lettuce (chopped roughly)
- 2 tablespoons of red onion (finely chopped)
- Optional: chopped green onion, black pepper, lemon juice
- 5 oz canned tuna

Instructions

1. Using a bowl of medium size. Mix some of the ingredients such as lime, pepper and chili lime
2. Then, add tuna and vegetables to the bowl and stir. You can serve with cucumber, celery or a bed of green

100. Brussels Sprouts and Bacon

Servings: 2

Prep + cook time: 5 minutes

Ingredients

- 6 oz bacon
- Salt
- 6 oz raw Brussels sprouts
- Pepper

Instructions

1. Prepare the oven by preheating it. Then, prepare the baking sheet with parchment

paper
2. Prepare Brussels sprouts in the pan
3. Use kitchen shears to cut the bacon into little pieces
4. Add the cut bacon, and Brussel sprouts into the baking sheet already prepared. Then, add pepper and salt
5. Bake for up to 45 minutes. Allow the Brussel sprouts to become brown before taking out of the oven.

101. Super Simple Chicken Cauliflower Fried Rice

Servings: 4

Prep + cook time: 20 minutes

Ingredients

- 1/2 teaspoon of sesame oil
- 1 small carrot (chopped)
- 1 tablespoon of avocado or coconut oil
- 1 small onion (finely sliced)
- 1/2 cup of snap peas (chopped)
- Half cup of red peppers cut finely
- Properly chopped tablespoon of garlic
- One tablespoon of garlic, properly chopped
- 1 teaspoon of salt
- 2 teaspoons of garlic powder
- chicken breasts, chopped and cooked
- 4 cups of rice cauliflower
- 2 large scrambled eggs
- Gluten-free soy sauce, one quarter cup size

Instructions

1. Gently season the chicken breasts with half a tablespoon of salt, Y tablespoon of pepper and half tablespoon of olive oil. Cook the chicken on any pan of your choice
2. To the pan, add coconut/olive oil/ avocado and sesame oil. Cut some onions and carrots and sauce and leave for up to 3 minutes
3. Next, add the rest of the vegetables, pepper/salt/garlic powder and then cook for extra 3 minutes

4. Put in fresh garlic coconut aminos or soy sauce and rice cauliflower; then stir
5. Add scrambled eggs and chicken and mix until they are well combined
6. Put off the heat and then stir in some green peas. Season again, though you can top it with sesame seeds if you like

102. Prep-Ahead Low-Carb Casserole

Servings: 5

Prep + cook time: 45 minutes

Ingredients

- 1 cooked and cubed chicken breast
- 4 cooked and crumbled strips of bacon
- Half cup of celery, chopped and ready
- 1/3 cup of mozzarella cheese
- 1 tablespoon of Italian seasoning
- Half cup of grated parmesan
- 3 whisked eggs
- ½ whipping cream

Instructions

1. Start by pre-heating the oven to at least above 350 degrees.
2. Use a non-stick cooking spray to spray a casserole dish
3. Combine all the ingredients, leaving out the only mozzarella with a mixing bowl. Continue mixing until properly mixed
4. Pour out the mixture into a casserole dish. You can top it with mozzarella.
5. Allow baking for up to 35 minutes. Then, increase the heat and allow to boil until the mozzarella turns to a golden brown
6. Allow it to cool before serving

103. BBQ Pulled Beef Sando

Servings: 5

Prep + cook time: 12 minutes

Ingredients

- 3lbs boneless chuck roast

- 2 tablespoon of pink Himalayan salt
- 2 tablespoon of garlic powder
- 1 tablespoon of powder
- Apple cider vinegar
- 2 tablespoon of coconut amino
- Half cup of bone broth
- 1/4 cup of melted Kerry gold butter
- 1 tablespoon of black pepper
- 1 tablespoon of smoked paprika
- tablespoon of tomato paste

Instructions

1. Trim the fat from the beef and slice it into two huge pieces
2. Mix salt, onion, paprika, black pepper, and garlic. Next is to rub the mixture on the beef and then put the beef in a slow cooker
3. Use another bowl to melt butter. Then, add a tomato paste, coconut aminos, and vinegar and pour it all over the beef. Next is to add the bone broth into the slow cooker by pouring it around the beef
4. Cook for about 10 minutes. After that, take out the beef and increase the temperature of the cooker so that the sauce can thicken. Tear the beef before adding it to the slow cooker with the sauce.

104. Stuffed peppers

Servings: 1

Prep + cook time: 35 minutes

Ingredients:

- 1 tbsp. bacon fat
- 1 tsp. chili powder
- ½ onion
- 7 baby Bella mushrooms
- ¼ cup packed cilantro
- Salt and pepper
- 4 poblano peppers
- 1 tomato

- 1 tsp. cumin
- 1 lb. ground pork

Directions:

1. Broil the peppers in the oven for around 8-10 minutes. Grill them.
2. Brown the bacon fat pork and season with salt, pepper, cumin, and chili.
3. Add diced onion and gritty garlic in the mixture. Mix all together and add the champagne cut. When all the fat in the bowl is drained, remove the coriander and tomatoes chopped. Twelve minutes of cooking time.
4. In the peppers, put the meat and cook at 350 ° F for eight minutes.

105. Glazed salmon

Servings: 2

Prep + cook time: 30 minutes

Ingredients

- 1 tbsp. Sugar-free ketchup 1 tbsp. rice vinegar
- 1 tbsp. red boat fish sauce
- 2 tsp. garlic minced
- 2 tbsp. white wine
- 10 oz. salmon filet
- 2 tbsp. soy sauce
- 2 tsp. Sesame oil 1 tsp. ginger, minced

Directions:

1. In a pan, add all the ingredients and marinate the salmon in an oven for 1015minutes, except the ketchup, sesame oil, and white wine.
2. Apply sesame oil to the smoke in a high heat pot and bring the filet down on the side of the body.
3. Cook on both sides until crisp (4 minutes on both sides). Clear the glaze from the meat.
4. Fill the marinade with ketchup and white wine.
5. In the oven, cook 5 minutes, or until glaze is through.

106. Coconut shrimp

Servings: 3

Prep + cook time: 60 minutes

Ingredients:

For the Coconut Shrimp:
- 2 egg whites
- 1 lb. Peeled and deveined shrimp
- cup unsweetened coconut flakes
- tbsp. coconut flour

For the Sweet Chili Dipping Sauce:
- ¼ tsp. red pepper flakes
- 1 medium diced red chili
- 1 ½ tsp. rice wine vinegar
- 1 tbsp. lime juice
- ½ cup sugar-free apricot preserves

Directions:

1. Whisk the egg's white till it is fluffy. Prepare the coconut flour and coconut flakes in two different bowls.
2. Soak shrimp in coconut flour, and then add white eggs, and then flakes of coconut. Put the shrimp on a grated baking sheet. Bake for 15 minutes at a temperature of 400°F. Turn and broil until browned and crispy for about thirty-five minutes.
3. Combine all the ingredients for the dipping sauce to make the sauce.

107. Shrimp salad

Servings: 4

Prep + cook time: 20 minutes

Ingredients

- 3 endives, leaves separated
- 1-pound shrimp, peeled and deveined
- 1 tablespoon lemon juice
- tablespoon tarragon, chopped
- tablespoons lime juice
- tablespoons mayonnaise
- tablespoons parsley, chopped

- 2 tablespoons olive oil
- ½ cup sour cream
- Salt and black pepper to the taste
- teaspoon lime zest 2 teaspoons mint, chopped

Directions:

1. Mix the shrimp and the olive oil in a bowl, and add it to the baking sheet, then scatter the shrimp over a pan.
2. Place shrimp in the oven and bake for 10 minutes at 400 degrees F.
3. Flip lemon, flip again and leave for now. Apply lime juice.
4. Put the mayo in a bowl of sour cream, lime zest, citrus juice, sugar, pepper, tarragon, mint, and parsley.
5. Chop shrimp and add salad dressing and throw with endive leaves to fill.
6. Serve immediately.

108. Little Portobello pizza

Servings: 1

Prep + cook time: 11 minutes

Ingredients

- 1½ oz. Monterey jack
- 9 spinach leaves
- 3 Portobello mushrooms
- 1½ oz. cheddar cheese
- Olive oil
- 1½ oz. mozzarella
- 12 pepperoni slices
- 3 tomato slices
- 3 tsp. pizza seasoning

Directions

1. Through cleaning them and cutting the gills and the stalks, dress the Portobello mushrooms.
2. Sprinkle with the seasoning of olive oil and bread, and add the other ingredients, except the pepperoni. Cook 6 minutes at 450 ° F. Add the slices of pepperoni and

grill until crumbly.

109. Duck and Eggplant Casserole

Servings: 4

Prep + cook time: 45 minutes

Ingredients

- 1-pound ground duck meat
- 1 ½ tablespoons ghee, melted
- 1/3 cup double cream
- 1/2-pound eggplant, peeled and sliced
- 1 ½ cups almond flour
- Salt and black pepper, to taste
- 1/2 teaspoon fennel seeds
- 1/2 teaspoon oregano, dried
- 8 eggs

Directions

1. Mix the almond flour with salt, black, fennel seeds, and oregano. Fold in one egg and the melted ghee and whisk to combine well.
2. Press the crust into the bottom of a lightly-oiled pie pan. Cook the ground duck until no longer pink for about 3 minutes, stirring continuously.
3. Whisk the remaining eggs and double cream. Fold in the browned meat and stir until everything is well incorporated. Pour the mixture into the prepared crust. Top with the eggplant slices.
4. Bake for about 40 minutes. Cut into four pieces.

110. Spicy Breakfast Sausage

Servings: 4

Prep + cook time: 15 minutes

Ingredients:

- 4 chicken sausages, sliced
- 1 chili pepper, minced
- cup shallots, diced
- 1/4 cup dry white wine

- teaspoons lard, room temperature
- teaspoon garlic, minced
- Spanish peppers, deveined and chopped
- 2 tablespoons fresh coriander, minced
- 2 teaspoons balsamic vinegar
- 1 cup pureed tomatoes

Directions:

1. In a frying pan, warm the lard over a moderately high flame.
2. Then, sear the sausage until well browned on all sides; add in the remaining ingredients and stir to combine.
3. Allow it to simmer over low heat for 10 minutes or until thickened slightly.

111. Classic Chicken Salad

Servings: 4

Prep + cook time: 20 minutes

Ingredients:

- 1 medium shallot, thinly sliced
- 1 tablespoon Dijon mustard
- tablespoon fresh oregano, chopped
- 1/2 cup mayonnaise
- cups boneless rotisserie chicken, shredded
- 2 avocados, pitted, peeled and diced Salt and
- black pepper, to taste 3 hard-boiled eggs, cut into quarters

Directions:

- Toss the chicken with the avocado, shallots, and oregano.
- Add in the mayonnaise, mustard, salt, and black pepper; stir to combine.

112. Creamed Sausage with Spaghetti Squash

Servings: 4

Prep + cook time: 20 minutes

Ingredients:

- 1 ½ pound cheese & bacon chicken sausages, sliced
- 8 ounces' spaghetti squash
- 1/2 cup green onions, finely chopped
- 2/3 cup double cream
- 1 Spanish pepper, deveined and finely minced
- garlic clove, pressed
- teaspoons butter, room temperature
- 1 ¼ cups cream of onion soup
- Sea salt and ground black pepper, to taste.

Directions:

1. Melt the butter in a saucepan over a moderate flame. Then, sear the sausages until no longer pink about 9 minutes. Reserve.
2. In the same saucepan, cook the green onions, pepper, and garlic until they've softened.
3. Add in the spaghetti squash, salt, black pepper and cream of onion soup; bring to a boil.
4. Reduce the heat to medium-low and fold in the cream; let it simmer until the sauce has reduced slightly or about 7 minutes. Add in the reserved sausage and gently stir to combine.

113. Chicken Fajitas with Peppers and Cheese

Servings: 4

Prep + cook time: 15 minutes

Ingredients:

- 1 Habanero pepper, deveined and chopped
- 4 banana peppers, deveined and chopped
- 1 teaspoon Mexican seasoning blend
- tablespoon avocado oil
- garlic cloves, minced
- 1 cup onions, chopped
- 1-pound chicken, ground
- 1/3 cup dry sherry
- Salt and black pepper, to taste

- 1/2 cup Coria cheese, shredded

Directions:

1. In a skillet, heat the avocado oil over a moderate flame.
2. Sauté the garlic, onions, and peppers until they are tender and aromatic or about 5 minutes.
3. Fold in the ground chicken and continue to cook until the juices run clear.
4. Add in the dry sherry, Mexican seasonings, salt, and pepper.
5. Continue to cook for 5 to 6 minutes more or until cooked through.

114. Crispy Chicken Drumsticks

Servings: 4

Prep + cook time: 50 minutes

Ingredients

- 4 chicken drumsticks
- 1/4 teaspoon ground black pepper, or more to the taste
- 1 teaspoon dried basil
- 1 teaspoon dried oregano
- 1 tablespoon olive oil
- 1 teaspoon paprika
- Salt, to your liking

Directions

1. Pat dry the chicken drumsticks and rub them with olive oil, salt, black pepper, paprika, basil, and oregano.
2. Preheat your oven to 410 degrees F. Coat a baking pan with a piece of parchment paper.
3. Bake the chicken drumsticks until they are browned on all sides for 40 to 45 minutes.

115. Chicken Fillet with Brussels Sprouts

Servings: 4

Prep + cook time: 20 minutes

Ingredients:

- 3/4-pound chicken breasts, chopped into bite-sized pieces

- 1/2 teaspoon ancho Chile powder
- 1/2 teaspoon whole black peppercorns
- 1/2 cup onions, chopped
- cup vegetable broth
- tablespoons olive oil
- 1 ½ pound Brussels sprouts, trimmed and cut into halves
- 1/4 teaspoon garlic salt
- clove garlic, minced
- tablespoons port wine

Directions:

1. Heat 1 tablespoon of the oil in a frying pan over medium-high heat. Sauté the Brussels sprouts for about 3 minutes or until golden on all sides. Salt to taste and reserve.
2. Heat the remaining tablespoon of olive oil—Cook the garlic and chicken for about 3 minutes.
3. Add in the onions, vegetable broth, wine, Ancho Chile powder, and black peppercorns; bring to a boil. Then, reduce the temperature to simmer and continue to cook for 4 to 5 minutes longer.
4. Add the reserved Brussels sprouts back to the frying pan.

116. Chicken Breasts with Mustard Sauce

Servings: 4

Prep + cook time: 25 minutes

Ingredients:

- 1/4 cup vegetable broth
- Salt and pepper, to taste
- 1/2 cup fresh parsley,
- 1/2 cup heavy whipped cream
- 1/2 cup onions, chopped
- 2 garlic cloves, minced
- 1/4 cup Marsala wine
- 2 tablespoons brown mustard

- 1 tablespoon olive oil
- 1-pound chicken breasts, butterflied

Directions:
1. Heat the oil in a frying pan over a moderate flame. Cook the chicken breasts until no longer pink or about 6 minutes; season with salt and pepper to taste and reserve.
2. Cook the onion and garlic until it is fragrant or about 5 minutes. Add in the wine to scrape the bits that may be stuck to the bottom of your frying pan.
3. Pour in the broth and bring to boil. Fold in the double cream, mustard, and parsley.

117. Chinese-Style Cabbage with Turkey

Servings: 4

Prep + cook time: 45 minutes

Ingredients:
- pound turkey, ground
- slices smoked bacon, chopped
- 1 pound Chinese cabbage, finely chopped
- 1 tablespoon sesame oil
- 1/2 cup onions, chopped
- teaspoon ginger-garlic paste
- ripe tomatoes, chopped
- 1 teaspoon Five-spice powder
- Coarse salt and ground black pepper, to taste

Directions:
1. Heat the oil in a wok over a moderate flame. Cook the onions until tender and translucent.
2. Now, add in the remaining ingredients and bring to a boil. Reduce the temperature to medium-low and partially cover.
3. Reduce the heat to medium-low and cook an additional 30 minutes, crumbling the turkey and bacon with a fork.

118. Easy Turkey Meatballs

Servings: 4

Prep + cook time: 25 minutes

Ingredients:

For the Meatballs:

- 1/3 cup Colby cheese, freshly grated
- 3/4-pound ground turkey
- 1/3 teaspoon Five-spice powder
- 1 egg

For the Sauce:

- 1/3 cups water
- 1/3 cup champagne vinegar
- tablespoons soy sauce
- 1/2 cup Swerve
- 1/2 cup tomato sauce, no sugar added
- 1/2 teaspoon paprika 1/3 teaspoon guar gum

Directions:

1. Thoroughly combine all ingredients for the meatballs. Roll the mixture into balls and sear them until browned on all sides.
2. In a saucepan, mix all of the sauce ingredients and cook until the sauce has thickened, whisking continuously.
3. Fold the meatballs into the sauce and continue to cook, partially covered, for about 10 minutes.

119. Chicken with Mediterranean Sauce

Servings: 6

Prep + cook time: 15 minutes

Ingredients:

- 1 stick butter
- ½ pounds of chicken breasts
- teaspoons red wine vinegar
- ½ tablespoons olive oil
- 1/3 cup fresh Italian parsley, chopped
- tablespoon green garlic, finely minced
- 2 tablespoons red onions, finely minced Flaky sea salt and ground black pepper, to

taste

Directions:

1. In a cast-iron skillet, heat the oil over a moderate flame. Sear the chicken for 10 to 12 minutes or until no longer pink. Season with salt and black pepper.
2. Add in the melted butter and continue to cook until heated through. Stir in the green garlic, onion, and Italian parsley; let it cook for 3 to 4 minutes more.
3. Stir in the red wine vinegar and remove from heat.

120. Easy Roasted Turkey Drumsticks

Servings: 4

Prep + cook time: 1 hour 40 minutes

Ingredients:

- 2 turkey drumsticks
- 1 ½ tablespoon sesame oil 1 tablespoon poultry seasoning
- For the Sauce:
- 1-ounce Cottage cheese
- 1-ounce full-fat sour cream
- small-sized avocado, pitted and mashed
- tablespoons fresh parsley, finely chopped
- 1 teaspoon fresh lemon juice
- 1/3 teaspoon sea salt

Directions:

1. Pat the turkey drumsticks dry and sprinkle them with the poultry seasoning.
2. Brush a baking pan with the sesame oil.
3. Place the turkey drumsticks on the baking pan.
4. Roast in the preheated oven at 350 degrees F for about 1 hour 30 minutes, rotating the pan halfway through the cooking time.
5. In the meantime, make the sauce by whisking all the sauce ingredients.

121. Herbed Chicken Breasts

Servings: 8

Prep + cook time: 40 minutes

Ingredients:

- 4 chicken breasts, skinless and boneless
- 1 Italian pepper, deveined and thinly sliced
- 10 black olives, pitted
- ½ cups vegetable broth
- garlic cloves, pressed
- 2 tablespoons olive oil
- 1 tablespoon Old Sub Sailor
- Salt, to taste

Directions:

1. Rub the chicken with the garlic and Old Sub Sailor; salt to taste. Heat the oil in a frying pan over moderately high heat.
2. Sear the chicken until it is browned on all sides, about 5 minutes.
3. Add in the pepper, olives, and vegetable broth and bring it to boil. Reduce the heat simmer and continue to cook, partially covered, for 30 to 35 minutes.

122. Cheese and Prosciutto Chicken Roulade

Servings: 2

Prep + cook time: 35 minutes

Ingredients:

- 1/2 cup Ricotta cheese
- 4 slices of prosciutto
- 1-pound chicken fillet
- 1 tablespoon fresh coriander, chopped
- Salt and ground black pepper, to taste pepper
- 1 teaspoon cayenne pepper

Directions:

1. Season the chicken fillet with salt and pepper. Spread the Ricotta cheese over the chicken fillet; sprinkle with the fresh coriander.
2. Roll up and cut into 4 pieces. Wrap each piece with one slice of prosciutto; secure with kitchen twine.
3. Place the wrapped chicken in a parchment-lined baking pan. Now, bake in the preheated oven at 385 degrees F for about 30 minutes.

123. Boozy Glazed Chicken

Servings: 4

Prep + cook time: 60 minutes

Ingredients:

- 2 pounds' chicken roomettes
- 2 tablespoons ghee, at room temperature
- Sea salt and ground black pepper, to taste
- teaspoon Mediterranean seasoning mix
- vine-ripened tomatoes, pureed
- 3/4 cup rum
- tablespoons coconut aminos
- A few drops of liquid Stevia
- 1 teaspoon Chile peppers, minced
- 1 tablespoon minced fresh ginger
- teaspoon ground cardamom
- 2 tablespoons fresh lemon juice, plus wedges for serving

Directions:

1. Toss the chicken with the melted ghee, salt, black pepper, and Mediterranean seasoning mix until well coated on all sides.
2. In another bowl, thoroughly combine the pureed tomato puree, rum, coconut aminos, Stevia, Chile peppers, ginger, cardamom, and lemon juice.
3. Pour the tomato mixture over the chicken drumettes; let it marinate for 2 hours. Bake in the preheated oven at 410 degrees F for about 45 minutes.
4. Add in the reserved marinade and place under the preheated grill for 10 minutes.

124. Festive Turkey Rouladen

Servings: 5

Prep + cook time: 30 minutes

Ingredients

- 2 pounds' turkey fillet, marinated and cut into 10 pieces
- 10 strips prosciutto

- 1/2 teaspoon chili powder
- 1 teaspoon marjoram
- sprig rosemary, finely chopped
- tablespoons dry white wine
- 1 teaspoon garlic, finely minced
- 1 ½ tablespoons butter, room temperature
- 1 tablespoon Dijon mustard
- Sea salt and freshly ground black pepper, to your liking

Directions:

1. Start by preheating your oven to 430 degrees F.
2. Pat the turkey dry and cook in hot butter for about 3 minutes per side. Add in the mustard, chili powder, marjoram, rosemary, wine, and garlic.
3. Continue to cook for 2 minutes more. Wrap each turkey piece into one prosciutto strip and secure it with toothpicks.
4. Roast in the preheated oven for about 30 minutes.

125. Pan-Fried Chorizo Sausage

Servings: 4

Prep + cook time: 20 minutes

Ingredients:

- 16 ounces smoked turkey chorizo
- 1 ½ cups Asiago cheese, grated
- 1 teaspoon oregano
- 1 teaspoon basil
- 1 cup tomato puree
- 4 scallion stalks, chopped
- 1 teaspoon garlic paste
- Sea salt and ground black pepper, to taste
- 1 tablespoon dry sherry
- tablespoon extra-virgin olive oil
- tablespoons fresh coriander, roughly chopped

Directions:

1. Heat the oil in a frying pan over moderately high heat. Now, brown the turkey chorizo, crumbling with a fork for about 5 minutes.
2. Add in the other ingredients, except for cheese; continue to cook for 10 minutes more or until cooked through.

126. Chinese Bok Choy and Turkey Soup

Servings: 8

Prep + cook time: 40 minutes

Ingredients:

- 1/2-pound baby Bok choy, sliced into quarters lengthwise
- 2 pounds' turkey carcass
- 1 tablespoon olive oil
- 1/2 cup leeks, chopped
- celery rib, chopped
- carrots, sliced
- 6 cups turkey stock
- Himalayan salt and black pepper, to taste

Directions:

1. In a heavy-bottomed pot, heat the olive oil until sizzling.
2. Once hot, sauté the celery, carrots, leek, and Bok choy for about 6 minutes.
3. Add the salt, pepper, turkey, and stock; bring to a boil.
4. Turn the heat to simmer. Continue to cook, partially covered, for about 35 minutes.

127. Italian-Style Turkey Wings

Servings: 6

Prep + cook time: 60 minutes

Ingredients:

- 2 tablespoons sesame oil
- 1-pound turkey wings
- 1/2 cup marinara sauce
- tablespoon Italian herb mix
- tablespoons balsamic vinegar

- 1 teaspoon garlic, minced
- Salt and black pepper, to taste

Directions:

1. Place the turkey wings, Italian herb mix, balsamic vinegar, and garlic in a ceramic dish. Cover and let it marinate for 2 to 3 hours in your refrigerator. Rub the sesame oil over turkey wings.
2. Grill the turkey wings on the preheated grill for about 1 hour, basting with the reserved marinade. Sprinkle with salt and black pepper to taste.

128. Easy Chicken Tacos

Servings: 4

Prep + cook time: 20 minutes

Ingredients:

- 1-pound ground chicken
- 1 ½ cups Mexican cheese blend
- tablespoon Mexican seasoning blend
- teaspoons butter, room temperature
- 2 small-sized shallots, peeled and finely chopped
- 1 clove garlic, minced
- cup tomato puree
- 1/2 cup salsa
- slices bacon, chopped

Directions:

1. Melt the butter in a saucepan over a moderately high flame. Now, cook the shallots until tender and fragrant.
2. Then, sauté the garlic, chicken, and bacon for about 5 minutes, stirring continuously and crumbling with a fork. Add the in Mexican seasoning blend.
3. Fold in the tomato puree and salsa; continue to simmer for 5 to 7 minutes over medium-low heat; reserve.
4. Line a baking pan with wax paper. Place 4 piles of the shredded cheese on the baking pan and gently press them down with a wide spatula to make "taco shells."
5. Bake in the preheated oven at 365 degrees F for 6 to 7 minutes or until melted. Allow these taco shells to cool for about 10 minutes.

DESSERT

129. Greek-Style Cheesecake

Servings: 6

Prep + cook time: 1 hour 35 minutes

Ingredients:

- 2 cups almond meal
- 6 tablespoons butter, melted
- 1/2 teaspoon cinnamon
- 2 tablespoons Greek-style yogurt
- 10 ounces' cream cheese softened
- 2 cups confectioner's Swerve
- 2 eggs

Directions:

1. Mix the almond meal, butter, and cinnamon until well blended.
2. Press the mixture into a parchment-lined baking pan.
3. Then, whip the Greek-style yogurt, cream cheese, and confectioner's Swerve until well combined. Fold in the eggs, one at the time, and mix well after each addition.
4. Pour the filling over the crust in the baking pan. Bake in the preheated oven at 330 degrees F for about 30 minutes.
5. Run a sharp paring knife between the cheesecake and the baking pan and allow it to sit on the counter for 1 hour.
6. Cover loosely with plastic wrap and refrigerate overnight. Serve well-chilled and enjoy!

130. Caramel Chocolate Pudding

Servings: 3

Prep + cook time: 1 hour 15 minutes

Ingredients:

- 2 ounces' cream cheese, at room temperature
- 1/2 cup double cream
- 1 teaspoon caramel extract

- 4 tablespoons cocoa powder, unsweetened
- 1/2 cup Swerve
- A pinch of salt
- A pinch of grated nutmeg

Directions:

1. In a large bowl, whip the cream cheese and
2. double cream until firm peaks form.
3. Fold in the caramel extract, cocoa powder, Swerve, salt, and nutmeg. Blend until well mixed.
4. Cover the bowl with a lid and refrigerate at least 1 hour. Bon appétit!

131. Old-Fashioned Penuche Bars

Servings: 10

Prep + cook time: 45 minutes

Ingredients:

- 1/2 stick butter
- 2 tablespoons tahini (sesame paste)
- 1/2 cup almond butter
- teaspoon Stevia
- ounces baker's chocolate, sugar-free
- A pinch of salt
- A pinch of grated nutmeg
- 1/2 teaspoon cinnamon powder

Directions:

1. Microwave the butter for 30 to 35 seconds. Fold in the tahini, almond butter, Stevia, and chocolate.
2. Sprinkle with salt, nutmeg, and cinnamon; whisk to combine well. Scrape the mixture into a parchment-lined baking tray.
3. Transfer to the freezer for 40 minutes. Cut into bars and enjoy!

132. Easiest Keto Cheesecake Ever

Servings: 6

Prep + cook time: 35 minutes

Ingredients:

- 3/4 cup coconut flour
- 1/3 cup butter, at room temperature
- 16 ounces' cream cheese, at room temperature
- 6 ounces' sour cream
- 1/2 cup Erythritol

Directions:

1. To make the crust, thoroughly combine the coconut flour with butter. Scrape the coating into the bottom of a lightly greased baking pan; transfer the pan to your refrigerator.
2. Then, make the filling by mixing the cream cheese, sour cream, and Erythritol. Pour the mixture over the prepared crust.
3. Bake in the preheated oven at 450 degrees F for 10 minutes; reduce temperature to 360 degrees F and bake an additional 20 minutes.
4. Serve well chilled and enjoy!

133. Chocolate Pudding

Servings: 1

Prep + cook time: 50 minutes

Ingredients:

- 3 tbsp. chia seeds
- 1 cup unsweetened almond milk
- 1 scoop cocoa powder
- ¼ cup fresh raspberries
- ½ tsp honey

Directions:

1. Mix all of the ingredients in a large bowl.
2. Let rest for 15 minutes but stir halfway through.
3. Stir again and refrigerate for 30 minutes. Garnish with raspberries.
4. Serve!

134. Cranberry Cream Surprise

Servings: 2

Prep + cook time: 30 minutes

Ingredients:

- cup mashed cranberries
- ½ cup Confectioner's Style Swerve
- tsp natural cherry flavoring
- 2 tsp natural rum flavoring 1 cup organic heavy cream

Directions:

1. Combine the mashed cranberries, sweetener, cherry, and rum flavorings.
2. Cover and refrigerate for 20 minutes.
3. Whip the heavy cream until soft peaks form.
4. Layer the whipped cream and cranberry mixture.
5. Top with fresh cranberries, mint leaves or grated dark chocolate.
6. Serve!

135. Coconut Dream

Servings: 2

Prep + cook time: 1+ day

Ingredients:

- 1 can unsweetened coconut milk
- Berries of choice
- Dark chocolate

Directions:

1. Refrigerate the coconut milk for 24 hours.
2. Remove it from your refrigerator and whip for 2-3 minutes.
3. Fold in the berries.
4. Season with the chocolate shavings.
5. Serve!

136 Keto Sorbet

Servings: 2

Prep + cook time: 25 minutes

Ingredients:

- 10 tablespoons Lemon
- 1 cup frozen blackberries
- 1 cup frozen raspberries
- 1 tablespoon of Stevia
- Fat water [you can use regularly filtered, but fat water is better]

Directions:

1. Place lemon, blackberries, raspberries, stevia and water in a blender
2. Blend till smooth
3. Keep in the freezer to harden

137. White Chocolate Berry Cheesecake

Servings: 4

Prep + cook time: 10 minutes **Ingredients:**

- 8 oz. cream cheese, softened
- 2 oz. heavy cream
- ½ tsp Splenda
- 1 tsp raspberries
- 1 tbsp. Da Vinci Sugar-Free syrup, white chocolate flavor

Directions

1. Whip together the ingredients to a thick consistency.
2. Divide into cups.
3. Refrigerate.
4. Serve!

138. Coconut Pillow

Servings: 4

Prep + cook time: 1-2 days **Ingredients:**

- 1 can unsweetened coconut milk
- Berries of choice
- Dark chocolate

Directions:

1. Refrigerate the coconut milk for 24 hours.
2. Remove it from your refrigerator and whip for 2-3 minutes.
3. Fold in the berries.
4. Season with the chocolate shavings.
5. Serve!

139. Coffee Surprise

Servings: 1

Prep + cook time: 5 minutes **Ingredients:**
- 2 heaped tbsp. flaxseed, ground
- 100ml cooking cream 35% fat
- ½ tsp cocoa powder, dark and unsweetened
- 1 tbsp. goji berries Freshly brewed coffee

Directions:
1. Mix the flaxseeds, cream, and cocoa and coffee.
2. Season with goji berries.
3. Serve!

140. Chocolate Cheesecake

Servings: 4

Prep + cook time: 60 minutes

Ingredients:
- 4 oz. Cream cheese
- ½ oz. heavy cream
- 1 tsp Stevia Glycerite
- 1 tsp Splenda
- 1 oz. Enjoy Life mini chocolate chips

Directions:
1. Combine all the ingredients except the chocolate to a thick consistency.
2. Fold in the chocolate chips. Refrigerate in serving cups.
3. Serve!

141. Almond Crusty

Servings: 3

Prep + cook time: 60 minutes

Ingredients:

- 2 cups keto almond flour
- 4 tsp melted butter
- 2 large eggs
- ½ tsp salt

Directions:

1. Mix the almond flour and butter.
2. Add in the eggs and salt and combine well to form a dough ball.
3. Place the dough between two pieces of parchment paper. Roll out to 10" by 16" and ¼ inch thick.
4. Serve!

142. Cheesecake Cups

Servings: 1

Prep + cook time: 10 minutes

Ingredients:

- 8 oz. cream cheese, softened
- 2 oz. heavy cream
- 1 tsp Stevia Glycerite
- 1 tsp Splenda
- 1 tsp vanilla flavoring (Frontier Organic)

Directions:

1. Combine all the ingredients.
2. Whip until a pudding consistency is achieved.
3. Divide into cups.
   1. Refrigerate until served!

143. Strawberry Shake

Servings: 1

Prep + cook time: 5 minutes

Ingredients:

- 3/4 cup coconut milk (from the carton)
- ¼ cup heavy cream
- 7 ice cubes
- 2 tbsp. sugar-free strawberry Torani syrup
- ¼ tsp Xanthan Gum

<u>Directions:</u>

2. Combine all the ingredients into a blender.
3. Blend for 1-2 minutes.
4. Serve!

SOUP

144. Cream of Red Bell Pepper Soup

Servings: 4

Prep + cook time: 30 minutes

Ingredients

- 2 ½ pounds of red bell peppers
- 4 tablespoons of coconut oil, melted
- 2 shallots, finely chopped
- medium garlic cloves, peeled and minced
- cups of homemade low-sodium vegetable stock
- 2 teaspoons of red wine vinegar
- ½ teaspoon of cayenne pepper
- 1 teaspoon of fine sea salt
- 1 teaspoon of freshly cracked black pepper
- ½ cup of heavy cream

Directions

1. Press the "Sauté" function on your Instant Pot and add the coconut oil. Once hot, add the bell peppers, shallots, and garlic cloves. Sauté until softened, stirring occasionally.
2. Add the remaining ingredients except for the heavy cream.
3. Lock the lid and cook at high pressure for 3 minutes. When the cooking is done, quickly release the tension and carefully remove the cover. Use an immersion blender to blend the soup until smooth. Stir in the heavy cream and adjust the seasoning if necessary.
4. Serve and enjoy!

145. Stuffed Pepper Soup

Servings: 6

Prep + cook time: 35 minutes

Ingredients:

- 1 pound of lean ground beef 2 tablespoons of coconut oil
- small onion, finely chopped

- large red bell peppers, seeds removed and chopped
- 1 (28-ounce) can of diced tomatoes
- (14.5-ounce) can of tomato sauce
- cups of homemade low-sodium chicken stock
- 2 cups of cauliflower rice
- 1 teaspoon of garlic powder
- 1 teaspoon of fine sea salt
- 1 teaspoon of freshly cracked black pepper

Directions.

1. Press the "Sauté" function on your Instant Pot and add the coconut oil, ground beef, bell peppers, and onions. Cook until the meat has browned and vegetables have softened, stirring frequently.
2. Add the remaining ingredients and stir until well combined.
3. Lock the lid and cook at high pressure for 15 minutes.
4. When the cooking is done, naturally release the pressure and carefully remove the lid.
5. Stir the soup again and adjust the seasoning if necessary. Serve and enjoy!

146. Shiitake Mushroom and Asparagus Soup

Servings: 4

Prep + cook time: 35 minutes

Ingredients:

- 1 pound of asparagus, trimmed and cut into bite-sized pieces
- 1 pound of shiitake mushrooms, sliced
- 4 cups of baby spinach
- 4 tablespoons of coconut oil, melted
- 4 cups of homemade low-sodium chicken or vegetable stock
- 1 bay leaf
- 1 cup of heavy cream (more as needed)
- ¼ cup of fresh parsley, finely chopped
- 1 lemon, juiced
- 1 teaspoon of fine sea salt

- 1 teaspoon of freshly cracked black pepper

Directions:

1. Press the "Sauté" setting on your Instant Pot and add the coconut oil. Once hot, add the onions and garlic cloves. Sauté until translucent, stirring frequently.
2. Add the chopped mushrooms and asparagus. Saute for 3 minutes or until softened, stirring frequently.
3. Stir in the remaining ingredients except for the heavy cream. Lock the lid and cook at high pressure for 15 minutes. When the cooking is done, allow for a full original release pressure method and carefully remove the cover.
4. Stir in the heavy cream and adjust the seasoning if necessary.
5. Serve and enjoy!

147. Green Chile Chicken Soup

Servings: 6

Prep + cook time: 40 minutes

Ingredients:

- 3 boneless, skinless chicken breasts
- red bell pepper, seeds removed and chopped
- tablespoons of coconut oil, melted
- 1 onion, finely chopped
- celery stalks, chopped
- garlic cloves, peeled and minced
- 4 cups of homemade low-sodium chicken stock
- (16-ounce) jar of salsa verde
- (4-ounce) cans of diced green chiles, undrained
- 1 tablespoon of ground cumin
- 1 tablespoon of oregano
- 1 teaspoon of fine sea salt
- 1 teaspoon of freshly cracked black pepper
- ¼ cup of fresh cilantro, finely chopped

Directions:

1. Press the "Sauté" function on your Instant Pot and add the coconut oil. Once hot, add the chicken breasts and sear on both sides until brown.

2. Gently stir in the remaining ingredients. Lock the lid and cook at high pressure for 15 minutes. When the cooking is done, allow for a full natural release method. Carefully remove the cover.
3. Transfer the chicken to a cutting board and shred using two forks. Stir the shredded chicken into the soup and adjust the seasoning if necessary. Serve and enjoy!

148. Egg Drop Soup

Servings: 4

Prep + cook time: 15 minutes

Ingredients:

- cups of homemade low-sodium chicken stock
- large organic eggs, beaten
- 3 fresh scallions, chopped
- 1 teaspoon of toasted sesame oil
- 1 tablespoon of fresh ginger, minced
- 1 teaspoon of garlic powder
- 1 teaspoon of fine sea salt
- 1 teaspoon of freshly cracked black pepper 1 teaspoon of arrowroot powder or xanthan gum
- A drop of yellow food coloring.

Directions:

1. Add all the ingredients inside your Instant Pot except for the arrowroot powder and give a good stir.
2. Lock the lid and cook at high pressure for 3 minutes. When the cooking is done, naturally release the tension and carefully remove the cover. Stir in the yellow food coloring and arrowroot powder.
3. Cook until the liquid thickens, stirring occasionally.
4. Serve and enjoy!

149. Vegetable Cream Soup

Servings: 6

Prep + cook time: 35 minutes

Ingredients:

- 1 pound of cauliflower florets

- 1 pound of broccoli florets
- bunch of kale or spinach, roughly chopped
- celery ribs, chopped
- 4 tablespoons of extra-virgin olive oil
- 2 medium garlic cloves, minced
- 1 medium red onion, roughly chopped
- 10 cups of homemade low-sodium vegetable stock
- 1 cup of heavy cream (more as needed)
- 1 teaspoon of fine sea salt
- 1 tablespoon of Dijon mustard
- 1 tablespoon of fresh parsley, finely chopped

Directions:

1. Press the "Sauté" function on your Instant Pot and add the olive oil. Once hot, add the onions and garlic cloves. Sauté until translucent, stirring frequently.
2. Add the celery, cauliflower florets, and broccoli florets. Cook for 2 minutes, stirring frequently.
3. Add the remaining ingredients except for the heavy cream inside your Instant Pot. Lock the lid and cook at high pressure for 15 minutes. When the cooking is done, naturally release the tension and carefully remove the cover.
4. Use an immersion blender to puree the soup until smooth. Gently stir in the heavy cream and adjust the seasoning if necessary. Serve and enjoy!

150. Beef and Mushroom Soup

Servings: 4

Prep + cook time: 25 minutes

Ingredients:

- 1 pound of ground beef
- a pound of mushrooms, sliced
- tablespoons of coconut oil, melted
- 1 small onion, finely chopped
- 4 garlic cloves, peeled and minced
- 1 teaspoon of fine sea salt
- 1 teaspoon of freshly cracked black pepper 2 cups of homemade low-sodium beef

broth

Directions:

1. Press the "Sauté" function on your Instant Pot and add the coconut oil. Once the coconut oil is hot, add the ground beef, onions, and garlic. Cook until the brown, stirring occasionally. Add the remaining ingredients and lock the lid. Cook at high pressure for 12 minutes. When the cooking is done, naturally release the tension and carefully remove the cover. Stir the soup again and adjust the seasoning if necessary. Serve and enjoy!

151. Columbian Creamy Avocado Soup

Servings: 4

Prep + cook time: 20 minutes **Ingredients:**

- 4 tablespoons of avocado oil
- 1 shallot, finely chopped
- 1 garlic clove, minced
- 4 cups of homemade low-sodium chicken stock
- 4 medium ripe avocados, peeled and mashed
- tablespoon of freshly squeezed lime juice
- cups of heavy cream
- 1 teaspoon of fine sea salt
- 1 teaspoon of freshly cracked black pepper
- ¼ cup of fresh cilantro, chopped

Directions

2. Press the "Sauté" setting on your Instant Pot and add the avocado oil. Once hot, add the chopped shallots and minced garlic. Sauté for 3 minutes, stirring frequently.

3. Add the chicken stock, lime juice, avocados, and seasonings. Lock the lid and cook at high pressure for 3 minutes. When the cooking is done, naturally release the tension and remove the cover.

4. Use an immersion blender to puree the soup until smooth. Stir in the heavy cream and fresh cilantro. Serve and enjoy!

152. Chicken Avocado Soup

Servings: 4

Prep + cook time: 20 minutes

Ingredients:

- 2 pounds of boneless, skinless chicken thighs
- 1 green onion, finely chopped
- 1 jalapeno pepper, seeds remove and chopped
- 4 cups of homemade low-sodium chicken stock
- 2 tablespoons of extra-virgin olive oil
- 6 garlic cloves, peeled and minced
- 2 teaspoons of ground cumin
- ½ cup of fresh cilantro, chopped
- 2 limes, freshly squeezed juice
- large avocados, pitted, peeled and mashed

Directions:

1. Press the "Sauté" setting on your Instant Pot and add the olive oil. Once hot, add the chicken thighs and sear for 4 minutes per side or until brown.
2. Add the remaining ingredients except for the heavy cream and avocados. Lock the lid and cook at high pressure for 8 minutes. When the cooking is done, quickly release the tension and remove the cover.
3. Transfer the chicken to a cutting board and shred using two forks.
4. Use an immersion blender to blend the contents inside your Instant Pot. Stir in the mashed avocados, heavy cream, and shredded chicken. Serve and enjoy!

153. Hot Avocado Curry with Shrimp

Servings: 2

Prep + cook time: 20 minutes

Ingredients:

- ½ pound of shrimp, peeled and deveined
- 2 cups of homemade low-sodium chicken stock
- (14-ounce) can of coconut milk
- avocados, ripe, pitted, peeled and cut into quarters
- ½ teaspoon of cayenne pepper
- 1 teaspoon of fine sea salt
- 1 tablespoon of freshly squeezed lime juice

Directions:

1. In a blender, add all the ingredients except for the shrimp. Blend until smooth and creamy.
2. Pour in the mixture inside your Instant Pot along with the shrimp.
3. Lock the lid and cook at high pressure for 3 minutes. When the cooking is done, quickly release the tension and remove the cover. Adjust the seasoning if necessary. Serve and enjoy!

154. Lamb and Herb Bone Broth

Servings: 8

Prep + cook time: 1 hour 30 minutes

Ingredients:

- 1 pound of lamb bones
- 1 large onion, quartered
- 3 medium carrots, cut into chunks
- celery stalks, roughly chopped
- whole garlic cloves
- fresh sprigs of rosemary
- fresh sprigs of thyme
- 8 cups of water

Directions:

1. Add all the ingredients inside your Instant Pot. Lock the lid and cook at high pressure for 50 minutes. When the cooking is done, naturally release the tension and remove the cover.
2. Strain the liquid through a fine-mesh strainer. Transfer the cash to mason jars. Refrigerate and use as needed.

SNACKS

155. Stuffed Mini Peppers

Servings: 6

Prep + cook time: 25 minutes

Ingredients:

- 3/4-pound ground beef
- 1/2 cup onion, chopped
- 2 garlic cloves, minced
- 12 mini peppers, deveined
- 1/2 cup cheddar cheese, shredded

Directions:

1. Heat a lightly oiled sauté pan over a moderate flame.
2. Brown the ground beef for 3 to 4 minutes, crumbling with a fork.
3. Stir in the onions and garlic; continue to sauté an additional 2 minutes or until tender and aromatic.
4. Cook the peppers in boiling water until just tender or approximately 7 minutes.
5. Arrange the stuffed peppers on a tinfoil-lined baking pan. Divide the beef mixture among the peppers. Top with the shredded cheddar cheese.
6. Bake in the preheated oven at 360 degrees F for approximately 17 minutes. Serve at room temperature.
7. Bon appétit!

156. Homemade Wings in Spicy Tomato Sauce

Servings: 6

Prep + cook time: 50 minutes

Ingredients:

- 3 pounds' chicken wings
- Sea salt and ground black pepper, to taste
- 1/2 teaspoon paprika 1/2 teaspoon cayenne pepper
- Sauce:
- 2 vine-ripe tomatoes

- onion
- garlic cloves
- 1 teaspoon chili pepper

Directions:

1. Start by preheating your oven to 400 degrees F.
2. Set a wire rack inside a rimmed baking sheet. Season the chicken wings with salt, black pepper, paprika, and cayenne pepper. Bake the wings approximately 45 minutes or until the skin is crispy. To make the sauce, puree all ingredients in your food processor.

157. Oven-Baked Cheesy Zucchini Rounds

Servings: 6

Prep + cook time: 20 minutes

Ingredients:

- 2 tablespoons olive oil
- 2 eggs
- 1/2 teaspoon smoked paprika
- Sea salt and ground black pepper, to taste
- 2 pounds' zucchini, sliced into rounds
- 1/2 cup Romano cheese, shredded

Directions:

1. Begin by preheating an oven to 420 degrees F. Coat a rimmed baking sheet with a Silpat mat or parchment paper.
2. In a mixing bowl, whisk the olive oil with eggs. Add in the paprika, salt, and black pepper. Now, dip the zucchini slices into the egg mixture.
3. Top with the shredded Romano cheese.
4. Arrange the zucchini rounds on the baking sheet; bake for 15 minutes until they are golden. Serve at room temperature.

158. Holiday Prawn Sticks

Servings: 4

Prep + cook time: 15 minutes

Ingredients:

- 2 tablespoons olive oil
- 1-pound king prawns, deveined and cleaned
- Sea salt and ground black pepper, to taste
- 1 teaspoon garlic powder
- 1 tablespoon fresh sage, minced
- teaspoon fresh rosemary
- tablespoons fresh lime juice
- 2 tablespoons cilantro, chopped
- 2 bell peppers, diced
- 1 cup cherry tomatoes
- Bamboo skewers

Directions

1. Heat the olive oil in a wok over moderately high heat.
2. Now, cook the prawns until they have turned pink. Stir in the seasonings and cook an additional minute, stirring frequently.
3. Remove from the heat and toss with the lime juice and fresh cilantro. Tread the prawns onto bamboo skewers, alternating them with peppers and cherry tomatoes.
4. Serve on a serving platter.

159. Deviled Eggs with Peppers and Cheese

Servings: 10

Prep + cook time: 15 minutes

Ingredients:

- 10 eggs
- 1/4 cup sour cream
- 1/4 cup red roasted pepper, chopped
- 2 tablespoons olive oil
- 1 teaspoon stone-ground mustard
- 1 garlic clove, minced
- Sea salt, to taste
- 1 teaspoon red pepper flakes

Directions:

1. Arrange the eggs in a saucepan. Pour in water (1-inch above the eggs) and bring to a boil. Heat off and let it sit, covered, for 9 to 10 minutes.
2. When the eggs are cool enough to handle, peel away the shells; rinse the berries under running water. Separate egg whites and yolks.
3. Mix the egg yolks with the sour cream, roasted pepper, olive oil, mustard, garlic, and salt. Stuff the eggs, arrange on a beautiful serving platter, and garnish with red pepper flakes. Enjoy!

160. Ranch Chicken Wings

Servings: 4

Prep + cook time: 15 minutes **Ingredients:**

- 2 pounds' chicken wings, pat dry
- Nonstick cooking spray
- Sea salt and cayenne pepper, to taste
- Ranch Dressing:
- 1/4 cup sour cream
- 1/4 cup buttermilk
- 1/2 cup mayonnaise
- 1/2 teaspoon lemon juice
- 1 tablespoon fresh parsley, minced
- clove garlic, minced
- tablespoons onion, finely chopped
- 1/4 teaspoon dry mustard
- Sea salt and ground black pepper, to taste

Directions:

1. Start by preheating your oven to 420 degrees F.
2. Spritz the chicken wings with a cooking spray. Sprinkle the chicken wings with salt and cayenne pepper. Arrange the chicken wings on a parchment-lined baking pan.
3. Bake in the preheated oven for 50 minutes or until the wings are golden and crispy.
4. In the meantime, make the dressing by mixing all of the above ingredients. Serve with warm wings.

161. Colby Cheese-Stuffed Meatballs

Servings: 8

Prep + cook time: 25 minutes

Ingredients:

- 1/2-pound ground pork
- 1-pound ground turkey
- 1 garlic clove, minced
- 4 tablespoons pork rinds, crushed
- 2 tablespoons shallots, chopped
- 4 ounces' mozzarella string cheese, cubed
- 1 ripe tomato, pureed
- Salt and ground black pepper, to taste

Directions:

1. In a mixing bowl, thoroughly combine all ingredients except for the cheese. Shape the mixture into bite-sized balls.
2. Press 1 cheese cube into the center of each ball.
3. Place the meatballs on a parchment-lined baking sheet. Bake in the preheated oven at 350 degrees F for 18 to 25 minutes. Bon appétit!

162. Cheese and Artichoke Dip

Servings: 10

Prep + cook time: 25 minutes

Ingredients:

- 10 ounces canned artichoke hearts, drained and chopped
- 6 ounces' cream cheese
- 1/2 cup Greek-style yogurt
- 1/2 cup mayo 1/2 cup water
- 2 cloves garlic, minced
- 20 ounces Monterey-Jack cheese, shredded

Directions:

1. Start by preheating your oven to 350 degrees F.
2. Combine all of the ingredients, except for the Monterey-Jack cheese. Place the mixture in a lightly greased baking dish.

3. Top with the shredded Monterey-Jack cheese. Bake in the preheated oven for 17 to 22 minutes or until bubbly. Serve warm.

163. Italian Cheese Crisps

Servings: 4

Prep + cook time: 10 minutes

Ingredients:

- 1 cup sharp Cheddar cheese, grated
- 1/4 teaspoon ground black pepper
- 1/2 teaspoon cayenne pepper
- 1 teaspoon Italian seasoning

Directions:

1. Start by preheating an oven to 400 degrees F. Line a baking sheet with a parchment paper.
2. Mix all of the above ingredients until well combined.
3. Then, place tablespoon-sized heaps of the mixture onto the prepared baking sheet.
4. Bake at the preheated oven for 8 minutes, until the edges start to brown. Allow the cheese crisps to cool slightly; then, place them on paper towels to drain the excess fat. Enjoy!

164. Paprika Cheese Dipping Sauce

Servings: 10

Prep + cook time: 10 minutes

Ingredients:

- 4 ounces' feta cheese
- 1 cup Asiago cheese, shredded
- 1 cup double cream 1 tablespoon paprika

Directions:

1. Melt the cheese and cream in a saucepan over medium-low heat.
2. Transfer to a serving bowl and top with paprika.
3. Serve with fresh celery sticks if desired. Enjoy!

VEGETARIAN KETO RECIPES

165. Generous Green Bean Fries

Servings: 4

Prep + cook time: 12 minutes

Ingredients:

- 1 pound of fresh green beans, trimmed and washed 2/3 cups of finely grated parmesan cheese 1 large egg
- ½ teaspoon of sea salt (more to taste)
- ¼ teaspoon of freshly cracked black pepper (more to taste)
- ½ teaspoon of smoked or regular paprika Directions:

Directions:

1. Preheat your oven to 400 degrees Fahrenheit.
2. On a plate, add the grated Parmesan cheese, sea salt, black pepper, and paprika. Mix until well combined.
3. In a bowl, add the egg and whisk. For each green: Add the green beans to the egg bowl and remove any excess.
4. Then coat each green bean with the parmesan cheese mixture.
5. Place the green beans on a greased baking sheet and spread evenly.
6. Place inside your oven and bake for 10 minutes or until golden color. Enjoy!

166. Traditional Roasted Asparagus

Servings: 3

Prep + Cook Time: 20 minutes

Ingredients

- 1 large bunch of asparagus, trimmed
- 2 tablespoons of olive oil, coconut oil, or avocado oil
- Freshly squeezed juice from ½ medium-sized lemon
- 1 teaspoon of sea salt
- 1 teaspoon of freshly cracked black pepper
- 1 tablespoon of fresh oregano, finely chopped Directions:
- Preheat your oven to 425 degrees Fahrenheit. Line the asparagus on a lined baking

sheet.

- Sprinkle sea salt, black pepper, olive oil, lemon juice, and freshly chopped oregano over the asparagus. Toss until well coated. Place the baking sheet inside your oven and bake for 10 minutes.
- Divide the asparagus among containers and enjoy!

167. King-Style Roasted Bell Pepper Soup

Servings: 3

Prep + Cook Time: 25 minutes

Ingredients

- 4 red bell peppers, chopped
- 4 tablespoons of olive oil
- 4 garlic cloves, minced
- 1 large red onion, chopped
- ¼ cup of finely grated parmesan cheese
- 2 celery stalks, chopped
- 4 cups of homemade low-sodium vegetable broth
- 1 teaspoon of freshly cracked black pepper
- 1 cup of heavy cream
- 1 teaspoon of sea salt

Directions:

1. Preheat your oven to 400 degrees Fahrenheit.
2. In a large bowl, add the chopped red bell peppers with 2 tablespoons of olive oil. Stir until well coated together.
3. Transfer the red bell peppers to a baking sheet and place it inside your oven.
4. Bake the red bell peppers inside your oven for 8 to 10 minutes. Carefully remove from the oven and set aside.
5. Heat the remaining 2 tablespoons of olive oil in a large pot over medium-high heat.
6. Once hot, add the onion, garlic, and celery. Saute for 8 minutes, stirring occasionally.
7. Add the roasted red bell peppers and chicken stock. Bring to a boil.
8. Cover with a lid and reduce the heat. Allow simmering for 5 minutes.
9. Use an immersion blender to puree the soup until smooth. Season with sea salt and

black pepper.
10. Stir in the heavy cream and bring to a boil. One begins to boil, remove from the heat.
11. Ladle the soup into container bowls and sprinkle with parmesan cheese.
12. Serve and enjoy!

168. Tastes Like Heaven Garlic and Mustard Brussel Sprouts

Servings: 3

Prep + Cook Time: 30 minutes

Ingredients

- 1 pound of fresh Brussel sprouts, trimmed and halved
- 1 tablespoon of low-sodium coconut aminos
- 1 tablespoon of Dijon mustard
- 2 garlic cloves, finely minced
- 2 tablespoons of olive oil
- 1 teaspoon of sea salt
- 1 teaspoon of freshly cracked black pepper

Directions:

1. Preheat your oven to 400 degrees Fahrenheit.
2. In a large bowl, add the Brussel sprouts, coconut aminos, Dijon mustard, minced garlic, olive oil, sea salt, and black pepper. Stir until well coated together. Place the Brussel sprouts on a lined baking sheet.
3. Place the baking sheet inside your oven and bake for 20 minutes or until cooked through.
4. Transfer to containers and enjoy!

169. Rockstar Creamy Mashed Cauliflower

Servings: 3

Prep + Cook Time: 20 minutes

Ingredients

- 1 large cauliflower head, chopped
- ¼ cup of sour cream
- ¼ cup of heavy cream

- 4 tablespoons of feta cheese
- 4 tablespoons of black olives, pitted and sliced
- 1 teaspoon of sea salt
- 1 teaspoon of freshly cracked black pepper
- 1 tablespoon of fresh parsley, finely chopped

Directions:

1. In a medium-sized pot, add water and bring to a boil over medium-high heat. Add the chopped cauliflower and allow to boil for 10 minutes.
2. Once done, remove from the heat and drain.
3. Return the chopped cauliflower to the pot along with the sour cream, heavy cream, sea salt, and freshly cracked black pepper. Use an immersion blender to blend until smooth.
1. Stir in the black olives and feta cheese. Transfer to containers and serve!

170. Appetizing Kale Chips

Servings: 4

Prep + Cook Time: 10 minutes

Ingredients

- 1 large bunch of kale, washed and torn
- 1 teaspoon of crushed red pepper flakes
- 1 teaspoon of garlic powder
- ½ teaspoon of onion powder
- 1 teaspoon of sea salt
- 3 tablespoons of coconut oil or olive oil
- 2 tablespoons of finely grated parmesan cheese

Directions:

2. Preheat your oven to 350 degrees Fahrenheit.
3. Line a cookie sheet with parchment paper.
4. In a large bowl or plate, add the torn kale pieces and drizzle the coconut oil and seasonings. Gently stir until well combined. Place the kale on the cookie sheet and spread evenly.
5. Place the cookie sheet inside your oven and bake for 8 minutes or until crunchy. Transfer the kale chips to a bowl.

KEEPING TRACK OF YOUR KETO DIET

Keeping track of your Keto weight loss plan is something this is vital and will pass a long way towards your success.

The first factor that you have probably observed is that the eBook has already talked a little about monitoring what you are doing with measuring your ketones. This is something this is crucial, but there is such a whole lot greater to the diet than simply casting off carbs and increasing your protein and high fats content. This is alas an oversimplification of the food, but that's the wrong information, the good news is while you maintain track of the eating regimen you may be able to determine the relationships among the specific forms of food which you are ingesting and how it affects not just how you get into the nation of ketosis however how you feel while you eat these ingredients.

The aim of the food regimen is with a purpose to shed pounds and feel excellent, so in case you are losing weight. Still, you aren't feeling perfect, then something is inaccurate, and it wishes to be fixed so that it why monitoring what you are doing is so very important. Make sure which you are detailed for your monitoring of what you do, so that you may be sure that you have become the most from your Keto Diet. Focusing on matters just like the percent along with the foods you ate and what times is an excellent place to start.

Naturally, there are questions about a way to track your progress, but the good news is the techniques that can be out there for monitoring your progress come right down to repetition and being detailed. The more you can add, the higher you'll do. Now, earlier than we get into an extended discussion about the things to the song and a way to track them, what you need to understand is that there are a ton of apps out there to help you hold tune of your development on the Keto Diet and assist you in making sure that you aren't straying out of doors the traces with how you're running your sole ration.

The good news is that these apps can pass to your smartphone, and you could bring them around with you to have you ever in a better role for making sure that you are sticking with your food regimen. There are some matters which are vital to music, though, and they're signposts for how well you're doing on the Keto Diet.

Weight Loss

The most critical issue that you can track with the Keto Diet is your weight loss. This is the essential factor of the eating regimen and the remaining quit aim. There are several approaches that you may tune your weight loss, but the first component you want to do is get a scale. The excellent information is you do not wish to a level that does all sorts of such things as to measure frame fat and what now not, as a substitute, you may get a scale that will display your weight. These scales are relatively cheap and are at every unmarried primary store.

Once you've got your scale, the next aspect of doing is to weigh yourself. The key to considering your self is to do so every single day at the same time and under identical circumstances. The pleasant manner to track your weight is to weigh yourself in the morning while you wake up, but after you have long gone to the bathroom. This is when you are at your most correct weight due to the fact your body has gotten rid of the maximum of its excess weight.

Check Your Weight

There are numerous things to do here. You could file your weight at the app that you chose to music your progress on the Keto Diet, or you could maintain a chart. One factor this is virtually useful is the social promotion issue of how you are losing weight. Posting your weight each day on social media will get human beings that are on your lifestyles to rally around you and offer encouragement. It also facilitates you to live on the pinnacle of your game.

The remaining thing which you need is to be in a role in which you want to get out of the food plan. So maintaining the tune of your weight is especially important, due to the fact it guarantees which you are sticking with the weight-reduction plan and making sure the food plan is doing what you need it to do - maintaining you healthy and losing weight.

As you use the programs to track your weight, track other modifications as nicely. Take your measurements. What are your waist length and your chest-length? This is where lousy fat receives stored, so in case you recognize what your size is. You do your measurements every couple weeks, that is another way to offer yourself the effective reinforcement you need to make sure that you are doing what wishes to be completed to lose the burden and keep it off while getting on the Keto Diet.

Tracking Your Food

This is something else this is important - you've got to maintain track of what you devour with the Keto Diet. This matters because as you eat the food, you also are going to be trying out your stages of ketones for your frame. When you do a food diary, this is an exquisite manner to make sure that you are doing the proper ranges of calories in conjunction with the exclusive grams of food that you want to consume. There are so many various things to do with a food diary, but while you keep a food diary, what finally ends up going on is which you can correlate how you are feeling and your stages of ketones with what you are ingesting. This in flip makes your time at the Keto Diet that much more productive - you're able to lose weight with greater efficiency, and in turn that make it so that you can easily hold yourself faithful to the eating regimen. Having a meals journal is something this is genuinely smooth to do, and it's miles observed on many of the Keto Diet apps.

Tracking Your Ketones

The other component that human beings at the Keto Diet want to do is stay abreast of where their numbers are. Now in terms of testing yourself, doing stuff like taking a blood check is something which you should now not do every day because you'll not see a whole lot of variance. However, if you want to ensure that each day you're performing some bit higher, it's miles straightforward to use the equipment along with the breath analyzer and the urine strips. These gear make it so clean to check your tiers of ketones, see in case you are in ketosis, and at the give up of the day, ensure which you are doing what is essential to preserve yourself on this state together with the food which you are eating and the substances you are drinking.

That being said, the preliminary foray into ketosis isn't the whole issue, so that requires quite a few patience. With all of the different Keto Diet apps which can be obtainable, you may make sure to input the readings and some of the one of a kind devices are even capable of integrating with the apps, which makes them that much more ambitious on the subject of retaining tune of all the different things that you are doing.

The bottom line is that so long as you are getting the numbers that you want to look and that they're heading within the proper direction, you could rest assured that it will be quite simple to get to the factor where your body is burning your fats cells as an alternative of looking for the one of a kind glycogen stores - due to the fact the one's glycogen stores aren't there.

When it involves monitoring what you do, it's miles always better to be disciplined and vigilant together with your monitoring. This is the most straightforward manner to make sure that what you are doing is generating results. The worst aspect could be if you are attempting to maintain the music of stuff, but at the equal time, you aren't able to correlate the records with the outcomes.

The Keto Diet does require a large quantity of cohesion with all the distinct elements, and that is why this is not the very best of diets, but when you are maintaining tune of everything which you are doing, what finally ends up occurring is that the food regimen will become a rewarding endeavor and the signposts that you get from the tracking are matters that genuinely keep you engaged with the weight loss program and pushing yourself to more heights for weighing that you could lose alongside being that lots healthier. So, find a Keto Diet app that you like and get started right away with tracking all the different elements of the eating regimen.

NEGATIVE MOMENTS AND OVERCOMING THEM

It is not news that the keto diet has some undesirable side consequences. Despite its exceptional blessings, there are nevertheless a lot of things researchers don't know approximately each the benefits and side outcomes of keto weight loss program. It is pretty smooth to look at why the keto food regimen has gained over so many human beings seeking to gain from one in all its many benefits. Although the keto weight-reduction plan may be very tempting, it does have some acknowledged downsides. This is despite that inside a long time, there are lots of unknown consequences of keto food plans on the frame.

Keeping in step with all the guidelines and hints of the keto weight loss program can be hard for a protracted period. Many experts advise against preserving its restrictive recommendations. They propose that you may observe the weight loss plan while balancing the needs of your body with the purpose of you following the eating regimen. Cutting carbohydrates from your diet with the aid of taking much less than 50 grams in keeping with day for an extended period may be very annoying and taxing for anyone, and sticking to this for the long term could have many adverse outcomes on the frame. Below are some of the possible brief term outcomes of sticking to keto eating regimen:

When getting commenced on a keto eating regimen, you may limit your carb intake to between 20-30 grams per day. This is to permit your body to go into ketosis. This also can be finished via restricting your carb intake to underneath 50 according to day, though it depends on the sort of keto diet you comply with.

Limiting your carb consumption to as low as this will be very difficult for your body, in particular at first. Consuming an eating regimen wealthy in fat and coffee in carbs, you cast off many other foods such as maximum dairy, many results, entire grains, starchy greens, and legumes (basically all sugar) out of your meals. This can be difficult for your body and, once in a while, uncomfortable.

In the fast term, earlier than you begin seeing any benefit of sticking to the food regimen, you may experience the keto flu. The keto flu is a nasty side impact that happens due to the withdrawal of your frame from the use of glucose as its principal supply of power to the use of fats to generate the body's energy desires. Your structure makes use of this time to regulate to the keto eating regimen. Again, the precis of signs of keto flu include:

- Headache
- Fatigue
- Irritability
- Having problems focusing or mind fog
- Dizziness
- Lack of motivation
- Nausea
- Sugar craving
- Muscle cramps

Another foremost drawback to having keto flu is the amount of fluid and electrolyte loss from your body. Generally, the keto diet causes some multiplied diploma of fluid and electrolyte loss. However, during the primary few weeks of fixing to the food plan, you'll revel in a higher increased frequency of urination with loss of electrolytes. The loss of water and electrolyte is the motive of most of the awful signs of keto flu.

How to Deal with Keto Flu

The symptoms of keto flu generally tend to disappear with time, as your body adapts to the food plan. However, you may assist yourself cope higher with the signs and symptoms by using those remedies:

Increasing intake of salt and water

Loss of salt is primarily responsible for the lack of water. So, by growing your intake of salt and water, you could significantly lessen the signs and symptoms of keto flu or even cast off them.

Eat extra fats

This may sound a little funny. However, in case you retain feeling some aspect results of the keto flu even after growing your consumption of water and electrolyte, you have to try increasing your fat intake. When you abruptly restrict your intake of carbs without a boom in fat consumption, you may place your frame in a consistent country of starving, making you sense miserable, worn-out, and hungry. A proper keto meal ought to have enough fats, so you don't move hungry after lunch. You need to be capable of the pass without consuming for several hours while having sufficient energy to hold you are going

Reduce your physical activity

Although you may feel very lively with your change to the keto lifestyle, doing an excessive amount of at the early levels of keto food regimen should worsen the symptoms of keto flu. You need to keep off those worrying physical activities probably.

Another way to prepare for the keto flu is by mentally making ready yourself for the food plan. You need to realize that a keto diet is the most effective temporary and gained be the norm for long.

Long Term Impact of Keto Diet Plan

Limiting your consumption to approximately 50 grams in step with day, or even much less, means which you are keeping away from many unhealthy foods like delicate sugar and white bread. However, it also the method you're saying goodbye to several fines and wholesome foods not appropriate to keto weight loss program because they could serve as resources of carbohydrate. According to some researches, the restrictive nature of the keto weight loss program prevents you from ingesting masses of critical fruits and vegetables, which might be ordinarily wholesome for the frame. Fruits and veggies are wealthy in vitamins, antioxidants, and minerals; so, removing means, you won't be getting enough nutrients.

Cutting returned on the carbs approach, you are also significantly limiting the amount of fiber you get due to the fact entire grains contain one of the most significant sources of fiber. Lack of enough fiber within the weight-reduction plan can cause digestion issues such as diarrhea and constipation. It additionally results in weight gain, bloating, and now and again, growth LDL cholesterol and blood pressure.

It may also have an effect on your athletic performance

Keto additionally has a significant impact on your athletic performance. At first, you may find it tough to carry out your exercise routines, particularly high- intensity workouts, because the frame is on ketosis limits the potential of the structure to perform at an ideal level.

Relaxing the policies can cause weight regain

Keto weight-reduction plan can be so strict; as a result, there are many variations to the same old keto weight loss program. Also, there are many versions for every level of the diet. For the primary stage, which covers the first 3 months, it includes going with a keto weight loss program containing minimal carb and having a few cheat days. It involves you retaining an eye fixed for three amounts of fats and carbs consumption to hold your body in ketosis. Sometimes, many people can tweak their keto diet to a higher comfortable version, which involves little tracking of carbs. This is on occasion called lazy keto or keto cycling. The drawback of doing this is that it leaves space to regain weight.

Keto remains an excellent jump-start toward weight loss, but for many human beings, they can't stick to it for long. Many instances, people have a tendency to go into ketosis to lose weight, and while they arrive out, they fall lower back into their horrific habits and gain weight. Sometimes, they hold ongoing lower back and forth, dropping weight and gaining it again. This kind of weight fluctuations can be irritating and are related to an expanded threat of early death.

Losing weight with keto food plan additionally manner dropping a few muscle mass, and because keto weight loss plan is a high-fat containing diet, while you benefit weight again, you are more likely to gain even higher fat than muscle. This will result in an even slower fee of metabolism for you. This has quite a few negative results for your frame's metabolism and affects your capability to lose weight in the future.

It may also harm blood vessels

Ketogenic weight-reduction plan has masses of blessings, especially when it comes to your cardiovascular health. According to some studies, in cheat times or when you decide to pop out of ketosis to your regular food plan, you could emerge as undoing some of the blessings of keto food regimen when you all of the sudden cross returned to a standard weight-reduction policy wealthy in carbs. At the same time, on high fats, it can cause harm to blood vessels.

TIPS AND TRICKS FOR KETO WEIGHT LOSS

Although the leading cause of obese is menopause for ladies in their 50s, different factors additionally contribute to weight benefit and that they include:

- Stress
- Depression
- Lack of sleep
- Not consuming sufficient food
- The slowing fee of metabolism

So, if you are attempting to lose some weight and you want to upload something extra even as on keto eating regimen, below are the excellent tips:

Be Extra Lively

The extra we boost in age, the more we tend to be much less lively for lots of motives. You should also be retired and have lots of time at your disposal, or maybe your kids are all grown up and are now not within the house. Or perhaps you could just have pains and aches hold you from shifting around. Irrespective of the motives, menopausal ladies usually tend to be much less energetic due to the vast adjustments they pass through.

The above reasons are all valid when it comes to matters that keep you from exercising. However, it's miles essential to recognize that wholesome loss of weight at any age requires using. So, being energetic even at the age of fifty is useful for each of your body and mind. We may want to simply attempt to circulate a little bit extra around each day, perhaps a 30-minutes exercising or maybe only some minutes of jogging.

Build Up Muscle

As girls of over 50 years get older, they tend to lose muscle- it's far changed with fats. This fat is mostly saved inside the mid-section, otherwise called the abdomen. When you build muscle groups, you reduce the amount of fat stored in your body. Building up muscle mass additionally has a super way of burning off some calories without setting on any weight. The muscles make use of meals to grow, and to perform this function; they burn calories. Muscles also burn extra energy than fats.

Avoid Sugary Liquids

Sugary drinks, ranging from energy drinks, your favorite soda, and fruit juices, are wealthy in unnecessary energy that increases your weight when you're looking to lose a few. The calories contained in sugary drinks are called negative energy. They do no longer have any nutritional blessings; they do no longer fill you, yet they nonetheless add for your body's caloric count. Another aspect sugary liquids do is that because of the brought sugars, they increase your frame's tendency to store fats, especially in your abdomen.

The highly famous soda drink does several harm than merely the ones you've heard of. It also harms your

- brain
- bones
- heart
- teeth

Instead of damaging your fitness with these sugary drinks, you can replace them with water. You will make your life so an awful lot better by using being wholesome and taking one step toward attaining your ideal frame weight. Doing that is one of the easiest ways of dropping weight for girls of over 50 years.

Eat Greater Veggies

Eating vegetables can never be under-envisioned because it has many benefits to the body. You can upload them on your meals, as lots of them are delicious. So, all you need to do is to eat a few delightful greens to lose weight.

As cited earlier, menopause results in weight advantage because of how it affects your urge for food and hormones. With the keto food regimen, which enables you to grow your urge for food for meals, you need to recognition on consuming meals that help weight loss. Get high on authentic ingredients rich inadequate nutrients and occasional in calories.

That will make you get healthier and lose a few weight.

When seeking to shed pounds, the vegetable is one of the high dietary supplements to eat, as it's miles low in calories and excessive in vitamins; in reality, veggies are delicious.

Consume Extra Culmination

Fruits are the second meals institution after veggies that you have to consume while seeking to shed pounds. Although some result are wealthy in sugar and shouldn't be eaten in high quantity, especially when on keto weight loss program and trying to lose weight, there are some extraordinary keto-friendly fruits you could eat. Some result with low sugar include:

- blueberries
- raspberries
- strawberries
- cranberries
- watermelon
- clementines

Control Your Quantities

It isn't news that the charge of our body's metabolism reduces each decade. So, once you recover from the age of 50, you could now not consume as you probably did for your teenage days. Therefore, consuming healthy foods is one of the most critical factors of dropping weight, even though being capable of manage portions is essential.

Even if you devour all the healthy meals available, you don't expect your weight to drop much like that. You also have to recall the fee of your body's metabolism. You ought to preserve a near watch on the range of wholesome foods you consume and match it with the slower charge of your frame's metabolism. This weight loss tip is essential for each woman above 50 to recognize.

Eat Breakfast

Without a doubt, the essential meal of the day is breakfast. It is one of the reasons you go beforehand to keep your weight-reduction plan all day or go out of it. Taking breakfast affords your body with enough power for the day. It also prevents you from binge ingesting during the day. The blessings of eating breakfast cannot be overemphasized. If you don't devour breakfast, you turn out to be feeling lousy and starving during the day. When the time comes for lunch and dinner, you end up eating uncontrollably. You will eat extra than standard and stuff your frame with unnecessary energy. To avoid this, all you need to do is to devour your breakfast. Although making breakfast within the morning may be a touch tricky, doing so has masses of benefits. You can prepare in advance so that as quickly as you get out of bed, you won't be beaten with what you have to do to get the breakfast ready.

Eat When You're Hungry

It is not a wholesome move to bypass out breakfast, mainly while you are attempting to lose a few weight. However, it is also very harmful to skip any meal while you get those starvation pangs. When you are hungry, it manner your body needs those vitamins but denying your body the vitamins isn't beneficial. Similar to skipping breakfast is skipping out any meal, which can also bring about binge consuming later.

Sometimes, being on a keto weight loss plan approach, you will have a difficult time identifying what to devour, but you may always prepare ahead and get something ready. It is essential to consume while hungry to keep away from ruining your weight loss plans.

Eat Less

Of course, the weight loss manner you do ought to devour much less. With a keto weight loss plan, ingesting much less is not a great deal of a problems. The Keto food regimen energizes and makes you less hungry all through the day. You also have to recall the fact that your frame's metabolism is slower; so, consuming less is beneficial mainly in case you want to lose a few weight.

Eating less food is exceptional for many people. However, you might need to keep in mind eating about 1600 calories in line with day in case you are active. If you are not so energetic on the opposite hand, you might want to don't forget ingesting about 1200 energy in line with day. Irrespective of your activity, you might need to reduce your calorie intake to help you lose a few weight. However, recall getting sufficient vitamins for your frame.

Stay Hydrated

Even without being on a keto diet, staying hydrated is a vital part of being wholesome. To place it simply, you have to drink enough water.

Staying hydrated lets, you lose weight in several approaches:

- It enables in preserving you away from overeating
- It keeps you far from eating when you are not hungry at the same time as preserving you energized and boosting your metabolism
- It enables you in burning fats specifically for women over the age of fifty

All you have to do is drink water each time you get the chance, and you will see the wonders it does for your frame.

"If you enjoyed the contents of this book, bear in mind to leave your opinion with a review. In addition to being precious to me, your sincere opinion might be very beneficial for different readers who, such as you, have determined to improve their well-being."

CONCLUSION

It's in no way too past due to take rate of your health, and it's in no way too late to begin something new to help get you there, like with the keto diet.

Ok, maybe there's an age you reach while you just sense too vintage. But, that's now not where you're prompt. Gaining too much weight? Feeling specifically unproductive too often?

Then, trying out the keto diet might be the first element you've ever executed for yourself. What's even greater unusual is that those you like and the people you have to have interaction with regularly will also gain from your desire to go keto.

Losing unnecessary weight, feeling the munchies way less, and having extra stable strength will make anybody happier. And feeling glad is communicable!

These recipes are easy and brief to prepare, a number of them the use of ingredients already for your kitchen. Use the meal plan to manual you, and real good fortune on a healthier, happier, more productive you.

I want to depart you with some beautiful irony to mull over as you begin: you are by no means too old to look and feel young!

BONUS EXTRA RECIPES

Ketogenic Recipes

BREAKFASTS

171. Breakfast Egg Rolls

Preparation Time: 10 minutes

Yield: 4 Servings

Ingredients

- 1 tsp minced ginger
- 4 1/2 cups packaged coleslaw mix (shredded cabbage and carrots)
- 3 medium cooked scallions
- 3 Tbsp low sodium soy sauce
- 1 1/2 tsp sesame oil
- 1 pound uncooked ground chicken breast (can sub ground pork, turkey, or turkey sausage)
- 1 16 oz package of Egg Roll Wrappers (I only used 8 of them)
- 1 egg

Directions

1. Brown the sausage/meat in a medium non-stick skillet until cooked all the way through and then add the ginger.
2. Add soy sauce and sesame oil.
3. Add a full bag of coleslaw, stir until coated with sauce.
4. Add chopped scallions, mix thoroughly and cook on medium-high heat until the coleslaw has reduced by half.
5. Set the egg roll mixture aside.
6. Lay egg roll wrap in front of you so that it looks like a diamond.
7. Place 3 tablespoons of filling in the center of egg roll wrapper.
8. Brush each edge with egg wash.
9. Fold the bottom point up over filling and roll once.
10. Fold in the right and left points.
11. Finish rolling.
12. Set aside and repeat with remaining filling.
13. Heat Air Fryer to (370°F).
14. Set your stuffed egg rolls on the bottom of the air fryer basket and fry for 7 minutes or until they are golden brown.

Nutritional Information

Calories: 181
Fat: 4g
Carbs: 18g
Protein: 8g

172. Keto Air Fryer Fish Sticks

Preparation Time: 20 minutes
Yield: 2 Servings

Ingredients

- 1 lb white fish such as cod

Desserts

- 1/4 cup mayonnaise
- 2 tbsp Dijon mustard
- 2 tbsp water
- 1 1/2 cups pork rind panko such as Pork King Good
- 3/4 tsp cajun seasoning
- Salt and pepper to taste

Directions

1. Spray the air fryer rack with non-stick cooking spray (I use avocado oil spray).
2. Pat the fish dry and cut into sticks about 1 inch by 2 inches wide (how you can cut it will depend a little on what kind of fish you by and how thick and full it is).
3. In a small shallow bowl, whisk together the mayo, mustard, and water.
4. In another shallow bowl, whisk together the pork rinds and Cajun seasoning. Add salt and pepper to taste (both the pork rinds and seasoning could have a fair bit of salt, so dip a finger in to taste how salty it is).
5. Working with one piece of fish at a time, dip into the mayo mixture to coat and then tap off the excess. Dip into the pork rind mixture and toss to coat. Place on the air fryer rack.
6. Set to Air Fry at 400F and bake 5 minutes, then flip the fish sticks with tongs and cook another 5 minutes. Serve immediately.

Nutritional Information

Calories: 263
Fat: 16g
Carbs: 1g
Protein: 26g

173. Low Carb Mozzarella Sticks

Preparation Time: 15 minutes
Yield: 2 Servings

Ingredients

- 12 Mozzarella sticks string cheese, cut in half
- 2 large eggs beaten
- 1/2 cup Almond flour
- 1/2 cup Parmesan cheese the powdered kind
- 1 teaspoon Italian seasoning
- 1/2 teaspoon Garlic
- Salt

Instructions

- In a bowl, combine almond flour, Parmesan cheese, Italian seasoning, and garlic salt.
- In a separate bowl, whisk eggs.
- One at a time coat your mozzarella

stick halves in egg and then toss in the coating mixture. As you finish, place them in a resealable container if you have to make more than 1 layer place parchment paper between the layers of mozzarella sticks.

- Freeze mozzarella sticks for 30 minutes.
- Remove from freezer and place in Philips AirFryer.
- Set to 400 degrees F and cook for 5 minutes.
- Open air fryer and let stand for 1 minute before moving low carb mozzarella sticks to a plate.

Nutritional Information

Calories: 382
Fat: 27g
Carbs: 1g
Protein: 31g

174. Homemade Sausage Rolls

Preparation Time: 25 minutes
Yield: 4 Servings

Ingredients

- 225 g Almond Flour
- 100 g Butter
- 1 Tbsp Olive Oil
- 300 g Sausage Meat
- 1 Medium Egg beat
- 1 Tsp Mustard
- 1 Tsp Parsley
- Salt & Pepper

Instructions

1. Start by making your pastry. Place the flour, the seasoning, and the butter into a mixing bowl and using the rubbing in method, rub the fat into the flour until you have a mixture that resembles bread crumbs. Add the olive oil and a little water (a bit at a time) and using your hands make the mixture into a flaky dough. Knead the pastry as you mix it so that it becomes lovely and smooth.
2. Roll out the pastry onto a worktop and create a square shape of the bread. Using a teaspoon (or your fingers), rub the mustard into the cake. Place the sausage meat in the center and brush the edges of the pastry with egg. Roll up the sausage rolls and then divide them into portions. Brush the tops and sides of the sausage rolls with more eggs.
3. Slash the top of the sausage rolls with a knife so that they have the chance to breathe.
4. Cook in the Air fryer at 160c for 20 minutes and then for a further 5

Desserts

minutes at 200c so that you can have that lovely crunchy pastry.

5. Serve.

Nutritional Information

Calories: 545
Fat: 45g
Carbs: 25g
Protein: 18g
Easy Air Fryer Omelette
Preparation Time: 15 minutes
Yield: 2 Servings

Ingredients

- 2 eggs
- 1/4 cup milk
- Pinch of salt
- Fresh meat and vegetables, diced (I used red bell pepper, green onions, ham, and mushrooms)
- 1 teaspoon McCormick Good Morning Breakfast Seasoning - Garden Herb
- 1/4 cup shredded cheese (I used cheddar and mozzarella)

Instructions

1. In a small bowl, mix the eggs and milk until well combined.
2. Add a pinch of salt to the egg mixture.
3. Add your vegetables to the egg mixture.
4. Pour the egg mixture into a well-greased 6"x3" pan.
5. Place the pan into the basket of the air fryer.
6. Cook at 350F Fahrenheit for 8-10 minutes.
7. Halfway through cooking, sprinkle the breakfast seasoning onto the eggs and sprinkle the cheese over the top.
8. Use a thin spatula to loosen the omelet from the sides of the pan and transfer to a plate.
9. Garnish with extra green onions, optional

Nutritional Information

Calories: 274
Fat: 20g
Carbs: 3g
Protein: 16g

175. Air Fryer Tofu Scramble

Preparation Time: 30 minutes
Yield: 3 Servings

Ingredients

- 1 block tofu - chopped into 1" pieces
- 2 tablespoons soy sauce
- 1 tablespoon olive oil
- 1 teaspoon turmeric
- 1/2 teaspoon garlic powder
- 1/2 teaspoon onion powder

- 1/2 cup chopped onion
- 1 tablespoon olive oil
- 4 cups broccoli florets

Instructions

1. In a medium-sized bowl, toss together the tofu, soy sauce, olive oil, turmeric, garlic powder, onion powder, and onion. Set aside to marinate.
2. Add the tofu, reserving any leftover marinade. Set the tofu to cook at 370 for 15 minutes, and start the air fryer.
3. While the tofu is cooking, toss the broccoli in the reserved marinade. If there isn't enough to get it all over the broccoli, add a little bit of extra soy sauce. Be careful not to let the broccoli dry out. When there are 5 minutes of cooking time remaining, add the broccoli to the air fryer.

Nutritional Information

Calories: 150
Fat: 5g
Carbs: 5g
Protein: 10g

176. Air Fryer Hard Boiled Eggs

Preparation Time: 15 minutes
Yield: 6 Servings

Ingredients

- 6 eggs

Directions

1. Place the eggs onto the air fryer rack giving the eggs enough room so the air will circulate the egg.
2. Cook the eggs in the air fryer for 15 minutes at 260 degrees F.
3. Remove the eggs and place the eggs into an ice water bath for 10 minutes.
4. Notes:
5. Never skip the water bath; it helps stop the cooking process and also makes them easier to peel.

Nutritional Information

Calories: 26
Fat: 4g
Carbs: 0g
Protein: 5g

177. Fried Cheesecake Bites

Preparation Time: 25 minutes
Yield: 4 Servings

Ingredients

- 8 ounces cream cheese
- 1/2 cup erythritol
- 2 Tablespoons cream, divided
- 1/2 teaspoon vanilla extract
- 1/2 cup almond flour
- 2 Tablespoons erythritol

Desserts

Instructions

1. Allow the cream cheese to sit on the counter for 20 minutes to soften.
2. Fit a stand mixer with the paddle attachment.
3. Mix the softened cream cheese, 1/2 cup erythritol, vanilla, and 2 Tablespoons heavy cream until smooth.
4. Scoop onto a parchment paper-lined baking sheet.
5. Freeze for about 30 minutes, until firm.
6. Mix the almond flour with the 2 Tablespoons erythritol in a small mixing bowl.
7. Dip the frozen cheesecake bites into 2 Tablespoons cream, then roll into the almond flour mixture.
8. Place in an air fryer set at 350 for 5 minutes.
9. Alternatively, you can bake them in the oven for 8 minutes to achieve that crispy outside coating.

Nutritional Information

Calories: 80
Fat: 7g
Carbs: 2g
Protein: 2g

178. Air Fryer Fried Parmesan Zucchini

Preparation Time: 30 minutes
Yield: 6 Servings

Ingredients

- 2 medium zucchini
- 1 large egg
- 1/2 cup grated parmesan cheese
- 1/4 almond flour
- 1/2 teaspoon garlic powder
- 1 teaspoon Italian seasoning
- avocado oil spray or another cooking oil spray

Instructions

1. Slice zucchini into 1/4 to 1/3 of inch slices.
2. Beat egg well in a separate bowl.
3. Combine grated parmesan cheese, almond flour, garlic powder, and Italian seasoning in another bowl.
4. Dip zucchini slice in egg then dip it in the parmesan cheese mixture. Set on parchment-lined air fryer tray.
5. Repeat until the air fryer tray is full. Lightly spray-coated zucchini with avocado oil spray.
6. Set air fryer to 370F for 8 minutes.
7. Remove the tray and flip zucchini slices. Spray with avocado oil and

cook for another 8 minutes.

8. Repeat process with the second batch of zucchini.
9. Serve warm.

Nutritional Information

Calories: 92
Fat: 5g
Carbs: 4g
Protein: 6g

179. Keto Creamed Spinach

Preparation Time: 15 minutes

Yield: 2 Servings

Ingredients

- 1 10 ounces package frozen spinach thawed
- 1/2 cup chopped onion
- 2 teaspoons minced garlic
- 4 ounces cream cheese diced
- 1 teaspoon pepper
- 1 teaspoon salt
- 1/2 teaspoon ground nutmeg
- 1/4 cup shredded Parmesan cheese

Instructions

1. Grease a 6-inch pan and set aside.
2. In the medium bowl, combine spinach, onion, garlic, cream cheese dices, salt, pepper, and nutmeg. Pour into greased pan.
3. Set an air fryer to 350°F for 10 minutes. Open and stir the spinach to mix the cream cheese through the spinach.
4. Sprinkle the Parmesan cheese on top. Set air fryer to 400°F for 5 minutes or until the cheese has melted and browned.

Nutritional Information

Calories: 273
Fat: 23g
Carbs: 8g
Protein: 8g

LUNCHES

180. Air Fried Cauliflower Recipe with Sriracha

Preparation Time: 25 minutes
Yield: 4 Servings

Ingredients

- 1 small head of cauliflower (about 1 1/2 lbs. - 680g), cut into bite-sized pieces
- 2 Tablespoons olive oil
- 1 teaspoon sesame oil
- 1 Tablespoon soy sauce
- 1 Tablespoon rice vinegar
- 2 Tablespoons sriracha or any hot sauce

Directions

1. In a large bowl, combine olive oil, sesame oil, soy sauce, rice vinegar, and hot sriracha sauce.
2. Add cauliflower and toss with the marinade. Keep stirring the cauliflower so that it completely soaks up all the marinade (there shouldn't be any marinade pooling at the bottom of the bowl still).
3. Pour cauliflower into the air fryer basket and spread evenly in the basket.
4. Air Fry 360°F for 15-20 minutes, shake or gently turn halfway.
5. Serve warm and enjoy.

Nutritional Information

Calories: 155
Fat: 11g
Carbs: 10g
Protein: 5g

181. Keto Air Fryer Double Cheeseburger

Preparation Time: 15 minutes
Yield: 4 Servings

Ingredients

- 1/2 lb ground beef (or two pre-made beef patties)
- 2 slices cheese of choice
- 1 pinch pink Himalayan salt
- 1 pinch fresh ground black pepper
- 1 pinch onion powder

Directions

1. Form two 1/4 pound hamburger patties (if not using pre-made ones)
2. Lightly salt, pepper, and onion powder the hamburger patties
3. Place into your air fryer and set to 370°F for 12 minutes
4. At the 6 minute mark, flip the hamburgers

5. When the air fryer finishes, place the cheese onto the hamburger patties and shut the drawer for one minute

6. Remove the patties, stack, and devour!

Nutritional Information

Calories: 670
Fat: 50g
Carbs: 0g
Protein: 39g

182. Air Fryer Pork Chops & Broccoli

Preparation Time: 15 minutes
Yield: 4 Servings

Ingredients

- 2 5 ounce bone-in pork chops
- 2 tablespoons avocado oil, divided
- 1/2 teaspoon paprika
- 1/2 teaspoon onion powder
- 1/2 teaspoon garlic powder
- 1 teaspoon salt, divided
- 2 cups broccoli florets
- 2 cloves garlic, minced

Directions

1. Preheat air fryer to 350 degrees. Spray basket with non-stick spray.
2. Drizzle 1 tablespoon of oil both sides of the pork chops.
3. Season the pork chops on both sides with the paprika, onion powder, garlic powder, and 1/2 teaspoon of salt.
4. Place pork chops in the air fryer basket and cook for 5 minutes.
5. While pork chops are cooking, add the broccoli, garlic, remaining 1/2 teaspoon of salt, and remaining tablespoon of oil to a bowl and toss to coat.
6. Open the air fryer and carefully flip the pork chops.
7. Add the broccoli to the basket and return to the air fryer.
8. Cook for 5 more minutes, stirring the broccoli halfway through.
9. Carefully remove the food from the air fryer and serve.

Nutritional Information

Calories: 283
Fat: 30g
Carbs: 12g
Protein: 40g

183. Air Fryer Tuna Patties

Preparation Time: 15 minutes
Yield: 4 Servings

Ingredients

- 2 cans of tuna packed in water
- 1 and 1/2 tablespoon almond flour

Desserts

- 1 and 1/2 tablespoons mayo
- 1 teaspoon dried dill
- 1 teaspoon garlic powder
- 1/2 teaspoon onion powder
- Pinch of salt and pepper
- Juice of 1/2 lemon

Instructions

1. Combine all ingredients in a bowl and mix well
2. Tuna should be still wet, but able to form into patties - add a tablespoon of almond flour if it's not dry enough to form
3. Form into 4 patties
4. Heat to 400 degrees F.
5. Place patties in a single layer in the basket and cook for 10 minutes. Add 3 minutes if you'd like them crispier

Nutritional Information

Calories: 130
Fat: 4g
Carbs: 5g
Protein: 15g

184. Air Fryer Carne Asada

Preparation Time: 10 minutes
Yield: 4 Servings

Ingredients

- 2 medium limes juiced
- 1 medium orange peeled and seeded
- 1 cup cilantro
- 1 jalapeno diced
- 2 tablespoons vegetable oil
- 2 tablespoons vinegar
- 2 teaspoons ancho chile powder
- 1 teaspoon Splenda or 2 teaspoon sugar
- 1 teaspoon salt
- 1 teaspoon cumin seeds
- 1 teaspoon coriander seeds
- 1.5 pounds skirt steak

Directions

1. Place all ingredients except the skirt steak into a blender and mix until you get a smooth sauce.
2. Cut the skirt steak into four pieces and place it into a zip-top plastic bag.
3. Pour the marinade on the steak and let the meat marinate for 30 minutes or up to 24 hours in the refrigerator.
4. Set your air fryer to 400F and place the steaks into the air fryer basket. Depending on the size of your air fryer, you may have to do this in two batches.

5. Cook for 8 minutes, or until your steak has reached an internal temperature of 145F. It is critical not to overcook skirt steak not to toughen the meat.
6. Let the steak rest for 10 minutes. Don't rush this stage.
7. Slice the steak against the grain (this part is essential) and serve.

Nutritional Information

Calories: 330
Fat: 19g
Carbs: 1g
Protein: 37g

185. Healthy Eggplant Parmesan

Preparation Time: 25 minutes
Yield: 4 Servings

Ingredients

- 1 large eggplant mine was around 1.25 lb
- 1/2 cups pork rind panko such as Pork King Good
- 3 tbsp finely grated parmesan cheese
- salt to taste
- 1 tsp Italian seasoning mix
- 3 tbsp whole wheat flour
- 1 egg + 1 tbsp water
- olive oil spray
- 1 cup sugar-free marinara sauce
- 1/4 cup grated mozzarella cheese
- fresh parsley or basil to garnish

Directions

1. Cut eggplant into roughly 1/2" slices. Rub some salt on both sides of the slices and leave it for at least 10-15 mins.
2. Meanwhile, in a small bowl, mix the egg with water and flour to prepare the batter.
3. In a medium shallow plate combine pork rind panko, parmesan cheese, Italian seasoning blend, and some salt. Mix thoroughly.
4. Now apply the batter to each eggplant slice evenly. Dip the battered slices in the mix to coat it evenly on all sides.
5. Place eggplant slices on a clean and dry flat plate and spray oil on them.
6. Preheat the Air Fryer to 360F. Then put the eggplant slices on the wire mesh and cook for about 8 min.
7. Top the fried air slices with about 1 tablespoon of marinara sauce and lightly spread fresh mozzarella cheese on it. Cook the eggplant for another 1-2 min or until the cheese melts.

Desserts

8. Serve warm.

Nutritional Information

Calories: 217
Fat: 11g
Carbs: 19g
Protein: 12g

186. Air Fryer Radish Hash Browns

Preparation Time: 20 minutes
Yield: 4 Servings

Ingredients

- 1 pound Radishes washed
- 1 medium Yellow/Brown Onion
- 1 teaspoon Garlic Powder
- 1 teaspoon Granulated Onion Powder
- 3/4 teaspoon Pink Himalayan Salt (or Sea Salt)
- 1/2 teaspoon Paprika
- 1/4 teaspoon Freshly Ground Black Pepper
- 1 Tablespoon Pure Virgin Coconut Oil

Directions

1. Wash Radishes thoroughly and cut off roots. Trim steams, leaving 1/4-1/2 inch.
2. Use a Food Processor or Mandolin and slice the Radishes and Onions.
3. Add Coconut Oil and mix well. Grease Air Fryer Basket.
4. Add Radishes and Onions to Air Fryer Basket.
5. Cook at 360 degrees for 8 minutes, shaking a few times.
6. Dump Radishes and Onions back into Mixing Bowl. Add Seasonings to Radishes and Onions and cook at 400 degrees for five minutes, shaking halfway through.

Nutritional Information

Calories: 83
Fat: 4g
Carbs: 4g
Protein: 6g

187. Air Fryer Chicken Quesadilla

Preparation Time: 15 minutes
Yield: 4 Servings

Ingredients

- Zero Carb Soft Taco Shells
- Chicken Fajita Strips
- 1/2 cup sliced green peppers
- 1/2 cup sliced onions (I use the frozen fajita blend)
- Shredded Mexican Cheese
- Salsa (optional)
- Sour Cream (optional)

Directions

1. Preheat Air Fryer on 370 degrees for about 3 minutes.
2. Spray pan lightly with vegetable oil.
3. Place 1 soft taco shell in pan.
4. Place shredded cheese on the shell. (you can use as much or as little as you'd like.)
5. Layout fajita chicken strips so they are in a single layer.
6. Put your onions and green peppers on top of your chicken.
7. Add more shredded cheese.
8. Place another soft taco shell on top and spray lightly with vegetable oil.
9. (I put the rack that came with the air fryer on top of the shell to hold it in place. If you don't, the fan will suck it up. Trust me on this one!)
10. Set timer for 4 minutes.
11. Flip over carefully with a large spatula.
12. Spray lightly with vegetable oil and place rack on top of the shell to hold it in place.
13. Set timer for 4 minutes.
14. If it's not crispy enough for you, leave in for a couple of extra minutes.
15. Remove and cut into 4 slices or 6 slices.
16. Serve with salsa and sour cream if desired.

Nutritional Information

Calories: 190
Fat: 16g
Carbs: 7g
Protein: 8g

188. Tomato Basil Scallops

Preparation Time: 15 minutes
Yield: 2 Servings

Ingredients

- 3/4 cup heavy whipping cream
- 1 tablespoon tomato paste
- 1 tablespoon chopped fresh basil
- 1 teaspoon minced garlic
- 1/2 teaspoon salt
- 1/2 teaspoon pepper
- 1 12 oz package frozen spinach thawed and drained
- 8 jumbo sea scallops
- vegetable oil to spray
- additional salt and pepper to season scallops

Directions

1. Spray a 7-inch heatproof pan, and place the spinach in an even layer at the bottom.
2. Spray both sides of the scallops with vegetable oil, sprinkle a little more salt and pepper on them, and place scallops in the pan on top of the spinach.
3. In a small bowl, mix the cream, tomato paste, basil, garlic, salt, and pepper and pour over the spinach and scallops.

Desserts

4. Set the air fryer to 350F for 10 minutes until the scallops are cooked through to an internal temperature of 135F, and the sauce is hot and bubbling. Serve immediately.

Nutritional Information

Calories: 359
Fat: 33g
Carbs: 6g
Protein: 9g

189. Air Fryer Keto Low Carb Fried Chicken

Preparation Time: 30 minutes
Yield: 6 Servings

Ingredients

- 2 1/2 lbs chicken drumsticks
- 1/4 cup Coconut flour
- 1/2 tsp Sea salt
- 1/4 tsp Black pepper
- 2 large Eggs
- 1 cup Pork rinds (2.25 oz)
- 1 tsp smoked paprika
- 1/2 tsp Garlic powder
- 1/4 tsp dried thyme

Directions

1. Stir the coconut flour, sea salt, and black pepper in a medium shallow bowl. Set aside.
2. In a second medium bowl, whisk together the eggs. Set aside.
3. In a third bowl, mix the crushed pork rinds, smoked paprika, garlic powder, and thyme.
4. Dredge the chicken pieces in the coconut flour mixture, dip in the eggs, shake off the excess, then press into the pork rind mixture. For best results, keep most of the third mixture in a separate bowl and add a little at a time to the container where you'll be coating the chicken. That way, it won't get clumpy too fast.
5. Preheat the air fryer at 400 degrees F (204 degrees C) for 5 minutes. Lightly grease the metal basket and arrange the breaded chicken on it in a single layer without touching.
6. Place the basket into the air fryer. Cook the fried chicken in the air fryer for 20 minutes, until it reaches an internal temperature of 165 degrees F (74 degrees C).

Nutritional Information
Calories: 274
Fat: 15g
Carbs: 3g
Protein: 28g

APPETIZERS AND SIDE DISHES

190. Air Fryer Zucchini Fries

Ingredients

- 2 zucchinis large
- 1/4 cup coconut flour
- 1 tablespoon nutritional yeast
- 1 teaspoon garlic powder
- 1 teaspoon onion powder
- 1/2 teaspoon salt
- 1/2 teaspoon Italian seasoning
- 1/4 teaspoon pepper

Directions

1. Preheat air fryer to 400 degrees.
2. Wash and dry zucchini. Cut the ends off and then cut each zucchini in half. Cut each half into 1/2-inch-thick wedges.
3. In a large mixing bowl, combine coconut flour, nutritional yeast, garlic powder, onion powder, salt, pepper, and Italian seasoning. Mix thoroughly.
4. Working in batches, toss zucchini wedges in coconut flour mixture until evenly coated.
5. Arrange zucchini wedges in a single layer in the fryer basket, skin side down. Do not overlap wedges. Depending on the size of your air fryer, you may need to work in batches.
6. "Fry" in the 400-degree air fryer for 15 minutes or until edges are crispy and golden brown (no longer than 20 minutes).
7. Serve with sugar-free ketchup, marinara or pizza sauce.

Nutritional Information

Calories: 213
Fat: 12g
Carbs: 12g
Protein: 13g

191. Roasted Turnips

Preparation Time: 10 minutes
Yield: 4 Servings

Ingredients

- 4 medium turnips
- 2 teaspoons avocado oil
- 1 1/2 teaspoon paprika
- 1 teaspoon of sea salt
- 1 teaspoon cracked pepper
- 2 teaspoons minced parsley

Directions

1. Preheat the air fryer to 390 degrees or the oven to 450 degrees.

Desserts

2. Peel and dice the turnips and place them in a medium mixing bowl.
3. Add the avocado oil, paprika, sea salt, and pepper to the bowl and toss to coat.
4. Spread the turnips in an even layer in the air fryer basket or on a large baking sheet.
5. Air fry for 10 minutes, shaking the basket once halfway through cooking
6. Sprinkle with parsley just before serving.

Nutritional Information

Calories: 51
Fat: 3g
Carbs: 9g
Protein: 1g

192. Keto Air-Fried Pickles

Preparation Time: 15 minutes
Yield: 4 Servings

Ingredients

- 1/2 cup crushed pork rinds
- 3 tablespoons Parmesan cheese
- 16 slices dill pickles
- 1/2 cup almond flour
- 1 large egg beaten
- 1 teaspoon olive oil cooking spray

Instructions

1. Mix crushed pork rinds with Parmesan cheese in one bowl. In a second bowl, add a whisked egg. In a third bowl, combine the almond flour.
2. Dredge each pickle in the almond flour, then in the egg, and finally in the pork rind mixture.
3. Place in a greased air fryer to form one single layer of breaded pickles.
4. Spray the tops with olive oil using an olive oil mister.
5. Set air fryer timer to 6 minutes at 370 degrees Fahrenheit.

Nutritional Information

Calories: 275
Fat: 19g
Carbs: 5g
Protein: 24g

193. Air-Fried Onion Rings

Preparation Time: 10 minutes
Yield: 2 Servings

Ingredients

- 1 Onion Sliced
- 1 1/4 cup Flour
- 1 tsp Baking Powder
- 1 Egg Beaten
- 1 cup + 1 tsp Milk
- 3/4 cup pork rind panko such as Pork King Good

- Seasonings of your choice

Instructions

1. Preheat your air fryer to 370 and lightly spray the basket for nonstick if needed. Set up a 'dredging' area by setting two shallow bowls side by side.

2. A shallow dish or pan may work for the second area instead of using a bowl. In a mixing bowl, mix the flour, baking powder, and seasonings. Mix in the egg and then the milk (or beer). We will divide this by transferring half of this mixture to the first bowl in our dredging area.

3. Now in the second bowl, or dredging area, place your pork rind panko. Using a fork, carefully take the first slice of onion and fully cover it with the contents of the first bowl- using a dredging technique. Then dip this piece into the pork rind panko.

4. Place the covered slices of onion into the fryer basket, being careful not to overlap if possible. When the first bowl runs out of its contents, simply refill it with the leftovers from the mixing bowl.

5. Tip- spray the onion rings with a bit of spray oil or something similar before placing the ring into the fryer. This will help them become crisp¬like.

6. Air fry the onion rings for 8 minutes and then flip them over. Continue to air fry for another 8 minutes or until done.

Nutritional Information

Calories: 411
Fat: 2g
Carbs: 12g
Protein: 5g

194. Air Fryer Avocado Fries

Preparation Time: 10 minutes
Yield: 2 Servings

Ingredients

- 1 avocado
- 1 egg
- 1/2 cup pork rind panko such as Pork King Good
- 1/2 teaspoon salt

Directions

1. Get a ripe but firm avocado. Cut in half and remove the pit. Cut avocado into wedges.

2. Beat the egg with salt in one bowl. Add panko into another bowl.

3. Dip wedges into the egg mixture, and then into the pork rind panko.

4. Place wedges into preheated to

Desserts

400F air fryer in a single layer for 8-10 minutes. Shake halfway through.

5. They are done when lightly brown.

Nutritional Information

Calories: 251
Fat: 17g
Carbs: 15g
Protein: 6g

195. Air-Fried Okra

Preparation Time: 15 minutes
Yield: 4 Servings

Ingredients

- 1 egg
- 1 cup skim milk
- 1 cup pork rind panko
- 1/2 teaspoon sea salt
- oil for misting or cooking spray

Directions

1. Remove stem ends from okra and cut in 1/2 inch slices.
2. In a medium bowl, beat together egg and milk. Add okra slices and stir to coat.
3. In a sealable plastic bag or container with lid, mix the pork rind panko and salt.
4. Remove okra from egg mixture, letting excess drip off, and transfer into a bag with pork rind panko. Be sure okra is well-drained before placing it in the pork rind panko. You may want to use a slotted spoon to lift a little okra at a time and let plenty of the egg wash drip off before putting it into pork rind panko.
5. Shake okra in crumbs to coat thoroughly.
6. Place all of the coated okra into the air fryer basket and mist with oil or cooking spray. Okra does not have to be in a single layer, and it isn't necessary to spray all sides at this point. A good spritz on top will do.
7. Cook at 390 F for 5 minutes. Shake basket to redistribute and give it another oil spritz as you shake.
8. Cook 5 more minutes. Shake and spray again. Cook for 2 to 5 minutes longer or until golden brown and crispy.

Nutritional Information

Calories: 241
Fat: 18g
Carbs: 15g
Protein: 4g

196. Baked Chicken Nuggets

Preparation Time: 25 minutes
Yield: 4 Servings

Ingredients

- 1 Pound Free-range boneless, skinless chicken breast
- Pinch sea salt
- 1 tsp Sesame oil
- 1/4 Cup Coconut flour
- 1/2 tsp ground ginger
- 4 Egg whites
- 6 Tbsp toasted sesame seeds
- A cooking spray of choice
- For the dip:
- 2 Tbsp Natural creamy almond butter
- 4 tsp coconut aminos (or GF soy sauce)
- 1 Tbsp Water
- 2 tsp Rice vinegar
- 1 tsp Sriracha, or to taste
- 1/2 tsp ground ginger
- 1/2 tsp Monkfruit (omit for whole30)

Directions

1. Preheat your air fryer to 400 degrees for 10 minutes.
2. While the air fryer heats, cut the chicken into nuggets (about 1-inch pieces) dry them off and place them in a bowl. Toss with salt and sesame oil until coated.
3. Place the coconut flour and ground ginger in a large Ziploc bag and shake to combine. Add the chicken and stir until coated.
4. Place the egg whites in a large bowl and add in the chicken nuggets, tossing until they are all well coated in the egg.
5. Place the sesame seeds in a large Ziploc bag. Shake any excess egg off the chicken and add the nuggets into the bag, shake until well coated.
6. GENEROUSLY spray the mesh air fryer basket with cooking spray. Place the nuggets into the basket, making sure not to crowd them, or they won't get crispy. Spray with a touch of cooking spray.
7. Cook for 6 minutes. Flip each nugget and spray for cooking spray. Then, cook an additional 5-6 minutes until no longer pink inside, with a crispy outside.
8. While the nuggets cook, whisk all the sauce ingredients together in a medium bowl until smooth.
9. Serve the nuggets with the dip and devour!

Nutritional Information

Calories: 250
Fat: 18g

Desserts

Carbs: 6g
Protein: 25g

197. Air Fryer Egg Cups

Preparation Time: 30 minutes
Yield: 4 Servings

Ingredients

- Non-stick cooking spray
- 4 large eggs
- 1 cup diced vegetables of choice
- 1 cup shredded cheese
- 4 Tbs half and half
- 1 Tbs chopped cilantro
- Salt and Pepper

Directions

1. Grease 4 ramekins
2. In a medium bowl, whisk eggs, vegetables, half the cheese, half and half, cilantro, and salt and pepper together.
3. Divide between the ramekins
4. Place ramekins in the air-fryer basket set the temperature to 300 degrees F for 12 minutes.
5. Top the cups with remaining cheese.
6. Set air-fryer to 400 degrees F, cook 2 minutes until cheese is melted and lightly browned.
7. Serve immediately.

Nutritional Information

Calories: 195
Fat: 12g
Carbs: 7g
Protein: 13g

198. Air Fryer Frittata

Preparation Time: 15 minutes
Yield: 4 Servings

Ingredients

- 2 large Eggs
- 1 Cup shredded chicken
- 1 tbsp chopped Spring Onions
- 1 tbsp chopped Bell Peppers
- 2 tbsp Cheddar cheese
- 1 tbsp Melted Butter
- Salt and pepper to taste

Instructions

1. Generously grease a 4-inch cake pan or a mini loaf pan (or any oven-safe pan that fits in your air-fryer basket) with butter.
2. Add the chopped up breakfast sausage in the greased pan and air fry at 350F for 5 minutes.
3. Meanwhile, in a medium-sized bowl, crack 2 eggs. Add salt and pepper and whisk it well.
4. Add the chopped spring onion, bell peppers, and mix well. Once the sausage is cooked, add the egg

mixture. Mix well with the sausages.

5. Sprinkle with cheddar cheese and air fry at 350 F for another 5 minutes.

6. Serve hot with fresh tomato salsa.

Nutritional Information

Calories: 380
Fat: 27g
Carbs: 2g
Protein: 31g

199. Air Fried Blooming Onion

Preparation Time: 15 minutes
Yield: 4 Servings

Ingredients

- 1 Onion
- 2.5 cups almond Flour
- 4 tsp Old Bay Seasoning
- 2 Eggs (Beaten)
- 1/2 Cup Milk

Instructions

1. Preheat your air fryer to 400 and prep your basket for nonstick if desired.

2. In a bowl, whisk together your flour and seasonings. Now, in another bowl, whip together the eggs and milk (or liquid of choice). First, pour the flour mixture over the onion and coat well.

3. It is a good idea to get your hands involved and move the onion around in the bowl to help coat it. Or, you could cover the pan with a plate or wrap and shake it to paint it. Lift the onion and stir the excess flour mixture off back into the bowl. Move the onion over to the other dish that contains the egg and milk and coat well.

4. Use a spoon or ladle to help you coat the entire onion. Sprinkle the remaining flour mixture over the onion, shake the onion out again, and then place it into your air fryer.

5. Air Fry this for 8-10 minutes or until crisp. Optional: For a bit of an oil taste, you can lightly spray your onion with a bit of olive or other oil before frying.

Nutritional Information

Calories: 267
Fat: 20g
Carbs: 15g
Protein: 4g

FISH AND SEAFOOD

200. Perfect Air Fried Salmon

Preparation Time: 25 minutes
Yield: 4 Servings

Ingredients

- 1/12-inches thick
- 2 teaspoons avocado oil or olive oil
- 2 teaspoons paprika
- generously seasoned with salt and coarse black pepper
- lemon wedges

Directions

1. Remove any bones from your salmon if necessary and let fish sit on the counter for an hour. Rub each fillet with olive oil and season with paprika, salt, and pepper.
2. Place fillets in the basket of the air fryer. Set air fryer at 390 degrees for 7 minutes for 1-1/2-inch fillets.
3. When the timer goes off, open basket and check fillets with a fork to make sure they are done to your desired doneness.
4. Notes: One of the beauties of the air fryer is that it's so easy to pop something back in for a minute if you want it cooked longer. You can also open it while it's preparing to make sure it's not overdone. I always set my timer for a little less so I can check on how things are coming along, so I don't overcook an item. Things cook so fast; sometimes a minute more is all it needs.
5. Times for cooking will vary for salmon based on the temperature of the fish and the size of your fillets. Always set your air fryer for a little less time than you think until you become more used to the timing of your appliance.

Nutritional Information

Calories: 237
Fat: 11g
Carbs: 1g
Protein: 34g

201. Air Fryer Salmon Cakes

Preparation Time: 7 minutes
Yield: 4 Servings

Ingredients

- 8 oz fresh salmon fillet (could be from frozen)
- 1 egg
- 1/8 teaspoon salt
- 1/4 teaspoon garlic powder
- 1 sliced lemon

Directions

1. Mince salmon in the bowl, add egg and spices.
2. Form little cakes. Preheat air fryer to 390. Lay sliced lemons on the bottom of the air fryer basket. Place cakes on top.
3. Cook for 7 minutes. Serve with your favorite dip, depending on your diet preferences.

Nutritional Information

Calories: 288
Fat: 13g
Carbs: 13g
Protein: 26g

202. Air Fryer Coconut Shrimp

Preparation Time: 25 minutes
Yield: 4 Servings

Ingredients

- 12 wild-caught XL shrimp
- 1/3 cup almond flour
- 2 large eggs, beaten
- 1/2 cup unsweetened shredded coconut
- 1 lime wedge
- 1 tablespoon extra virgin olive oil for brushing the basket. Tropical Dipping Sauce
- 4 teaspoons coconut aminos
- 1 cup pineapple juice
- 1 teaspoon raw honey
- 1/4 teaspoon ginger powder
- 1/2 teaspoon tapioca starch

Directions

1. Wash the shrimp and devein them. Make small slits in the belly of the shrimps, so they don't curl when cooked. Place almond flour on a plate, the eggs in a shallow bowl, and the shredded coconut on another plate. Dredge shrimp in the flour, dip in the egg and roll and coat with the shredded coconut. Refrigerate for 30 minutes.
2. Preheat the air fryer to 360°F.
3. Brush the basket with extra virgin olive oil. Place 6 shrimp in the basket, in a single layer, and set the timer for 7 minutes.
4. Meanwhile, in a small saucepan, bring the pineapple juice to a boil and then simmer on low heat until it's reduced to half. Add the rest of the ingredients and stir well. Take the pan off the heat and set aside.
5. When the timer goes off, take the shrimp out, place them on a plate, and cover. Put the rest of the shrimp in the basket and cook for 7 minutes. When the timer goes off, squeeze some lime juice on the

Desserts

shrimp, and serve immediately with the Tropical Dipping Sauce.

Nutritional Information

Calories: 250
Fat: 9g
Carbs: 13g
Protein: 20g

203. Air Fryer Crispy Fish

Preparation Time: 15 minutes
Yield: 4 Servings

Ingredients

- 1 1/4 lb. cod
- 2 large eggs
- 1 cup almond flour
- 1 tbsp. dried parsley
- 1/2 tsp. garlic powder
- 1/2 tsp. onion powder
- 1/4 tsp. salt

Instructions

1. 1 tbsp. arrowroot powder (organic cornstarch works too)
2. Directions
3. In a medium mixing bowl, beat the eggs with a whisk until well combined.
4. In a separate, medium mixing bowl, mix the almond flour, parsley, garlic powder, onion powder, salt, and arrowroot powder (or cornstarch). Combine thoroughly.
5. Dip the fish pieces into the egg and then roll in the coating, making sure to cover each part of the fish.
6. Place the fish pieces in a single layer in the basket of the air fryer. Set to 350 for 7 minutes. When done, flip the pieces of fish in the basked and repeat for another 7 minutes.

Nutritional Information

- Calories: 338
- Fat: 17g
- Carbs: 12g
- Protein: 35g

204. Air Fryer Parchment Fish

Preparation Time: 25 minutes
Yield: 2 Servings

Ingredients

- 2 5-oz cod fillets thawed
- 1/2 cup julienned carrots
- 1/2 cup julienned fennel bulbs or 1/4 cup julienned celery
- 1/2 cup thinly sliced red peppers
- 2 sprigs tarragon or 1/2 teaspoon dried tarragon
- 2 pats melted butter

- 1 tablespoon lemon juice
- 1 tablespoon salt divided
- 1/2 teaspoon pepper
- 1 tablespoon oil

Directions

1. In a medium bowl, combine melted butter, tarragon, 1/2 teaspoon salt, and lemon juice. Mix well until you get a creamy sauce. Add the julienned vegetable and mix well. Set aside.
2. Cut two squares of parchment large enough to hold the fish and vegetables.
3. Spray the fish fillets with oil and apply salt and pepper to both sides of the nets.
4. Lay one filet down on each parchment square. Top each fillet with half the vegetables. Pour any remaining sauce over the vegetables.
5. Fold over the parchment paper and crimp the sides to hold fish, vegetables, and sauce securely inside the packet. Place the containers inside the air fryer basket.
6. Set your air fryer to 350F for 15 minutes. Remove each packet to a plate and open just before serving.

Nutritional Information

Calories: 251
Fat: 12g
Carbs: 7g
Protein: 3g

205. Lemon Garlic Shrimp

Preparation Time: 10 minutes
Yield: 4 Servings

Ingredients

- 1 pound small shrimp, peeled with tails removed
- 1 Tablespoon olive oil
- 4 garlic cloves, minced
- 1 lemon, zested and juiced
- 1 pinch crushed red pepper flakes (optional)
- 1/4 cup parsley, chopped
- 1/4 teaspoon sea salt

Directions

1. Heat your air fryer to 400°F.
2. In a bowl, combine the shrimp, olive oil, garlic, salt, lemon zest, and red pepper flakes (if using). Toss to coat.
3. Transfer the shrimp to the basket of your fryer. Cook for 5-8 minutes, shaking the basket halfway through, or until the shrimp are cooked through.
4. Pour the shrimp into a serving

Desserts

bowl and toss with lemon juice and parsley. Season with additional salt to taste.

Nutritional Information

Calories: 120
Fat: 5g
Carbs: 4g
Protein: 16g

206. Coconut Curry Salmon Cakes

Preparation Time: 25 minutes
Yield: 4 Servings

Ingredients

- 1 lb Fresh Atlantic Salmon Side (half aside)
- 1/4 Cup Avocado, mashed
- 1/4 Cup Cilantro, diced + additional for garnish
- 1 1/2 tsp yellow curry powder
- 1/2 tsp Stonemill Sea Salt Grinder
- 1/4 cup + 4 tsp Starch, divided (40g)
- 2 SimplyNature Organic Cage Free Brown Eggs
- 1/2 cup SimplyNature Organic Coconut Flakes (30g)
- Organic Coconut Oil, melted (for brushing)
- For the greens:
- 2 tsp SimplyNature Organic Coconut Oil, melted
- 6 Cups SimplyNature Organic Arugula & Spinach Mix, tightly packed
- Pinch of Stonemill Sea Salt Grinder

Directions

1. Remove the skin from the salmon, dice the flesh, and add it into a large bowl.
2. Add in the avocado, cilantro, curry powder, sea salt, and stir until well mixed. Then, stir in 4 tsp of the tapioca starch until well incorporated.
3. Line a baking sheet with parchment paper. Form the salmon into 8, 1/4 cup-sized patties, just over 1/2 inch thick, and place them onto the pan. Freeze for 20 minutes, so they are easier to work with.
4. While the patties freeze, pre-heat your Air Fryer to 400 degrees for 10 minutes, rubbing the basket with coconut oil. Additionally, whisk the eggs and place them into a shallow plate. Place the remaining 1/4 cup of Tapioca starch and the coconut flakes in separate shallow dishes as well.
5. Once the patties have chilled, dip

one into the tapioca starch, making sure it's fully covered. Then, dip it into the egg, covering it entirely, and gently brushing off any excess. Finally, press just the top and sides of the cake into the coconut flakes and place it, coconut flake-side up, into the air fryer. Repeat with all cupcakes.

6. Gently brush the tops with a little bit of melted coconut oil (optional, but recommended) and cook until the outside is golden brown and crispy, and the inside is juicy and tender about 15 minutes. Note: the patties will stick to the Air Fryer basked a little, so use a sharp-edged spatula to remove them.

7. When the cakes have about 5 minutes left to cook, heat the coconut oil in a large pan on medium heat. Add in the Arugula and Spinach Mix, and a pinch of salt, and cook, continually stirring, until the greens JUST begin to wilt, only 30 seconds - 1 minute.

8. Divide the greens between 4 plates, followed by the salmon cakes.

9. Garnish with extra cilantro and devour!

Nutritional Information

Calories: 211
Fat: 6g
Carbs: 2g
Protein: 34g

207. Air Fryer Parmesan Shrimp

Preparation Time: 15 minutes

Yield: 4 Servings

Ingredients

- 2 pounds jumbo cooked shrimp, peeled and deveined
- 4 cloves garlic, minced
- 2/3 cup parmesan cheese, grated
- 1 teaspoon pepper
- 1/2 teaspoon oregano
- 1 teaspoon basil
- 1 teaspoon onion powder
- 2 tablespoons olive oil
- Lemon, quartered

Directions

1. In a large bowl, combine garlic, parmesan cheese, pepper, oregano, basil, onion powder, and olive oil.
2. Gently toss shrimp in the mixture until evenly coated.
3. Spray air fryer basket with non-stick spray and place shrimp in a basket.
4. Cook at 350 degrees for 8-10 minutes or until seasoning on

Desserts

shrimp is browned.

5. Squeeze the lemon over the shrimp before serving.

Nutritional Information

Calories: 102
Fat: 9g
Carbs: 4g
Protein: 5g

208. Keto Air Fryer Shrimp Scampi

Preparation Time: 15 minutes
Yield: 4 Servings

Ingredients

- 4 tablespoons butter
- 1 tablespoon lemon juice
- 1 tablespoon minced garlic
- 2 teaspoons red pepper flakes
- 1 tablespoon chopped chives or 1 teaspoon dried chives
- 1 tablespoon minced basil leaves plus more for sprinkling or 1 teaspoon dried basil
- 2 tablespoons chicken stock (or white wine)
- 1 lb. defrosted shrimp (21-25 count)

Directions

1. Turn your air fryer to 330F. Place a 6 x 3 metal pan in it and allow the oven to start heating while you gather your ingredients.
2. Place the butter, garlic, and red pepper flakes into the hot 6-inch pan.
3. Allow it to cook for 2 minutes, stirring once, until the butter has melted. Do not skip this step. This is what infuses garlic into the butter, which is what makes it all taste so good.
4. Open the air fryer, add all ingredients to the pan in the order listed, stirring gently.
5. Allow shrimp to cook for 5 minutes, stirring once. At this point, the butter should be well-melted and liquid, bathing the shrimp in spiced goodness.
6. Mix very well, remove the 6-inch pan using silicone mitts, and let it rest for 1 minute on the counter. You're doing this so that you make the shrimp cook in the residual heat, rather than allowing it accidentally overcook and get rubbery.
7. Stir at the end of the minute. The shrimp should be well-cooked at this point.
8. Sprinkle with additional fresh basil leaves and enjoy.

Nutritional Information

Calories: 221
Fat: 13g
Carbs: 1g
Protein: 23g

209. Tomato Mayonnaise Shrimp

Preparation Time: 10 minutes

Yield: 4 Servings

Ingredients

- 1 pound large 21-25 count peeled, tail-on shrimp
- 3 tablespoons mayonnaise
- 1 tablespoon ketchup
- 1 tablespoon minced garlic
- 1 teaspoon sriracha
- 1/2 teaspoon smoked paprika
- 1/2 teaspoon salt For Finishing
- 1/2 cup chopped green onions green and white parts

Directions

1. In a medium bowl, mix mayo, ketchup, garlic, sriracha, paprika, and salt.
2. Add the shrimp and toss to coat with the sauce.
3. Spray the air fryer basket. Place the shrimp into the greased basket.
4. Set air fryer to 325F for 8 minutes or until shrimp are cooked, tossing halfway through and spraying with oil again.
5. Sprinkle chopped onions before serving.

Nutritional Information

Calories: 196
Fat: 9g
Carbs: 2g
Protein: 23g

POULTRY FOOD

210. Air Fryer Chicken Wings with Buffalo Sauce

Ingredients

Wings:

- 2 pounds chicken wingettes
- 1 tablespoon olive oil or avocado oil
- 1/2 teaspoon garlic powder
- 1/2 teaspoon salt
- extra oil for greasing

Buffalo Sauce:

- 1/3 cup hot pepper sauce I used Frank's Red Hot
- 1/4 cup butter ghee for paleo
- 1 tablespoon white vinegar
- 1/8 teaspoon ground chipotle pepper or cayenne pepper

Directions

Wings:

1. In a large bowl, rub olive oil on chicken wings and then sprinkle on the garlic powder and salt.
2. Rub inside of air fryer basket with a little more olive oil, avocado oil, or coconut oil.
3. Place chicken wings in a single layer in the basket.
4. Cook wings at 360°F for 25 minutes.
5. Flip wings over. Then increase the temperature to 400°F and cook for 4 more minutes.
6. Sauce:
7. While wings are cooking in the air fryer, combine hot sauce, butter, vinegar, and ground pepper in a small pot.
8. Bring sauce to a boil on medium heat while whisking everything together. Remove from heat and set aside.
9. 8.   When wings are done, add them to the sauce and coat each piece evenly.
10. Serve with blue cheese dressing and celery.

Nutritional Information

Calories: 327
Fat: 28g
Carbs: 0g
Protein: 18g

211. Keto Thai Chili Chicken Wings

Preparation Time: 25 minutes

Yield: 2 Servings

Ingredients

- 16 chicken wings drummettes (party wings)
- the cooking spray I prefer to use olive oil or coconut oil
- 1/4 cup low-fat buttermilk
- 1/2 cup almond flour
- McCormicks Grill Mates Chicken Seasoning to taste
- Thai Chili Marinade
- 3 tbsp low-sodium soy sauce
- 1 tsp ginger I used ginger in a jar
- 3 garlic cloves
- 2 green onions
- 1 tsp rice wine vinegar
- 1 tbsp Sriracha This amount produces a mild/medium spice. For spicier wings, use more Sriracha.
- 1 tsp granulated erythritol sweetener
- 1 tbsp sesame oil

Directions

1. Thai Chili Marinade
2. Combine all of the ingredients in a blender. Blend for 45-60 seconds or until the mixture is of liquid consistency.
3. Chicken
4. Wash and pat dry the chicken. Place the chicken in a Ziploc bag and drizzle the buttermilk over the chicken. Season, the chicken with the chicken seasoning. Place the Ziploc bag in the fridge to marinate for at least 30 minutes. I prefer overnight.
5. Once the chicken has marinated, add the flour to a separate Ziploc bag. Add the chicken to the bag with the meal.
6. Shake to coat the chicken thoroughly.
7. Spray the Air Fryer pan with cooking oil. I love to use olive oil or coconut.
8. Using tongs, remove the chicken from the bag and place it on the air fryer pan. It's ok to stack the chicken on top of each other. Spray cooking oil over the top of the chicken.
9. Set the timer on the air fryer for 5 minutes at a temperature of 400 degrees.
10. Allow the chicken to cook for 5 minutes. Remove the pan and shake the chicken to ensure all of the pieces are fully cooked. You can also turn each piece of chicken onto the other side using tongs.
11. Allow the chicken to cook an

Desserts

   additional 5 minutes.

12. Remove the chicken from the pan. Glaze each piece of chicken with the Thai Chili marinade using a cooking brush.

13. Return the chicken to the Air Fryer. Cook for 7-10 minutes. I allowed my chicken to cook for 10 minutes. Use your judgment here. Each Air Fryer brand is different. You can check in on your chicken at the 5-minute mark to ensure it has fully cooked on the inside.

14. Cool before serving.

Nutritional Information

Calories: 202
Fat: 11g
Carbs: 10g
Protein: 12g

212. Keto Adobo Air Fried Chicken Thighs

Preparation Time: 20 minutes
Yield: 4 Servings

Ingredients

- 4 large chicken thighs
- 2 tbsp adobo seasoning
- 1 tbsp olive oil

Directions

1. Add olive oil to bag or plate and coat chicken in it.

2. Toss chicken thighs in adobo seasoning to coat.

3. Place chicken thighs in the air fryer basket, making sure they don't touch or crowd each other.

4. Set air fryer to 350 degrees and set the timer to 10 minutes.

5. After 10 minutes, flip the chicken to the other side and cook another 10 minutes.

6. The chicken will be golden brown and 165 degrees internal temperature at the end of cooking.

Nutritional Information

Calories: 359
Fat: 24g
Carbs: 1g
Protein: 36g

213. Jalapeno Popper Stuffed Chicken Breast

Preparation Time: 30 minutes
Yield: 4 Servings

Ingredients

- 4 chicken breasts 4oz
- 2 jalapenos
- 4 oz cream cheese
- 4 oz cheddar cheese
- 8 strips bacon

Directions

1. Butterfly chicken with a sharp knife, but don't cut all the way through.
2. Spread cream cheese evenly on the inside of the chicken breasts.
3. Divide jalapeno between the two chicken breasts. Top with the cheddar cheese. And close the chicken back up.
4. Wrap each chicken breast with 2 slices of bacon
5. Place chicken in the air fryer and turn air fryer on to 370 degrees for 20 minutes.

Nutritional Information

Calories: 354
Fat: 42g
Carbs: 2g
Protein: 62g

214. Herb-Marinated Chicken Thighs

Preparation Time: 35 minutes
Yield: 4 Servings

Ingredients

- 6-10 bone-in, skin-on chicken thighs
- 1/4 cup olive oil
- 2 T lemon juice
- 2 tsp. garlic powder
- 1 tsp. Spike Seasoning, or use any all-purpose herb blend.
- 1 tsp. dried basil
- 1/2 tsp. dried oregano
- 1/2 tsp. onion powder
- 1/2 tsp. Dried sage 1/4 tsp. black pepper

Directions

1. Trim some of the skin and most of the fat from the chicken thighs. (I used kitchen shears to trim the chicken.) I like to make short slits through the skin and into the meat, but that's not essential.
2. Mix olive oil, lemon juice, garlic powder, Spike Seasoning (or another seasoning blend), dried basil, dried oregano, onion powder, dried sage, and black pepper to make the marinade.
3. Put chicken thighs in a Ziploc bag or plastic container with a snap-tight lid, add the marinade and let the chicken marinate in the fridge at least 6 hours, or all day while you're at work.
4. When it's time to cook, drain the chicken well in a colander placed in the sink and discard marinade.
5. Arrange chicken top-side down in the air fryer basket or on a baking rack and let the chicken come to room temperature while you preheat the air fryer to 360F/185C

Desserts

(if needed) or preheat the oven to 400F/200C.

6. TO COOK IN AIR FRYER: Cook chicken top-side down in the preheated air fryer for 8 minutes. Then turn the chicken thighs over and cook about 6 minutes more. After six minutes, check the chicken to see if some pieces are getting too browned and rearrange the chicken thighs in the air-fryer basket if needed. (I switched some of the outside more-browned pieces to the inside, and I think some parts would have burned if I hadn't done that.) Cook about 6 minutes more or until the chicken is well-browned with crispy skin, and the internal temperature is at least 165F/75C.

7. Serve hot. If you want to use the air fryer and need to cook two batches for a larger family, keep the first batch warm in a 200F/100C oven while the second batch cooks.

Nutritional Information

Calories: 262
Fat: 10g
Carbs: 11g
Protein: 32g

215. Air Fryer Chicken Nuggets

Preparation Time: 20 minutes

Yield: 4 Servings

Ingredients

- 1 pound Chicken Breast, cut into bite-sized nugget shapes
- 3A cup Almond Flour
- ½ cup Ground Flax Seed
- 2 Eggs
- 1 tsp Garlic Powder
- 1 tsp Salt
- M tsp Ground Black Pepper
- 1 pinch Paprika
- 2 tsp Avocado Oil

Directions

1. Grease the bottom of your air fryer with avocado oil and preheat your air fryer to 400

2. Grab 2 medium-sized bowls: In one whisk the 2 eggs together. In another, add flours and spices and whisk until thoroughly combined.

3. Add 2-3 nuggets to bowl with beaten eggs and thoroughly coat before dredging in the breading mix, making sure all sides of chicken are covered. Set aside on a plate until all of them are covered.

4. Once all chicken nuggets are coated in egg and breading, place in your air fryer basket leaving

room in between each piece of chicken so that air has a chance to flow through and make them crispy.

5. Cook on one side for 10 minutes.
6. Using tongs, carefully flip the chicken nuggets to cook for 10 more minutes or until fully cooked through.

Nutritional Information

Calories: 232
Fat: 10g
Carbs: 3g
Protein: 25g

216. Bacon Wrapped Chicken Bites

Preparation Time: 10 minutes
Yield: 4 Servings

Ingredients

- 1.25 lbs (3) boneless skinless chicken breast, cut in 1-inch chunks (about 30 pieces)
- 10 slices center-cut bacon, cut into thirds
- optional, duck sauce or Thai sweet chili sauce for dipping

Instructions

1. Preheat the air fryer.
2. Wrap a piece of bacon around each piece of chicken and secure with a toothpick.
3. Air fry, in batches in an even layer 400F for 8 minutes, turning halfway until the chicken is cooked and the bacon is browned.
4. Blot on a paper towel and serve right away.

Nutritional Information

- Calories: 98
- Fat: 4g
- Carbs: 0g
- Protein: 16g

217. Air Fryer Chicken Parmesan

Preparation Time: 25 minutes
Yield: 4 Servings

Ingredients

- 1 lb. chicken breasts, pounded thin, sliced in half or 4 chicken cutlets at approx. 4 oz. each
- 3/4 cup blanched almond flour
- 2 tablespoons coconut flour
- 1 tablespoon Italian seasoning spice blend
- 1 teaspoon salt
- 1 teaspoon pepper
- 1 egg, whisked
- 4 slices fresh mozzarella cheese - omit if paleo/whole30
- 1/2 cup marinara sauce, plus more

Desserts

- to taste
- cooking spray

Directions

1. In a mixing bowl, combine almond flour, coconut flour, Italian spices, salt, and pepper. Whisk well to combine.
2. Add 1 whisked egg to another bowl.
3. Dip chicken cutlet into the egg wash, then dip into the almond flour breading. Make sure both sides are evenly coated with breading.
4. Spray each breast with cooking spray, and add to the basket of Air Fryer.
5. Cook 8-10 minutes at 350F. Using tongs, flip sides, and top with marinara and mozzarella, if using. Cook 4-6 more minutes, until chicken is cooked through (will read at 165F). Repeat if making in batches (depending on basket size).

Nutritional Information

Calories: 360
Fat: 20g
Carbs: 8g
Protein: 30g

218. Air Fryer Keto Chicken Meatballs

Preparation Time: 12 minutes
Yield: 20 Servings

Ingredients

- 1 pound ground chicken
- 1 large egg, beaten
- ½ cup Parmesan cheese, grated
- ½ cup pork rinds, ground
- 1 teaspoon garlic powder
- 1 teaspoon paprika
- 1 teaspoon kosher salt
- ½ teaspoon pepper

Breading

- ½ cup pork rinds, ground

Directions

1. Preheat Air Fryer to 400°
2. In a large bowl, combine chicken, egg, cheese, pork rinds (1/2 cup), garlic, paprika, salt, and pepper. Roll into 1½-inch balls.
3. Roll the meatballs in the ground pork rinds.
4. Coat the air fryer basket with cooking spray, add meatballs in a single layer and cook for 12 minutes, turning once.

Nutritional Information

Calories: 360

Fat: 20g
Carbs: 8g
Protein: 30g

219. Keto Southern Fried Chicken Tenders

Preparation Time: 25 minutes

Yield: 4 Servings

Ingredients

- 4 Chicken Breasts
- 5oz (150g) Almond Flour
- 1 Large Egg
- 1/2 Tbsp Cayenne Pepper
- 1/2 Tbsp Onion Salt
- 1/2 Tbsp Garlic Powder
- 1/2 Tbsp Dried Mixed Herbs
- 1 tsp Salt
- 1 tsp Black Pepper

Directions

1. Slice up your chicken into strips, about 5-6 pieces per breast. Lay your chicken strips out on a plate.
2. Mix all your dry ingredients, except for the almond flour. Make sure they are mixed well.
3. Using half of the spice mix, you want to coat the chicken evenly. You can do this by sprinkling it from a height of about two feet above the plate. Turn over the chicken and cover the other side.
4. Hold back half of your spice mix for the next step.
5. Combine your remaining spices with your almond flour in a bowl. In a separate bowl, whisk your egg well.
6. Now it's time to make your tenders! Take the chicken one piece at a time, and dunk it into the egg, and then dunk it straight into the almond flour mixture. You will want to roll it around in the flour to make sure it is evenly coated. I'd recommend using tongs or another utensil for this, as the mixture can get pretty sticky and messy on your fingers.
7. Place the coated chicken on a greased baking rack as you go.
8. When you have all your chicken coated, you will pop the baking tray into the oven at about 350 degrees F (180C) for 22 mins, turning halfway through (Be careful that the coating doesn't stick to the rack and come away from the keto fried chicken).

Nutritional Information

Calories: 365
Fat: 20g
Carbs: 4g
Protein: 38g

Desserts

220. Chicken Strips Recipe

Preparation Time: 25 minutes

Yield: 4 Servings

Ingredients

- 2 lbs boneless, skinless chicken tenderloins
- 1 cup almond flour
- 3 tbsp tapioca starch
- 1 1/2 tsp garlic salt
- 1 tsp salt
- 2 tsp Italian seasoning
- 1/2 tsp paprika
- 2 large eggs

Instructions

1. Mix almond flour, tapioca starch, garlic salt, salt, Italian seasoning, and paprika in a shallow bowl. In a separate bowl, whisk together the eggs.
2. Dip each chicken tenderloin in the eggs then dip in the almond flour mixture to coat. Repeat with all the fillets.
3. Place the prepared chicken strips in a single layer in the basket of your Air Fryer. Cook for 20 minutes at 360 degrees F. Check for doneness (ensure no pink in the center).
4. Serve with your favorite dipping sauce or pair with sweet potato fries.

Nutritional Information

Calories: 112
Fat: 6g
Carbs: 7g
Protein: 7g

221. Chick-Fil-A Copycat Recipe

Preparation Time: 25 minutes

Yield: 8 Servings

Ingredients

Keto *Fried* Chicken Tenders

- 8 Chicken Tenders
- 24oz Jar of Dill Pickles (you only need the juice)
- 3/4 Cup Now Foods Almond Flour
- 1 tsp Salt
- 1 tsp Pepper
- 2 Eggs, beaten
- 1 1/2 Cups pork panko (Bread Crumb Substitute)
- Nutiva Organic Coconut Oil for frying

Low Carb *Copycat* Chick-Fil-A Sauce

- 1/2 Cup Mayo
- 2 tsp Yellow Mustard
- 1 tsp Lemon Juice
- 2 tbs Honey Trees Sugar-Free

Honey

- 1 tbs Organicville BBQ sauce

Directions

1. Put chicken tenders and pickle juice in a large zip lock bag and marinate for at least 1 hour, preferably overnight.
2. In a small bowl, mix almond flour, salt, and pepper
3. Create an assembly line of three bowls, one with almond flour mixture, the second with the eggs and the third with the pork panko
4. Dredge the chicken in the almond flour mixture, then in the egg and finally in the pork panko until well coated
5. Set the air fryer to 375 F and cook the chicken for about 15 minutes.
6. Low Carb Copycat Chick-Fil-A Sauce
7. In a small bowl, combine all ingredients and stir until thoroughly combined

Nutritional Information

Calories: 193
Fat: 9g
Carbs: 5g
Protein: 26g

222. Crumbed Chicken Tenderloins

Preparation Time: 25 minutes
Yield: 4 Servings

Ingredients

- 1 egg
- 1/2 cup pork rind panko breadcrumbs
- 2 tablespoons vegetable oil
- 8 chicken tenderloins

Directions

1. Preheat an air fryer to 350 degrees F (175 degrees C).
2. Whisk egg in a small bowl.
3. Mix pork rind panko breadcrumbs and oil in a second bowl
4. until the mixture becomes loose and crumbly.
5. Dip each chicken tenderloin into the bowl of an egg; shake off any residual egg. Dip chicken into the crumb mixture, making sure it is evenly and thoroughly covered.
6. Lay chicken tenderloins into the basket of the air fryer. Cook until no longer pink in the center, about 12 minutes. An instant-read thermometer inserted into the center should read at least 165 degrees F (74 degrees C).

Nutritional Information

- Calories: 253
- Fat: 11g
- Carbs: 9g
- Protein: 26g

MEAT RECIPES

223. Air Fryer Steak with Garlic Butter

Preparation Time: 25 minutes

Yield: 2 Servings

Ingredients

- 2 8 oz Ribeye steak
- salt
- freshly cracked black pepper
- olive oil

Garlic Butter

- 1 stick unsalted butter softened
- 2 Tbsp fresh parsley chopped
- 2 tsp garlic minced
- 1 tsp Worcestershire Sauce
- 1/2 tsp salt

Directions

1. Prepare Garlic Butter by mixing butter, parsley garlic, Worcestershire sauce, and salt until thoroughly combined.
2. Place in parchment paper and roll into a log. Refrigerate until ready to use.
3. Remove steak from the fridge and allow to sit at room temperature for 20 minutes. Rub a little bit of olive oil on both sides of the steak and season with salt and freshly cracked black pepper.
4. Grease your Air Fryer basket by rubbing a little bit of oil on the basket. Preheat Air Fryer to 400 degrees Fahrenheit. Once preheated, place steaks in the air fryer and cook for 12 minutes, flipping halfway through.
5. Remove from air fryer and allow to rest for 5 minutes. Top with garlic butter.

Nutritional Information

Calories: 253
Fat: 11g
Carbs: 9g
Protein: 26g

224. Air Fryer Meatloaf

Preparation Time: 25 minutes

Yield: 4 Servings

Ingredients

- 1 cup pork rind panko breadcrumbs
- ¼ cup beef broth
- ½ cup chopped mushrooms
- ½ cup shredded carrots
- ½ cup chopped onions
- 2 cloves garlic

- 2 eggs lightly beaten
- 1 Tbsp Dijon-style mustard
- 1 Tbsp Worcestershire sauce
- ½ tsp kosher salt
- 2 lbs ground beef

For glaze
- ½ cup Heinz No Sugar Added Ketchup
- ¼ cup granulated erythritol sweetener
- 2 tsp dijon mustard

Directions

1. Add pork rind panko breadcrumbs and beef broth to a small bowl and stir until breadcrumbs are coated. Set aside.
2. Add mushrooms, carrots, onions, and garlic and process until finely chopped. Place in a large bowl.
3. Add ground beef, soaked breadcrumbs, Dijon-style mustard, Worcestershire sauce, and salt to a large bowl. Mix with hands until incorporated. Form into a loaf.
4. Preheat Air Fryer to 390 degrees.
5. Place meatloaf in Air Fryer and cook for 40-45 minutes.
6. While meatloaf is cooking, prepare the glaze by combining ketchup, granulated erythritol sweetener, and dijon mustard when there are about 5 minutes left on your timer, spread glaze over meatloaf in Air Fryer.
7. Remove and allow the meatloaf to rest for 10 minutes before slicing.

Nutritional Information

Calories: 407
Fat: 15g
Carbs: 9g
Protein: 30g

225. Air Fryer Ribeye with Coffee and Spice

Preparation Time: 35 minutes
Yield: 4 Servings

Ingredients

- 1 lb. ribeye steak
- 1 1/2 tsp. coarse sea salt
- 1 tsp. granulated erythritol sweetener
- 1/2 tsp. ground coffee
- 1/2 tsp. black pepper
- 1/4 tsp. chili powder
- 1/4 tsp. garlic powder
- 1/4 tsp. onion powder
- 1/4 tsp. paprika
- 1/4 tsp. chipotle powder
- 1/8 tsp. coriander
- 1/8 tsp. cocoa powder

Desserts

Directions

1. In a small bowl - add all spices. Using a whisk - combine spices, making sure to break up the brown sugar.

2. Sprinkle a generous amount of spice mix onto a plate. Lay one steak on top of spices. Then season steak liberally with the spice mix and rub into the meat evenly. Flip to make sure the other side is seasoned correctly as well.

3. Pick up steak and press all sides into the remaining spice mix on the plate so that none of the spices are wasted.

4. Let steak sit for at least 20 minutes to come to room temperature. This helps the steak cook evenly.

5. Meanwhile - Prepare the air fryer tray by coating with the oil to prevent sticking. Preheat air fryer to 390 degrees for at least 3 minutes.

6. Cook steak undisturbed for 9 minutes. Do not flip and do not open.

7. Once cook time is finished, remove from air fryer and let rest for at least 5 minutes before slicing.

Nutritional Information

Calories: 495
Fat: 32g
Carbs: 5g
Protein: 46g

226. Air Fryer Crispy Pork Belly

Preparation Time: 25 minutes

Yield: 4 Servings

Ingredients

- 1-pound pork belly
- 3 cups water
- 1 teaspoon salt
- 1 teaspoon pepper
- 2 tablespoons soy sauce
- 2 bay leaves
- 6 cloves garlic

Directions

1. Cut the pork belly into 3 thick chunks so that it cooks more evenly.

2. Place all ingredients into the inner liner of an Instant Pot or pressure cooker. Cook the pork belly at high pressure for 15 minutes. Allow the pot to sit undisturbed for 10 minutes and then release all remaining stress. Using a set of tongs, very carefully remove the meat from the pressure cooker. Allow the chicken to drain and dry for 10 minutes.

3. If you do not have a pressure cooker, place the ingredients into a saucepan, cover, and cook for 60 minutes, until a knife can be easily inserted into the skin-side of the pork belly. Remove the meat and allow the meat to drain and dry for 10 minutes.
4. Cut each of the three chunks of pork belly into 2 long slices.
5. Place the pork belly slices in the air fryer basket. Set the air fryer to 400°F for 15 minutes or until the fat on the pork belly has crisped up, and then serve.

Nutritional Information

Calories: 594
Fat: 30g
Carbs: 2g
Protein: 11g

227. Keto Beef Satay

Preparation Time: 25 minutes
Yield: 4 Servings

Ingredients

- 1 pound beef flank steak sliced thinly into long strips
- 2 tablespoons oil
- 1 tablespoon fish sauce
- 1 tablespoon soy sauce
- 1 tablespoon minced ginger
- 1 tablespoon minced garlic
- 1 tablespoon sugar
- 1 teaspoon Sriracha or other hot sauce
- 1 teaspoon ground coriander
- 1/2 cup chopped cilantro divided
- 1/4 cup chopped roasted peanuts

Directions

1. Place beef strips into a large bowl or a ziplock bag.
2. Add oil, fish sauce, soy sauce, ginger, garlic, sugar, Sriracha, coriander, and 1/4 cup cilantro to the beef and mix well. Marinate for 30 minutes or up to 24 hours in the refrigerator.
3. Using a set of tongs, place the beef strips in the air fryer basket, laying them side by side and minimizing overlap.
4. Leave behind as much of the marinade as you can and discard this marinade.
5. Set your air fryer to 400F for 8 minutes, flipping once halfway.
6. Remove the meat to a serving tray, top with remaining 1/4 cup chopped cilantro and the chopped roasted peanuts.
7. Serve with Easy Peanut Sauce.

Desserts

Nutritional Information

Calories: 594
Fat: 30g
Carbs: 2g
Protein: 11g

228. Air Fryer Bacon

Preparation Time: 10 minutes

Yield: 11 Servings

Ingredients

- 11 slices bacon, thick-cut

Directions

1. Divide the bacon in half, and place the first half in the air fryer.
2. Set the temperature at 400 degrees and set the timer to 10 minutes (possibly less time for thinner bacon).
3. Check it halfway through to see if anything needs to be rearranged (tongs are helpful!).
4. Cook remainder of the time. Check for the desired doneness.

Nutritional Information

Calories: 91
Fat: 8g
Carbs: 0g
Protein: 2g

229. Keto Air Fryer Meatloaf Sliders

Preparation Time: 25 minutes

Yield: 8 Servings

Ingredients

- 1 lb ground beef 80/20 fat
- 2 eggs beaten
- ½ C onion finely chopped
- 1 clove garlic minced
- ½ C blanched almond flour extra fine
- ½ C coconut flour
- ½ C ketchup
- ½ tsp sea salt
- ½ tsp black pepper
- 1 Tbsp Worcestershire Sauce
- 1 tsp Italian Seasoning See below
- ½ tsp Tarragon dried

Directions

1. In a large mixing bowl, combine all the ingredients and mix well. Make patties that are about 2" in diameter and about 1" thick. If you want to make thicker or thinner patties, make sure all of them are similar in size, so they cook properly at the same time.
2. Place the patties on a platter and refrigerate for 10 minutes for the flour to absorb the wet ingredients

and the patties to become firm.

3. Preheat the air fryer to 360°F.
4. Place as many patties you can fit in the basket and close. Set the timer for 10 minutes.
5. Check the patties halfway. When the timer goes off, take them out to a serving platter and cover until all the patties are cooked.
6. These sliders are perfect on your favorite paleo bread or biscuits (P.164) or lettuce wraps or with a side of spring greens.

Nutritional Information

- Calories: 228
- Fat: 16g
- Carbs: 6g
- Protein: 13g

230. Air Fried Spicy Bacon Bites

Preparation Time: 15 minutes
Yield: 4 Servings

Ingredients

- 4 strips of bacon
- 1/4 cup hot sauce
- 1/2 cup crushed pork rinds

Directions

1. Cut uncooked bacon slices into 6 even pieces and place in a bowl.
2. Add hot sauce to a bowl, ensuring both sides of the bacon get the sauce.
3. Dip bacon pieces into crushed pork rinds, coating both sides.
4. Cook in air fryer on 350F for 10 minutes, checking around 8 minutes to ensure it's not burning.

Nutritional Information

Calories: 120
Fat: 8g
Carbs: 0g
Protein: 7g

231. Keto Lasagna

Preparation Time: 30 minutes
Yield: 4 Servings

Ingredients

- 1 cup marinara sauce
- 1 zucchini sliced into long, thin slices

For *Meat* Layer

- 1 cup diced yellow or white onion
- 1 teaspoon minced garlic
- 1/2 pound bulk hot or mild Italian sausage

For *Cheese* Layer (mix all ingredients in a bowl)

- 1/2 cup ricotta cheese
- 1/2 cup shredded mozzarella cheese
- 1/2 cup shredded parmesan,

Desserts

- divided
- 1 egg
- 1/2 teaspoon garlic minced
- 1/2 teaspoon dried Italian seasoning
- 1/2 teaspoon black pepper

Directions

1. Using a mandolin, slice the zucchini into long, thin slices.
2. Spray a 7-inch springform pan with oil and arrange the zucchini in overlapping layers in the bottom of the pan.
3. Place 1/4 cup of marinara sauce on top of the zucchini and spread evenly.
4. In a large bowl, mix the onions, garlic, and Italian sausage. Layer the meat on top of the zucchini and spread evenly.
5. Pour the rest of the marinara sauce and spread it evenly.
6. Rinse the bowl you used earlier, and mix the ricotta and mozzarella and 1/4 of a cup of the Parmesan cheese.
7. Spread the cheese mixture on top of the meat.
8. Top with the remaining 1/4 cup parmesan cheese.
9. To recap, the layer is so: zucchini, sauce, meat, sauce, cheese mix, parmesan cheese.
10. Cover the pan with foil or a silicone lid.
11. Set the air fryer to 350F and bake for 20 minutes. Then, remove the foil and cook for another 8-10 minutes at 350F until the top is browned and bubbling.
12. Allow the lasagna to rest for 10 minutes before unclasping the springform pan to serve.

Nutritional Information

Calories: 375
Fat: 27g
Carbs: 8g
Protein: 17g

VEGETABLES

232. Three Cheese Stuffed Mushrooms

Preparation Time: 15 minutes

Yield: 6 Servings

Ingredients

- 8 oz large fresh mushrooms (I used Monterrey)
- 4 oz cream cheese (I used reduced-fat)
- ½ cup parmesan cheese shredded
- 1/8 cup sharp cheddar cheese shredded
- 1/8 cup white cheddar cheese shredded
- 1 teaspoon Worcestershire sauce
- 2 garlic cloves chopped
- salt and pepper to taste

Directions

1. Cut the stem out of the mushroom to prepare it for stuffing. I first chop off the stem and then make a circular cut around the area where the stem was. Continue to cut until you have removed excess mushroom.
2. Place the cream cheese in the microwave for 15 seconds to soften.
3. Combine the cream cheese, all of the shredded cheeses, salt, pepper, and Worcestershire sauce in a medium bowl. Stir to combine.
4. Stuff the mushrooms with the cheese mixture.
5. Place the mushrooms in the Air Fryer for 8 minutes on 370 degrees.
6. Allow the mushrooms to cool before serving.

Nutritional Information

Calories: 116
Fat: 8g
Carbs: 3g
Protein: 8g

233. Air Fryer roasted Asian broccoli

Preparation Time: 20 minutes

Yield: 4 Servings

Ingredients

- 1 Lb Broccoli, Cut into florets
- 1 1/2 Tbsp Peanut oil
- 1 Tbsp Garlic, minced
- Salt
- 2 Tbsp reduced-sodium soy sauce
- 2 tsp Stevia

Desserts

- 2 tsp Sriracha
- 1 tsp Rice vinegar
- 1/3 Cup Roasted salted peanuts
  Fresh lime juice (optional)

Directions

1. In a large bowl, toss together the broccoli, peanut oil, garlic, and season with sea salt. Make sure the oil covers all the broccoli florets. I like to use my hands to give each one a quick rub.
2. Spread the broccoli into the wire basket of your air fryer, in a single of a layer, as possible, trying to leave a little bit of space between each floret.
3. Cook at 400 degrees until golden brown and crispy, about 15 - 20 minutes, stirring halfway.
4. While the broccoli and peanuts cook, mix the stevia, soy sauce, sriracha, and rice vinegar in a small, microwave-safe bowl.
5. Once mixed, microwave the mixture for 10-15 seconds.
6. Transfer the cooked broccoli to a bowl and add in the soy sauce mixture. Toss to coat and season to taste with a pinch more salt, if needed.
7. Stir in the peanuts and squeeze lime on top (if desired.)
8. Devour!

Nutritional Information

Calories: 68
Fat: 4g
Carbs: 2g
Protein: 1g

234. Cauliflower Buffalo Wings

Preparation Time: 15 minutes
Yield: 4 Servings

Ingredients

- 1 head cauliflower cut into small bites
- cooking oil spray
- 1/2 cup buffalo sauce
- 1 tablespoon butter melted
- salt and pepper to taste

Directions

1. Spray the air fryer basket with cooking oil.
2. Add the melted butter, buffalo sauce, and salt and pepper to taste to a bowl. Stir to combine.
3. Add the cauliflower bites to the air fryer. Spray with cooking oil. Cook for 7 minutes on 400 degrees.
4. Open the air fryer and place the cauliflower in a large mixing bowl. Drizzle the butter and buffalo

mixture throughout. Stir.

5. Add the cauliflower back to the air fryer. Cook for an additional 7-8 minutes on 400 degrees until the cauliflower wings are crisp. Every air fryer brand is different. Be sure to use your judgment to assist with optimal cook time.

6. Remove the cauliflower from the air fryer.

Nutritional Information

Calories: 101
Fat: 7g
Carbs: 4g
Protein: 3g

235. Air Fryer Herbed Brussels Sprouts

Preparation Time: 10 minutes

Yield: 4 Servings

Ingredients

- 1 lb. brussels sprouts (cleaned and trimmed)
- 1/2 tsp. dried thyme
- 1 tsp. dried parsley
- 1 tsp. garlic powder (Or 4 cloves, minced)
- 1/4 tsp. salt
- 2 tsp. oil

Directions

1. Place all ingredients in a medium to a large mixing bowl and toss to coat the brussels sprouts evenly.
2. Pour them into the food basket of the air fryer and close it up.
3. Set the heat to 390 F. and the time to 8 minutes. This setting roasts them nicely on the outside while leaving the insides a beautifully cooked al dente.
4. Cool slightly and serve.

Nutritional Information

Calories: 79
Fat: 2g
Carbs: 12g
Protein: 4g

236. Cilantro Ranch Sweet Potato Cauliflower Patties

Preparation Time: 20 minutes

Yield: 7 Servings

Ingredients

- 1 medium to large sweet potato, peeled
- 2 cup cauliflower florets
- 1 green onion, chopped.
- 1 tsp minced garlic
- 2 tbsp organic ranch seasoning mix or paleo ranch seasoning (dairy-free)
- 1 cup packed cilantro (fresh)
- 1/2 tsp chili powder

Desserts

- 1/4 tsp cumin
- 2 tbsp arrowroot starch or gluten-free flour of choice
- 1/4 cup ground flaxseed
- 1/4 cup sunflower seeds (or pumpkin seeds)
- 1/4 tsp Kosher Salt and pepper (or to taste)
- Dipping sauce of choice

Directions

1. Cut your peeled sweet potato into smaller pieces. Place in a food processor or blender and pulse until the larger pieces are broken up.
2. Add in your cauliflower, onion, and garlic and pulse again.
3. Add in you sunflower seeds, flaxseed, arrowroot (or flour), cilantro, and remaining seasonings. Pulse or place on medium until a thick batter is formed. See the blog for pictures.
4. Place batter in a larger bowl. Scoop 1/4 cup of the mixture out at a time and form into patties about 1.5 inches thick. Place on the baking sheet.
5. Repeat until you have about 7-10 patties.
6. Chill in the freeze for 10 minutes so the patties can set.
7. Once set, Place cauliflower patties (4 at a time) in the air fryer at 360 to 370F for 18 minutes, flipping halfway. If your patties are extra thick, they could take closer to 20 minutes.

Nutritional Information

Calories: 85
Fat: 3g
Carbs: 9g
Protein: 3g

237. Air-Fried Asparagus

Preparation Time: 15 minutes

Yield: 2 Servings

Ingredients

- 1/2 bunch of asparagus, with bottom 2 inches trimmed off
- Avocado or Olive Oil in an oil mister or sprayer
- Himalayan salt
- Black pepper

Directions

1. Place trimmed asparagus spears in the air-fryer basket. Spritz spears lightly with oil, then sprinkle with salt and a tiny bit of black pepper.
2. Place basket inside air-fryer and bake at 400° for 10 minutes.

3. Serve immediately.

Nutritional Information

Calories: 45
Fat: 3g
Carbs: 3g
Protein: 2g

238. Cauliflower Tater Tots

Preparation Time: 15 minutes

Yield: 4 Servings

Ingredients

- 1 large head of cauliflower separated into large florets
- 2 large Eggs
- 1/4 cup Coconut Flour
- 1 tsp Garlic Powder
- 1 tsp Onion Powder
- Coconut Oil spray or mist
- 1 tsp dried Parsley
- Salt and Pepper to taste

Directions

1. Separate the cauliflower into large florets.
2. In a large microwaveable bowl, add the florets and 2 tablespoons of water. Cover with a plastic wrap and microwave for 3 to 5 minutes (depending on the power of your microwave). The floret should be tender but not mushy. Initially microwave for 3 minutes. If underdone, microwave for another minute or two. Drain well.
3. Combine the florets in a chopper or food processor and process till it resembles grains of rice. Pour it in a bowl.
4. Add the beaten eggs, coconut flour, garlic powder, onion powder, dried parsley, salt, and pepper. Mix well.
5. Take a small amount of the mix and shape it like tater tots. Chill the cauliflower tots for 30 minutes.
6. Liberally grease the air fryer basket. Place the cauliflower tots in a single layer and spray with coconut oil or mist.
7. Air fry at 400 F for 12 minutes.
8. Serve hot with Paleo Ketchup or condiment of choice.

Nutritional Information

Calories: 142
Fat: 11g
Carbs: 3g
Protein: 7g

239. Air Fryer Pumpkin French Fries

Preparation Time: 15 minutes

Yield: 4 Servings

Ingredients

- 250g Pumpkin

Desserts

- 1 Tsp Thyme
- 1 Tbsp Mustard
- Salt & Pepper
- Tomato Ketchup optional

Directions

1. Peel the pumpkin, remove the seeds and slice into French Fries.
2. Place them in the Airfryer at 390 degrees for 15 minutes.
3. Halfway through, shake and season with the thyme, mustard, salt, and pepper.
4. Serve hot with tomato ketchup.

Nutritional Information

Calories: 142
Fat: 10g
Carbs: 6g
Protein: 3g

240. Air Fryer Keto Falafel

Preparation Time: 15 minutes
Yield: 4 Servings

Ingredients

- 1 cup (170g) brined lupini beans
- 1 1/2 cups (150g) thawed frozen broccoli
- 1/4 cup (60g) tahini
- 2 tbsp lemon juice
- 1 tbsp dried parsley
- 2 tsp cumin
- 2 tbsp ground chia seeds
- 1/2 tsp garlic powder
- 1/4 tsp onion powder 1/4 tsp allspice

Directions

1. Before you start, soak the lupini beans in hot water for between 30-60 minutes and then drain them. This should help to temper some of the overly briny flavors.
2. In a food processor, chop the beans and broccoli until they are in pieces about the size of a grain of rice (you can even go smaller if you have the patience!). Transfer this mixture to a medium-sized mixing bowl.
3. Add the tahini, lemon juice, and seasoning to the mixture and stir until thoroughly combined.
4. Stir in the ground chia seeds entirely and let the mixture sit for about 5 minutes so that the chia can absorb some liquid and a thick dough forms.
5. Shape the dough mixture into 12 patties - I started with a golfball-sized ball of dough, and then flattened them to be about 5cm (2 inches) across and 1cm (a little less

than 1/2 inch) thick.

6. Arrange the patties in your air fryer in a single layer, and cook at 350F(177C) for 14-15 minutes, depending on how crunchy you like them!

7. Enjoy while warm. To reheat these, I stuck them back in the air fryer for around 8 minutes at the same temp.

Nutritional Information

Calories: 188
Fat: 12g
Carbs: 5g
Protein: 11g

241. Keto Air Fryer Roasted Cauliflower with Tahini Sauce

Preparation Time: 25 minutes

Yield: 4 Servings

Ingredients

- 5 cups chopped cauliflower about 1 large head of cauliflower
- 6 cloves garlic peeled and chopped
- 4 tablespoons vegetable oil
- 1 teaspoon cumin-coriander blend
- 1/2 tsp salt

For *the* Sauce

- 2 tablespoons tahini sesame paste
- 2 tablespoons hot water
- 1 tablespoon fresh lemon juice
- 1 teaspoon minced garlic
- 1/2 teaspoon salt

Directions

1. Chop the cauliflower into evenly-sized florets and put them in a large bowl.

2. Cut each garlic clove into 3 pieces and smash them down with the side of your knife. Don't be shy about smashing the garlic. You want to expose as much of the garlicky surface area as possible so that it roasts well. Add this to the cauliflower.

3. Pour over the oil and add salt and the cumin-coriander blend. Mix well until the cauliflower is well-coated with the oil and the spices.

4. Turn your air fryer to 400F for 20 minutes and add the cauliflower, flipping once at the halfway mark.

5. Make The Sauce

6. While the cauliflower cooks, make the sauce. In a small bowl, add the Tahini, hot water, lemon juice, minced garlic, and salt.

7. As soon as you do this, you will see a curdled murky mess, and you'll wonder if you messed up. You haven't messed up. Just stir and keep stirring until you get a thick, creamy, smooth mix with the tahini

Desserts

    and water.

8. One the cauliflower is cooked, place it into a large serving bowl. Pour the tahini sauce over the cauliflower and mix well and then serve.

Nutritional Information

Calories: 207
Fat: 18g

DESSERTS

242. Chocolate Lava Cake

Preparation Time: 10 minutes
Yield: 4 Servings

Ingredients

- 1 egg
- 2 tablespoons cocoa powder
- 2 tablespoons water
- 2 tablespoons non-GMO erythritol
- 1/8 teaspoon Stevia
- 1 tablespoon golden flax meal
- 1 tablespoon coconut oil, melted
- 1/2 teaspoon aluminum-free baking powder
- dash of vanilla
- pinch of Himalayan salt

Directions

1. Whisk all ingredients in a two-cup glass Pyrex dish or ramekin.
2. Preheat air fryer at 350° for just a minute.
3. Place glass dish with cake mix into the air fryer and bake at 350° for 8-9 minutes.
4. Carefully remove dish with an oven mitt.
5. Let cool for a few minutes and then enjoy!

Nutritional Information

Calories: 173
Fat: 13g
Carbs: 4g
- Protein: 8g

243. Keto Chocolate Cake

Preparation Time: 20 minutes
Yield: 4 Servings

Ingredients

- 3 Eggs
- 1/3 cup Truvia
- 4 tablespoons butter
- 1/2 cup heavy whipping cream
- 1 teaspoon Vanilla extract
- 1/4 cup Coconut Flour
- 1 teaspoon baking powder
- 2 tablespoon unsweetened Cocoa powder
- 1/4 teaspoon salt

Frosting

- 4 tablespoons Cream cheese softened
- 4 tablespoons butter unsalted softened
- 1 tablespoon Truvia
- 1 teaspoon Vanilla extract

Desserts

Directions

1. Preheat the Breville Smart Oven Air or your regular oven to 350F degrees.
2. Grease a silicone flower cupcake mold or a 6-cup muffin pan and set aside.
3. In a large mixing bowl, melt the butter in the microwave for 30-60 seconds
4. Remove and stir in the Truvia into the butter.
5. Add in eggs, heavy whipping cream, and vanilla extract and beat with a mixer.
6. Stop the mixer and add in all the dry ingredients into the bowl.
7. Mix again until the batter is well-mixed and relatively smooth.
8. Coconut flours vary in absorbency. If the batter is thicker than regular cake batter, add in a little more heavy whipping cream and mix.
9. Pour the batter into the silicone flower cupcake mold pan (or 6-cup muffin pan). Bake for 20 minutes until the tops spring back lightly when touched and a toothpick inserted emerges clean.
10. Allow cooling
11. To make the Frosting
12. Beat together all four ingredients and spread on cooled cupcakes.

Nutritional Information

Calories: 296
Fat: 28g
Carbs: 5g
Protein: 4g

244. Air Fried Sweet Potato Dessert Fries

Preparation Time: 25 minutes
Yield: 4 Servings

Ingredients

- 2 medium sweet potatoes and yams peeled (see notes for low carb option)
- Half a tablespoon of coconut oil.
- 1 tablespoon arrowroot starch or cornstarch
- Optional 2 tsp melted butter (for coating)
- 1/4 cup coconut sugar or raw sugar
- 1 to 2 tablespoons cinnamon
- Optional powdered sugar for dusting (see notes for sugar-free option)
- Dipping Sauces -
- Dessert Hummus
- Honey or Vanilla Greek Yogurt

- Maple Frosting {vegan}

Directions

1. Peel your sweet potatoes and wash them with clean water, then dry.
2. Slice peeled sweet potatoes lengthwise, 1/2 inch thick.
3. Toss your sweet potato slices in 1/2 tbsp coconut oil and arrowroot starch (or cornstarch)
4. Place in the air fryer for 18 minutes at 370F. Shake halfway at 8-9 minutes.
5. Remove the fries from the air fryer and place it in a large bowl. Drizzle 2 tsp optional butter on top of chips. Then mix in cinnamon and sugar and toss fries together again.
6. Place on a plate to serve, sprinkle with powdered sugar.
7. Serve fries with a dipping sauce of choice. To store, keep chips wrapped in foil and fridge. Then reheat in the oven again to warm before serving. Should keep for 2-3 days.
8. For low sugar/carb options:
9. Replace the sweet potato with peeled jicama sticks (baking times are similar)
10. Use swerve sugar sweetener in place of powdered sugar and other sugars.

Nutritional Information
Calories: 181
Fat: 11g
Carbs: 6g
Protein: 6g

245. Easy Coconut Pie

Preparation Time: 45 minutes
Yield: 6 Servings

Ingredients

- 2 eggs
- 1 1/2 cups milk (you can use coconut milk or almond milk)
- 1/4 cup butter
- 1 1/2 tsp. vanilla extract
- 1 cup shredded coconut
- 1/2 cup Monk Fruit (or your preferred sugar)
- 1/2 cup coconut flour

Directions

1. In a large bowl, add in all the ingredients and using a wooden spoon stir until well blended.
2. Coat a 6" pie plate with nonstick spray and fill it with the batter.
3. Cook in the Air Fryer at 350 degrees for 10 to 12 minutes. Check the pie halfway through the cooking time to be sure it is not burning, give the plate a turn, use a

Desserts

toothpick to test for doneness. Continue to cook accordingly.

4. Toast ½ cup of shredded coconut either in the oven or in a small fry pan for garnish (*optional*)
5. Fresh pie and garnish with shredded coconut and powdered sugar.
6. Keep leftovers refrigerated.

Nutritional Information

Calories: 281
Fat: 16g
Carbs: 18g
Protein: 3g

246. Air Fried Cheesecake Bites

Preparation Time: 10 minutes
Yield: 4 Servings

Ingredients

- 8 ounces cream cheese
- 1/2 cup erythritol
- 2 Tablespoons cream, divided
- 1/2 teaspoon vanilla extract
- 1/2 cup almond flour
- 2 Tablespoons erythritol

Directions

1. Allow the cream cheese to sit on the counter for 20 minutes to soften.
2. Fit a stand mixer with the paddle attachment.
3. Mix the softened cream cheese, 1/2 cup erythritol, vanilla, and heavy cream until smooth.
4. Scoop onto a parchment paper-lined baking sheet.
5. Freeze for about 30 minutes, until firm
6. Mix the almond flour with the 2 Tablespoons erythritol in a small mixing bowl.
7. Dip the frozen cheesecake bites into 2 Tablespoons cream, then roll into the almond flour mixture.
8. Place in an air fryer for 5 minutes.

Nutritional Information

Calories: 90
Fat: 3g
Carbs: 16g
Protein: 1g

247. Chocolate Brownies

Preparation Time: 35 minutes
Yield: 4 Servings

Ingredients

- 1/2 cup sugar-free chocolate chips
- 1/2 cup butter
- 3 eggs
- 1/4 cup Truvia or another sweetener

- 1 tsp Vanilla extract

Instructions

1. In a microwave-safe bowl, melt butter and chocolate for about 1 minute. Remove and stir well. You want to use the heat within the butter and chocolate to melt the rest of the clumps. If you microwave until it's all melted, you've overcooked the chocolate. So get a spoon and start stirring. Add 10 seconds if needed but mix well before you decide to do that.
2. In a bowl, add eggs, sweetener, and vanilla and blend until light and frothy.
3. Pour the melted butter and chocolate into the bowl in a slow stream and beat again until it is well-incorporated.
4. Pour the mixture into greased springform container or cake pan and bake at 350F for 30-35 minutes until a knife inserted in the center emerges clean.
5. Serve with whipped cream if desired

Nutritional Information

Calories: 224
Fat: 23g
Carbs: 3g
Protein: 4g

248. Apple Cider Vinegar Donuts

Preparation Time: 10 minutes

Yield: 4 Servings

Ingredients

For the Muffins

- 4 large eggs
- 4 tbsp coconut oil melted
- 3 tbsp Truvia or any other stevia you like
- 2/3 cup apple cider vinegar
- 1 cup coconut flour
- 1 tsp cinnamon
- 1 tsp baking soda
- pinch salt

Instructions

1. Preheat oven to 350 F. Prepares a donut baking pan by spraying liberally with cooking spray or greasing well with coconut oil.
2. In a small bowl, whisk together the eggs, salt, stevia, apple cider vinegar, and melted coconut oil.
3. In a separate bowl, sift together cinnamon, baking soda, and coconut flour to disperse the dry ingredients well.
4. Add the dry ingredients to the wet ingredients until thoroughly combined. The batter will be a bit wet.

Desserts

5. Transfer the batter to the donut baking pan and scoop the mixture into the cavities. Use your fingers to spread the batter evenly in the hole.
6. Bake at 350 F for 10 minutes until golden around the edges.
7. Remove from the oven and cool in the baking 5-10 minutes before flipping onto a wire rack to remove. These must be cool before you remove; otherwise, they will fall apart. They need to be a bit hard!
8. Devour!

Nutritional Information

Calories: 179
Fat: 11g
Carbs: 9g
Protein: 6g

249. Air-Fried Spiced Apples

Preparation Time: 15 minutes

Yield: 4 Servings

Ingredients

- 4 small apples, sliced 2 tablespoons ghee or coconut oil, melted
- 1 cup granulated erythritol sweetener 1 teaspoon apple pie spice
- Directions
- Place the apples in a bowl. Drizzle with ghee or coconut oil and sprinkle with erythritol and apple pie spice. Stir to coat the apples evenly.
- Place the apples in the air-fryer basket.
- Set the air fryer to 350° for 10 minutes. Pierce the apples with a fork to ensure they are tender. If needed, place back in the air fryer for an additional 3-5 minutes.
- Serve with ice cream or whipped topping.

Nutritional Information

Calories: 112
Fat: 8g
Carbs: 2g
Protein: 3g

250. Air Fryer Brazilian Pineapple

Preparation Time: 25 minutes

Yield: 4 Servings

Ingredients

- 1 small pineapple peeled, cored and cut into spears
- 1/2 cup brown sugar
- 2 teaspoons ground cinnamon
- 3 tablespoons melted butter

Instructions

1. In a small bowl, mix brown sugar and cinnamon.
2. Brush the pineapple spears with the melted butter. Sprinkle cinnamon sugar over the spears, pressing lightly to ensure it adheres well.
3. Place the spears into the air fryer basket in a single layer. Depending on the size of your air fryer, you may have to do this in batches. Set fryer to 400°F for 10 minutes for the first batch (6-8 minutes for the next installment as your air fryer will be preheated). Halfway through, brush with any remaining butter.
4. Pineapple spears are done when they are heated through, and the sugar is bubbling.

Nutritional Information

Calories: 295
Fat: 11g
Carbs: 40g
Protein: 2g

251. Coconut-Encrusted Cinnamon Bananas

Preparation Time: 25 minutes
Yield: 4 Servings

Ingredients

- 4 ripe but firm Bananas cut into thirds
- 1/2 cup Tapioca Flour
- 2 large Eggs
- 1 cup Shredded Coconut Flakes
- 1 tsp Ground Cinnamon
- Coconut spray

Instructions

1. Cut each banana into thirds
2. Make an assembly line -
3. Pour the tapioca flour into a shallow dish.
4. Crack the eggs in another shallow bowl and whisk it lightly.
5. Combine the shredded coconut and the ground cinnamon in the third shallow dish. Mix well.
6. Dredge the bananas in tapioca flour and shake off the excess.
7. Dip it in the beaten eggs. Make sure it is completely coated in egg wash.
8. Roll the bananas in the cinnamon-coconut flakes to coat it thoroughly. Press it firmly to make sure the coconut flakes are adhering to the bananas. Keep them in a flat tray.
9. Liberally spray the air fryer basket with coconut oil.
10. Arrange the coconut-crusted bananas pieces in the fryer basket. Spray with more coconut spray.

Desserts

11. Air fry at 270F for 12 minutes
12. Dust with ground cinnamon and serve warm or at room temperature with a scoop of Low Carb ice-cream (optional).

Nutritional Information

Calories: 155
Fat: 11g
Carbs: 20g
Protein: 2g

VEGETABLE RECIPES OF KETO

BREAKFAST

252. Cauliflower Waffles

Preparation Time: 10 Minutes
Cooking Time: 10 Minutes
Servings: 4

Ingredients:

- ½ large head cauliflower, riced
- 1 cup mozzarella cheese, finely shredded
- 1 cup packed collard greens
- 1 egg
- 1/4 cup Parmesan cheese
- 1 tablespoon sesame seed
- 2 stalks green onion
- 2 tablespoons olive oil
- 2 teaspoons fresh thyme, chopped
- 1 teaspoon garlic powder
- ½ teaspoon ground black pepper
- ½ teaspoon salt

Directions:

1. Grind cauliflower florets with spring onion, collard veggies, and thyme in a meals processor.
2. Toss this combination with 1 cup Mozzarella cheese, egg, /4 cup Parmesan
3. Cheese. 1 tablespoon olive oil, 1 tablespoon sesame seeds, ½ teaspoon black pepper, ½ teaspoon salt, and 1 teaspoon garlic powder in a blending bowl.
4. Once the combination bureaucracy, an even mixture adds a ¼ cup of this batter inside the waffle iron.
5. Let the batter cook inside the iron as according to the machine's instructions.
6. Use the last batter to make more waffles.
7. Enjoy fresh.

Nutrition:

Calories: 203 Cal
Fat: 15.3 g
Carbs: 5 g

Protein: 14.6 g

Morning Bullet Coffee

Preparation Time: 10 Minutes
Cooking Time: 5 Minutes
Servings: 2

Ingredients:

- 1 oz. cacao butter
- 2 tablespoons coconut oil
- 2 tablespoons almond butter

Desserts

- 1/4 cup almond milk 2 cups of coffee, brewed

Directions:

1. Add cocoa butter, almond butter and coconut oil to a jug and warm them within the microwave for 20 seconds. Add almond milk and warmth greater for 30 seconds.
2. Stir in espresso and mix well using a handheld blender till foamy.
3. Serve fresh.

Nutrition:

Calories: 171 Cal Fat: 10.3 g Carbs: 7 g Protein: 14.3 g

253. Tofu Quiche Cups

Preparation Time: 10 Minutes
Cooking Time: 35 Minutes
Servings: 4

Ingredients:

- 1 (14 oz.) block extra firm tofu
- 3 tablespoon water
- 2 teaspoon garlic seasoning
- 1 tablespoon sugar- free ketchup
- 2 tablespoon dijon mustard
- 1 tablespoon lemon juice
- 1 tablespoon arrowroot powder
- 1/2 cup nutritional yeast
- 3.5 cups leafy greens

Directions:

1. Let your oven to preheat at 350 ranges F. Layer a muffin tin with muffin liners. Blend everything besides leafy veggies, in a blender until smooth. If the mixture is too thick, upload a few drops of water and blend again.
2. Stir in leafy veggies and mix till it forms an even aggregate. Divide the organized batter within the muffin tin and bake for 35 minutes until golden brown.
3. Enjoy warm and fresh.

Nutrition:

Calories: 231 Cal Fat: 14.3 g Carbs: 3.7 g Protein: 7.6 g

254. Cinnamon & Pecan Porridge

Preparation Time: 10 Minutes
Cooking Time: 5 Minutes
Servings: 2

Ingredients:

- 1/4 cup coconut milk
- 3/4 cup unsweetened almond milk
- 1/4 cup almond butter, roasted
- 1 tablespoon coconut oil
- 2 tablespoon whole chia seeds
- 2 tablespoon hemp seeds
- 1/4 cup pecans, chopped

- 1/4 cup unsweetened coconut, toasted
- 1/2 teaspoon cinnamon
- Stevia to taste

Directions:

1. Mix coconut milk with almond butter, almond butter and coconut oil in a saucepan. Cook the mixture on a simmer over medium warmness then add chia seeds, pecans, cinnamon, stevia, hemp seeds, and toasted coconut. Mix well and set it apart for 10 minutes approximately, then divide it in the serving bowls. Garnish with coconut shred.
2. Serve fresh.

Nutrition:

- Calories: 108 Cal Fat: 9 g
- Carbs: 2.7 g Protein: 6 g

255. Superfood Breakfast Bowl

Preparation Time: 10 Minutes
Cooking Time: 0
Servings: 1

Ingredients:

1. 1 cup almond milk
2. 2 tablespoon chia seeds
3. 1/4 cup protein powder
4. 5 tablespoon hemp seeds
5. 2 tablespoon unsweetened coconut flakes
6. ¼ cup mixed berries
7. 1 tablespoon pecans, chopped 1 tablespoon walnuts, chopped

Directions:

- Add protein powder, milk, hemp seeds, chia seeds and coconut to a mason
- jar.
- Seal the jar and mix well, then region the jar in the refrigerator for overnight.
- Garnish with chopped nuts and berries.
- Serve fresh.

Nutrition:

Calories: 231 Cal
Fat: 19.3 g
Carbs: 2.7 g
Protein: 32.6 g

256. Strawberry Chia Pudding

Preparation Time: 10 Minutes
Cooking Time: 0
Servings: 2

Ingredients:

- 1 ½ cup of coconut milk
- 2 cups strawberries, fresh
- ½ tablespoon almond butter
- 2 pinches sea salt

Desserts

- Stevia, to taste
- ½ cup chia seeds
- 1 tablespoon MCT coconut oil
- Garnish: 1 handful of berries
- 4 tablespoons keto granola

Directions:
1. Blend strawberries, coconut milk, salt and almond butter in a meals processor.
2. Add stevia to sweeten the mixture.
3. Spread the chia seeds in the bowl and pour the strawberry aggregate over chia seeds.
4. Refrigerate this bowl overnight until it thickens.
5. Garnish with your preferred berries.
6. Enjoy fresh.

Nutrition:
Calories: 118 Cal
Fat: 9.3 g
Carbs: 1.7 g
Protein: 12.6 g

257. Blueberry Coconut Porridge

Preparation Time: 10 Minutes
Cooking Time: 0
Servings: 2

Ingredients:
Porridge

- 1/4 cup ground flaxseed
- 1 cup almond milk 1 teaspoon cinnamon
- 1 teaspoon vanilla extract
- 1/4 cup coconut flour liquid stevia, to taste
- 1 pinch salt

Toppings

- ¼ cup blueberries
- 2 tablespoon butter
- 2 tablespoon pumpkin seeds
- 1 oz. shaved coconut

Directions:
1. Warm almond milk in a saucepan then provides flaxseed, salt, cinnamon, and coconut flour.
2. Mix nicely till smooth.
3. Cook till it bubbles.
4. Add vanilla extract and liquid stevia.
5. Mix properly then garnish with preferred toppings blueberries, cold butter, shaved coconut, and pumpkin seeds.
6. Serve fresh.

Nutrition:
Calories: 231 Cal
Fat: 13.3 g
Carbs: 4 g

Protein: 14.6 g

258. Raspberry Pancakes

Preparation Time: 10 Minutes
Cooking Time: 8 Minutes
Servings: 4

Ingredients:

- 1 teaspoon coconut flour
- 1/4 teaspoon baking powder
- 1/16 teaspoon Stevia
- 1/4 teaspoon cinnamon
- 1 tablespoon coconut oil 1 pinch salt
- 1/4 cup almond flour
- 1 tablespoon raspberries 2 tablespoons almond milk

Directions:

1. Blend all of the dry gadgets in a meals processor then add the wet ingredients.
2. Fold in raspberries and mix properly till smooth.
3. Warm-up a tablespoon of coconut oil in a flat pan and upload a dollop of raspberry batter.
4. Spread it into a pancake and cook for two minutes consistent with side.
5. Use the ultimate batter to make more pancakes.
6. Enjoy fresh.

Nutrition:
Calories: 91
Fat: 13.3g
Carbs: 7.3g
Protein: 22.6g

259. Raspberry Chia Pudding

Preparation Time: 10 Minutes
Cooking Time: 0
Servings: 1

Ingredients:

- 1 cup fresh raspberries
- 1 cup of coconut milk
- 1/2 cup almond milk
- 1/2 cup whole chia seeds
- 3 teaspoons unsweetened vanilla extract
- Stevia to taste

Directions:

1. Blend raspberries with water and coconut milk in a food processor.
2. Keep few raspberries aside for garnishing.
3. Add chia seeds, vanilla and occasional carb sweetener to the raspberry aggregate.
4. Mix nicely and refrigerate the pudding overnight.
5. Garnish with raspberries and serve fresh.

Nutrition:

Desserts

Calories: 153 Cal Fat: 5.3 g
Carbs: 4.4 g
Protein: 4.6 g

260. Chia Berry Yogurt Parfaits

Preparation Time: 10 Minutes
Cooking Time: 0
Servings: 2

Ingredients:

Chia *pudding*:

- 1/2 cup heavy cream
- 1/3 cup chia seeds
- 1/4 teaspoon vanilla powder
- 1/4 teaspoon ground cinnamon
- 2/3 cup water
- 1 tablespoon powdered Erythritol
- Layers:
- 1 cup full-fat yogurt 1 cup mixed frozen berries Coconut & seed crumble:
- 2 tablespoon pumpkin seeds
- 1/3 cup flaked coconut, toasted
- 2 tablespoon sunflower seeds

Directions:

1. Add all of the components for chia pudding to a jar and go away it within the fridge overnight.
2. Defrost the berries and crush them in a bowl to make a paste.
3. Prepare the crumble by using mixing all the elements in a separate bowl.
4. Assemble the parfaits via including layers of beaten berries and yogurt within the serving glass.
5. Serve fresh.

Nutrition:

Calories: 211 Cal
Fat: 14.3 g
Carbs: 5 g
Protein: 11.6g

261. Warm Quinoa Breakfast Bowl

Preparation Time: 5 Minutes
Cooking Time: 0
Servings: 4

Ingredients

- 3 cups freshly cooked quinoa
- 1 ⅓ cups unsweetened soy or almond milk
- 2 bananas, sliced
- 1 cup raspberries
- 1 cup blueberries
- ½ cup chopped raw walnuts
- ¼ cup maple syrup

Directions

1. Preparing the Ingredients
2. Divide the substances among four bowls, beginning with a base of ¾

cup quinoa, ⅓ cup milk, ½ banana, ¼ cup raspberries, ¼ cup blueberries, and 2 tablespoons walnuts.

3. Drizzle 1 tablespoon of maple syrup over the top of every bowl.

Nutrition:

Calories: 201 Cal
Fat: 15.3 g
Carbs: 3 g
Protein: 8.6 g

262. Banana Bread Rice Pudding

Preparation Time: 5 Minutes
Cooking Time: 50 Minutes
Servings: 4

Ingredients

- 1 cup of brown rice
- 1½ cups water
- 1½ cups nondairy milk
- 3 tablespoons sugar (omit if using sweetened nondairy milk)
- 2 teaspoons pumpkin pie spice or ground cinnamon
- 2 bananas
- 3 tablespoons chopped walnuts or sunflower seeds (optional)

Directions

1. In a medium pot, integrate the rice, water, milk, sugar, and pumpkin pie spice. Bring to a boil over excessive warmth, turn the warmth to low, and cowl the pot. Simmer, occasionally stirring, until the rice is tender and the liquid is absorbed. White rice takes approximately 20 minutes; brown rice takes about 50 minutes.

2. Smash the bananas and stir them into the cooked rice. Serve crowned with walnuts (if using). Leftovers will be refrigerated in an airtight box for up to five days.

Nutrition:

Calories: 479 Cal
Protein: 9 g
Fat: 13 g
Carbs: 86 g
Fiber: 7 g

263. Apple and Cinnamon Oatmeal

Preparation Time: 10 Minutes
Cook Time: 10 Minutes
Servings: 2

Ingredients

- 1¼ cups apple cider
- 1 apple, peeled, cored, and chopped
- ⅔ cup rolled oats
- 1 teaspoon ground cinnamon
- 1 tablespoon pure maple syrup or agave (optional)

Directions

1. Preparing the Ingredients.
2. In a medium saucepan, carry the apple cider to a boil over medium-

Desserts

excessive warmness. Stir inside the apple, oats, and cinnamon.

3. Bring the cereal to a boil and turn down warmth to low. Simmer till the oatmeal thickens, three to four minutes. Spoon into bowls and sweeten with maple syrup, if using. Serve hot.

Nutrition:

Calories: 216 Cal
Fat: 8.3 g
Carbs: 7 g
Protein: 9.6g

264. Cinnamon Muffins

Preparation Time: 15 Minutes
Cooking Time: 10 Minutes
Servings: 20

Ingredients:

- ½ cup coconut oil, melted
- ½ cup pumpkin puree
- ½ cup almond butter
- 1 tbsp. cinnamon
- 1 tsp baking powder
- 2 scoops vanilla protein powder
- ½ cup almond flour

Directions:

1. Preheat the oven to one hundred eighty C/ 350 F.
2. Spray a muffin tray with cooking spray and set aside.
3. Add all dry substances into the large bowl and mix properly.
4. Add moist substances and mix them until properly combined. Pour batter into the organized muffin tray and bake in preheated oven for 15 minutes.
5. Serve and enjoy.

Nutrition:

Calories: 80 Cal Fat: 7.1 g Carbs: 1.6 g Protein: 3.5 g

265. Chocolate Strawberry Milkshake

Preparation Time: 5 Minutes
Cooking Time: 0
Servings: 2

Ingredients:

- 1 cup ice cubes
- ¼ cup unsweetened cocoa powder
- 2 scoops vegan protein powder
- 1 cup strawberries
- 2 cups unsweetened coconut milk

Directions:

1. Add all elements into the blender and blend it till easy and creamy.
2. Serve at once and enjoy it.

Nutrition:

Calories: 221 Cal
Fat: 5.7 g
Carbs: 15 g
Protein: 27.7 g

MAIN DISHES

266. Creamy Brussels Sprouts Bowls

Preparation Time: 10 Minutes
Cooking Time: 30 Minutes
Servings: 4

Ingredients:

- 1 tablespoon olive oil
- 1-pound Brussels sprouts, trimmed and halved
- 1 cup coconut cream
- ½ teaspoon chili powder
- ½ teaspoon gram masala ½ teaspoon garlic powder
- A pinch of salt and black pepper
- 1 tablespoon lime juice

Directions:

1. In a roasting pan, combine the sprouts with the cream, chili powder and the opposite ingredients, toss, introduce in the oven at 380 degrees F and bake for 30 minutes.
2. Divide into bowls and serve for lunch.

Nutrition:

Calories: 219 Cal
Fat: 18.3 g
Fiber: 5.7 g
Carbs: 14.1 g
Protein: 5.4 g

267. Green Beans and Radishes Bake

Preparation Time: 10 Minutes
Cooking Time: 25 Minutes
Servings: 4

Ingredients:

- 2 tablespoons olive oil
- 1-pound green beans, trimmed and halved
- 2 cups radishes, sliced
- 1 cup coconut cream
- 1 teaspoon sweet paprika
- 1 cup cashew cheese, shredded
- Salt and black pepper to the taste
- 1 tablespoon chives, chopped

Directions:

1. In a roasting pan, integrate the green beans with the radishes and the other ingredients besides the cheese and toss. Sprinkle the cheese on top, introduce inside the oven at 375 ranges F and bake for 25 minutes. Divide the mixture between plates and serve.

Nutrition:

Calories: 130 Cal
Fat: 1 g
Fiber: 0.4 g

Desserts

Carbs: 1 g
Protein: 0.1 g

268. Green Goddess Buddha Bowl

Preparation Time: 10 Minutes
Cooking Time: 5 Minutes
Servings: 1

Ingredients:

- 2 cups fresh spinach
- 2 tablespoons avocado oil
- 4 broccoli spears ⅛ teaspoon salt
- ⅛ teaspoon freshly ground black pepper
- ⅓ cup frozen cauliflower rice, thawed
- 2 tablespoons shredded carrots
- ½ avocado, sliced
- 1 tablespoon almond butter, melted
- 1 tablespoon minced fresh cilantro

Directions:

1. Place the spinach within the bottom of a medium serving bowl. In a skillet over medium-excessive warmth, warmth the avocado oil. Add the broccoli and sauté for 2 to three mins. Season with the salt and pepper and transfer it to the bowl containing the spinach. Add the cauliflower rice to the skillet and cook dinner for 3 mins. Add it to the serving bowl. Top with the carrots and avocado.
2. Drizzle with the melted almond butter, sprinkle the cilantro on the pinnacle, and serve.

Nutrition:

Calories: 571
Cal Fat: 51 g
Protein: 9 g
Carbs: 19 g
Fiber: 11 g

269. Zucchini Sage Pasta

Preparation Time: 10 Minutes
Cooking Time: 5 Minutes
Servings: 1

Ingredients:

- 1 tablespoon grass-fed butter
- 1 tablespoon dried sage
- ¼ teaspoon ground nutmeg
- 1 zucchini, spiralizer
- 2 ounces' tofu, chopped
- 1 cup fresh spinach leaves ½ cup grated Parmesan cheese

Directions:

1. In a skillet over medium-excessive heat, melt the butter.
2. Add the sage and nutmeg and stir until fragrant, 1 to 2 minutes.
3. Stir within the zucchini and tofu, and cook dinner, stirring, for three to 4 minutes.

4. Next, add the spinach and cook for a further minute till the spinach wilts.
5. Remove from the heat and pinnacle with the Parmesan cheese.
6. Serve warm.

Nutrition:

Calories: 399 Cal
Fat: 27 g
Protein: 27 g
Carbs: 12 g
Fiber: 4 g

270. Broccoli Stir-Fry

Preparation Time: 5 Minutes
Cooking Time: 10 Minutes
Servings: 1

Ingredients:

- 1 cup fresh spinach
- 1 tablespoon coconut oil
- ½ cup broccoli florets
- 1 cup frozen cauliflower rice
- 2 ounces' seitan strips or cubes
- 1 tablespoon toasted sesame oil
- 1 tablespoon soy sauce
- ½ avocado, sliced

Directions:

1. In a dry, nonstick pan over medium heat, wilt the spinach leaves. Remove from the heat and transfer to a serving plate.
2. Turn the temperature up to medium-high, and inside the same skillet, soften the coconut oil. Add the broccoli and frozen cauliflower rice—Cook for 5 to 6 minutes or till tender.
3. Place the greens at the wilted spinach. Top with the seitan.
4. In a small bowl, mix the sesame oil and soy sauce.
5. Pour the dressing over the seitan and greens. Top with the avocado slices and revel in warm.

Nutrition:

Calories: 664 Cal
Fat: 44 g
Protein: 49 g
Carbs: 18 g
Fiber: 13 g

271. Kale and Cashew Stir-Fry

Preparation Time: 5 Minutes
Cooking Time: 5 Minutes
Servings: 1

Ingredients:

- 1 tablespoon coconut oil
- 1 cup frozen cauliflower rice (or pearls)
- ½ cup frozen stir-fry vegetables
- 1 cup de-stemmed and torn kale (small pieces)

Desserts

- 3 tablespoons tamari sauce or low-sodium soy sauce
- ⅓ cup chopped cashews

Directions:

1. In a skillet over medium warmth, melt the coconut oil. Add the cauliflower, stir-fry vegetables, and kale, and cook for 2 to 3 mins, or until soft however nevertheless crisp.
2. Pour within the tamari and toss the vegetables till they are lined with the sauce.
3. Transfer the stir-fry to a serving dish, top with the cashews, and enjoy.

Nutrition:

Calories: 523
Cal Fat: 35 g
Protein: 18 g
Carbs: 34 g
Fiber: 6 g

272. Tofu Green Bean Casserole

Preparation Time: 15 Minutes
Cooking Time: 25 Minutes
Servings: 1

Ingredients:

- Nonstick cooking spray
- 1 cauliflower head, chopped into florets
- 2 tablespoons coconut oil
- ¼ cup chopped onion
- 14 ounces' green beans, trimmed
- 1 tablespoon salt
- ¼ teaspoon freshly ground black pepper
- ¾ cup full-fat coconut milk
- 10 ounces' tofu
- 2 cups grated Parmesan cheese cup shredded mozzarella cheese

Directions:

1. Preheat the oven to 250°F. Grease a 9-by-13-inch casserole dish with cooking spray.
2. Put the cauliflower florets in a microwave-safe dish. Add 1 to two tablespoons of water and cowl the dish with plastic wrap— Microwave the cauliflower for 8 mins, or until smooth sufficient to mash.
3. While, the cauliflower is cooking, heat a skillet over medium warmness and soften the coconut oil. Add the onions and green beans, and cook until slightly tender and bright inexperienced.
4. Once the cauliflower is cooked, switch it to a high-powered blender. Add the salt, pepper, and coconut milk. Pulse until creamy.

5. Spread the cauliflower mash in an even layer within the prepared casserole dish. Place the inexperienced beans on the pinnacle of the mash, and then crumble the tofu on the pinnacle.
6. Cover with the Parmesan and mozzarella cheeses.
7. Bake the casserole for 15 mins. For a tacky bubbly crust, broil the casserole uncovered below a low heat for 1 to 2 mins.

Nutrition:

Calories: 297 Cal
Fat: 21 g
Protein: 18 g
Carbs: 9 g
Fiber: 3 g

273. Creamy Stuffed Peppers

Preparation Time: 10 Minutes
Cooking Time: 15 Minutes
Servings: 2

Ingredients:

- 2 green bell peppers, halved and deseeded
- 1 tablespoon olive oil ¼ cup chopped onion
- 1 teaspoon minced garlic
- 1 cup fresh spinach
- 12 ounces full-fat ricotta cheese 1 large egg
- 1 teaspoon dried basil
- 8 tablespoons grated Parmesan cheese

Directions:

1. Preheat the oven to 350°F. Line a baking sheet with aluminum foil.
2. Place the bell peppers at the baking sheet, cut-aspect up, and bake for 10 minutes. Set aside.
3. While the peppers are baking, set a skillet over medium-high heat and pour within the olive oil. Add the onion, garlic, and spinach and sauté for 2 mins, or till the spinach is wilted.
4. Transfer the combination to a mixing bowl. Stir inside the ricotta cheese, egg, and basil. Mix well.
5. Fill every pepper half with identical quantities of filling and top with 2 tablespoons of Parmesan cheese.
6. Return the peppers to the oven and bake for an additional 5 mins. Remove and serve.

Nutrition:

Calories: 546
Fat: 38g
Protein: 33g
Carbs: 18g
Fiber: 3g

Desserts

274. Zucchini Pizza Boats

Preparation Time: 10 Minutes
Cooking Time: 30 Minutes
Servings: 1

Ingredients:

- 1 medium zucchini, halved lengthwise and deseeded
- 2 tablespoons olive oil
- 2 garlic cloves, minced 1 cup fresh spinach
- 2 tablespoons low-sugar marinara sauce
- 8 ounces full-fat ricotta cheese

Directions:

1. Line a baking sheet with aluminum foil.
2. Place the zucchini, hollow-facet up, on the prepared baking sheet.
3. In a small skillet over medium-excessive warmth, heat the olive oil.
4. Add the garlic and stir for 1 to two mins or till fragrant; then upload the spinach and stir until it wilts.
5. Divide the spinach aggregate calmly between the zucchini halves. Top lightly with the marinara sauce and ricotta cheese.
6. Bake for 20 to 25 mins, or till the cheese is melted and the zucchini is tender.

Nutrition: Calories: 689 Cal Fat: 57 g
Protein: 28 g
Carbs: 16 g
Fiber: 3 g

275. Vegan Coconut Curry

Preparation Time: 15 Minutes
Cooking Time: 30 Minutes
Servings: 4

Ingredients:

- 2 tablespoons olive oil
- ½ yellow onion, diced
- 3 garlic cloves, minced
- ½ tablespoon minced fresh ginger
- 1 teaspoon gram masala
- 1 teaspoon curry powder
- 1 teaspoon ground cumin
- 1 (14-ounce) can dice, no-sugar-added tomatoes
- 3 (14-ounce) cans full-fat coconut milk
- 1 cauliflower head, cut into florets
- 2 large zucchinis, diced 1 cup chopped cashews

Directions:

1. In a stockpot over medium-excessive warmness, warm the olive oil. Add the onion and sauté for two to three minutes.

2. Stir in the garlic, ginger, gram masala, curry powder, cumin, and tomatoes—Cook for two minutes.

3. Pour inside the coconut milk and produce the mixture to a low simmer. Reduce the warmth to low and simmer for five mins. Stir in the cauliflower and zucchini and simmer for an additional 20 minutes.

4. Top with the chopped cashews and serve.

Nutrition:

Calories: 997 Cal
Fat: 89 g
Protein: 15 g
Carbs: 34 g
Fiber: 12 g

276. Chiles Rellenos

Preparation Time: 15 Minutes
Cooking Time: 50 Minutes
Servings: 8

Ingredients:

- Nonstick cooking spray
- 8 poblano chiles
- 1 tablespoon olive oil
- ½ onion, chopped
- 2 garlic cloves, minced
- 1 cup chopped button mushrooms
- 4 cups fresh spinach ½ cup sour cream
- ½ cup heavy (whipping) cream 16 ounces shredded pepper Jack cheese

Directions:

1. Preheat the oven to 450°F. Spray a baking dish with cooking spray.

2. Cut a slit down the length of each pepper and thoroughly scoop out and discard all the seeds and membranes. Cut some other slit horizontally at the top of the peppers to make a gap for the filling.

3. Place the peppers within the organized baking dish and cook dinner for about 20 mins, or until they begin to blister. Remove and set aside.

4. While the peppers are inside the oven, set a skillet over medium-high heat and pour in the olive oil. Add the onion, garlic, and mushrooms and cook dinner until fragrant, 2 to three mins. Add the spinach and cook dinner till wilted, 4 to five minutes.

5. Transfer the mushroom combination to a medium mixing bowl. Add the sour cream, heavy cream, and pepper Jack cheese, and stir until combined.

6. Remove the peppers from the oven

Desserts

and stuff every one with an equal amount of filling. Close with a toothpick.

7. Return the peppers to the oven for an additional 15 minutes, or until the cheese is melted. Serve heat.

Nutrition:

Calories: 341 Cal
Fat: 29 g
Protein: 16 g
Carbs: 4 g
Fiber: 1 g

277. Broccoli and Cauliflower Rice Casserole

Preparation Time: 5 Minutes
Cooking Time: 10 Minutes
Servings: 4

Ingredients:

- 2 tablespoons grass-fed butter
- 1 garlic clove, minced
- 3 cups frozen cauliflower rice
- 1 cup frozen broccoli rice
- ½ teaspoon salt
- ¼ teaspoon freshly ground black pepper
- 1 cup grated sharp cheddar cheese
- ¼ cup cream cheese, at room temperature 1 to 2 tablespoons heavy (whipping) cream

Directions:

1. In a medium skillet over medium-low heat, melt the butter. Add the garlic and sauté for 2 minutes or until fragrant. Add the cauliflower rice, broccoli rice, salt, and pepper.

2. Cook the combination for about 4 mins, and then remove from the warmth. Stir in the cheddar cheese and cream cheese and thin the combination to your favored consistency with the heavy cream.

3. Serve warm.

Nutrition:

Calories: 270 Cal
Fat: 22 g
Protein: 11 g
Carbs: 7 g
Fiber: 3 g

278. Cauliflower Fried Rice

Preparation Time: 2 Minutes
Cooking Time: 10 Minutes
Servings: 2

Ingredients:

- 1 tablespoon avocado oil
- 4 cups frozen cauliflower rice
- 1 cup frozen peas and carrots blend
- ½ tablespoon minced fresh ginger
- 2 tablespoons tamari sauce
- 2 tablespoons sesame oil 2 large eggs, beaten

- 2 scallions, finely chopped

Directions:

1. In a medium skillet over medium-high warmness, warm the avocado oil.
2. Add the cauliflower, peas and carrots, ginger, tamari sauce, and sesame oil. Cook until the vegetables are cooked thoroughly, 5 to 6 minutes.
3. Add the eggs and scramble them into the greens.
4. Divide the aggregate among 2 serving dishes and pinnacle with the scallions before serving.

Nutrition:

Calories: 362 Cal
Fat: 26 g
Protein: 14 g
Carbs: 18 g
Fiber: 8 g

279. Mexican Zucchini Hash

Preparation Time: 5 Minutes
Cooking Time: 10 Minutes
Servings: 4

Ingredients:

- 2 tablespoons avocado oil
- ½ onion, diced 2 garlic cloves, minced
- 4 large zucchinis, diced ½ teaspoon salt
- ¼ teaspoon freshly ground black pepper
- 1 teaspoon ground cumin
- 1 cup sliced button mushrooms
- 1 cup queso blanco cheese
- 2 avocados, diced
- 2 tablespoons chopped fresh cilantro

Directions:

1. In a large skillet over medium-excessive warmth, warm the avocado oil. Add the onion, garlic, and zucchini, and season with the salt, pepper, and cumin. Stir to mix.
2. Add the mushrooms and sauté for four to 6 mins, or till the greens are soft.
3. Remove from the warmth and pinnacle with the queso blanco, diced avocado, and cilantro. Serve warm.

Nutrition:

Calories: 401 Cal
Fat: 29 g
Protein: 12 g
Carbs: 23 g
Fiber: 10 g

280. Eggplant Lasagna

Preparation Time: 10 Minutes
Cooking Time: 1 Hour 10 Minutes
Servings: 4

Desserts

Ingredients:

- Nonstick cooking spray
- 1 large eggplant, cut into ⅛-inch-thick slices
- Salt
- 1½ cups full-fat ricotta cheese
- 1 large egg
- 1 (28-ounce) can whole tomatoes, drained
- 1 cup grated Parmesan cheese
- 2 cups shredded mozzarella cheese
- 2 tablespoons dried parsley

Directions:

1. Preheat the oven to 375°F. Grease an 8-with the aid of-8-inch baking dish with cooking spray.
2. Sprinkle the eggplant slices with salt. Allow them to sit for 15 minutes and then blot with a paper towel.
3. In a dry skillet over high heat, cook the eggplant slices for three mins on every side. Remove and set aside.
4. In a medium bowl, integrate the ricotta cheese and egg, and stir well. Set aside.
5. Crush a handful of tomatoes and area them inside the bottom of the prepared baking dish. Layer some slices of eggplant, a layer of cheese sauce, and any other layer of beaten tomatoes. Repeat this layering until the dish is full.
6. Sprinkle the Parmesan and mozzarella cheeses on the pinnacle, followed by using the parsley.
7. Cover the dish with aluminum foil and bake for 40 mins. Remove the foil and bake for an additional 10 minutes.
8. Remove the lasagna from the oven and let it take a seat for 5 mins earlier than slicing and serving.

Nutrition:

Calories: 439 Cal
Fat: 27g
Protein: 31g
Carbs: 18g
Fiber: 7g

281. Spaghetti Squash Bake

Preparation Time: 10 Minutes
Cooking Time: 30 Minutes
Servings: 4

Ingredients:

- Nonstick cooking spray
- 1 tablespoon grass-fed butter
- 5 garlic cloves, minced
- ½ cup of water
- 1 teaspoon seasoned vegetable

base
- 1 cup heavy (whipping) cream
- 4 cups cooked and shredded spaghetti squash
- ½ cup grated Parmesan cheese
- ½ cup shredded mozzarella cheese
- 2 tablespoons chopped fresh parsley 1 teaspoon freshly ground black pepper

Directions:
1. Preheat the oven to 350°F. Spray an 8-by-8-inch glass casserole dish with cooking spray.
2. In a medium saucepan over medium-low heat, melt the butter. Add the garlic and prepare dinner till fragrant, 2 to 3 minutes.
3. Add the water, vegetable base, and cream. Cook until well combined, and then remove from the heat.
4. Place the squash in the bottom of the organized dish. Pour the cream aggregate on pinnacle, and then pinnacle with the Parmesan and mozzarella cheeses, parsley, and pepper.
5. Bake for 20 mins and serve heat.

Nutrition:
Calories: 371 Cal Fat: 31g
Protein: 11g Carbs: 12g
Fiber: 1g

282. Cheesy Spinach Bake

Preparation Time: 10 Minutes
Cooking Time: 40 Minutes
Servings: 4

Ingredients:
- Nonstick cooking spray
- 2 tablespoons grass-fed butter
- 2 cups chopped onion
- 2 garlic cloves, minced
- 2 zucchinis, chopped into bite-size pieces
- 2 cups fresh spinach
- 3 eggs, beaten
- ¼ cup heavy (whipping) cream
- ½ teaspoon salt
- ¼ teaspoon freshly ground black pepper
- 1½ cups shredded mozzarella cheese
- ½ cup grated Parmesan cheese

Directions:
1. Preheat the oven to 350°F. Coat a 9-inch glass pie plate with cooking spray.
2. In a skillet over medium-excessive heat, melt the butter. Add the onion and garlic and sauté for two minutes.
3. Add the zucchini and cook for

Desserts

another four mins. Add the spinach and stir until wilted. Transfer the mixture to the organized pie plate and spread it lightly with a spatula.

4. In a small bowl, mix the eggs, cream, salt, and pepper collectively. Pour the aggregate over the vegetables.

5. Top with the mozzarella and Parmesan cheeses and bake for 30 to 35 minutes. Serve warm.

Nutrition:

Calories: 386 Cal
Fat: 30 g
Protein: 21 g
Carbs: 8g
Fiber: 2g

283. Fakeachini Alfredo

Preparation: Time: 15 Minutes
Cooking Time: 5 Minutes
Servings: 1

Ingredients:

- ½ tablespoon extra-virgin olive oil
- 1 teaspoon minced garlic
- ¼ teaspoon salt
- ¼ teaspoon garlic powder
- 1 wedge Laughing Cow Swiss cheese, cubed
- 1 to 2 tablespoons heavy (whipping) cream
- 3 tablespoons grated Parmesan cheese
- 2 ounces' seitan strips or cubes
- ⅓ cup cooked spaghetti squash
- 1 tablespoon chopped fresh parsley

Directions:

1. In a small saucepan over medium-low heat, heat the olive oil. Add the garlic, salt, and garlic powder and stir for 1 to 2 minutes or till fragrant.

2. Add the cubed cheese and stir until melted—thin the sauce to your desired consistency with the cream. Lower the heat and stir inside the Parmesan cheese.

3. Continue to stir until melted.

4. Add the seitan to the sauce.

5. Place the squash in a serving bowl, pour the sauce on the pinnacle, and sprinkle with the parsley.

Nutrition:

Calories: 452 Cal
Fat: 24 g
Protein: 52 g
Carbs: 7 g
Fiber: 3 g

284. Cheesy Cauliflower Mac 'N' Cheese

Preparation Time: 10 Minutes
Cooking Time: 30 Minutes
Serving: 6

Ingredients:

- Nonstick cooking spray
- 1 cauliflower head, chopped into small florets
- 8 ounces heavy (whipping) cream
- 4 ounces shredded sharp cheddar cheese
- 4 ounces grated Parmesan cheese
- 2 ounces' cream cheese 1 teaspoon salt ¼ teaspoon freshly ground black pepper

Directions:

1. Preheat the oven to 375°F. Spray an 8-by-8-inch baking dish with cooking spray. Place the cauliflower in a microwave-secure bowl and cook dinner for 3 minutes on excessive. Drain any extra liquid. In a small saucepan over medium heat, integrate the heavy cream, cheddar cheese, Parmesan cheese, cream cheese, salt, and pepper. Stir till properly combined, and then dispose of from the warmth. Pour the cheese sauce over the cauliflower and toss to coat. Transfer the aggregate to the organized baking dish and prepare dinner for 25 mins.

Nutrition:

Calories: 324
Fat: 28g
Protein: 13g
Carbs: 5g
Fiber: 1g

285. Margherita Pizza

Preparation Time: 10 Minutes
Cooking Time: 5 Minutes
Servings: 1

Ingredients:

- 1 tablespoon psyllium husk powder
- ¼ teaspoon salt
- ½ teaspoon dried oregano
- 2 large eggs
- 1 tablespoon avocado oil
- 3 tablespoons low-sugar marinara sauce
- 2 tablespoons grated Parmesan cheese
- ½ cup sliced mozzarella cheese
- 1 tablespoon chopped fresh basil

Directions:

2. Line a baking sheet with aluminum foil. Turn the oven to low broil.
3. Combine the psyllium husk powder, salt, oregano, and eggs in a blender. Blend for 30 seconds. Set aside.

Desserts

4. In a sauté pan or skillet, over high heat, warm the avocado oil. Pour the crust combination into the pan, spreading it out into a circle.

5. Cook until are browned, then turn the crust and cook dinner for a further minute.

6. Transfer the crust to the prepared baking sheet. Spread the marinara sauce over the pinnacle and cover with the Parmesan and mozzarella cheeses.

7. Broil until the cheese is melted and bubbling.

8. Top with the basil and enjoy.

Nutrition:

Calories: 545 Cal
Fat: 41 g
Protein: 32 g
Carbs: 12 g
Fiber: 8 g

APPETIZERS AND STARTERS

286. Keto Vegan Lasagna Rolls

Preparation Time: 20 Minutes
Cook Time: 20 Minutes
Servings: 10

Ingredients

Rolls;

- Pepper and salt to taste
- 1 teaspoon of coconut oil
- 1 zucchini
- 1 eggplant
- Half a cup of organic tomato sauce
- Cashew cheese;
- Water
- A pinch of salt
- A cup of raw cashews nuts
- Extras;
- Half a teaspoon of salt
- Half a teaspoon of garlic powder

Directions:

1. For the cashew cheese;
2. Add a pinch of sea salt right into a bowl of water, put the cashews in and permit them to soak for 8 hours or if you have the time, soak them overnight or for a complete day.
3. Drain the water from the cashew and vicinity them in a meals processor, add garlic powder and process till smooth, then season with a pinch or two of salt.
4. Blend again till the cashews come to be very creamy, if at this point they're too thick or pasty, you can skinny it out with some water.
5. Pour the creamy combination right into a jar and refrigerate.
6. For lasagna;
7. Cut the zucchini and eggplant lengthwise into thin strips.
8. Sprinkle some salt on one facet of the slices and set them apart to rest for approximately 10 minutes. This is to draw out extra moisture from the zucchini and eggplant strips.
9. Use a paper towel to pay the vegetable strips dry, to eliminate extra moisture.
10. Pour oil right into a medium-sized pan, set over medium warmth and permit to simmer for a minute, then upload the strips.
11. Fry on every aspect for two minutes, till they're gently browned. Repeat this technique for

Desserts

all of the strips then set aside.

12. Once they're ready, region the strips on a plate and scoop a few cashew cheeses in the middle of each strip.
13. Top with a pleasant drizzle of organic tomato sauce over each strip, sprinkle some salt and pepper and roll the strips.
14. Serve and enjoy.

Nutrition:

Calories: 97 Cal
Fat: 4 g
Fiber: 2 g
Carbs: 6 g
Protein: 2 g

287. Stuffed Avocados

Preparation Time: 15 Minutes
Cooking Time: 0
Servings: 6

Ingredients:

- Vegan Mayo
- 3 avocados (halved and seed removed)
- 1 jalapeño (seed removed and finely diced)
- 1 tablespoon of lemon juice
- Salt and pepper to taste
- 3 grape tomatoes (diced)
- A quarter teaspoon of garlic powder
- A quarter piece of cucumber (diced)
- 1 small red onion (diced)
- A quarter piece of orange bell pepper (cored and diced)

Directions:

1. Use the lemon juice to marinate the flash if the avocados to prevent them from browning. Put the cucumber, bell peppers, onions, tomatoes, garlic, jalapeño, and enough mayo right into a bowl, stir until nicely combined. Fill the avocados with the vegetable mixture, add a small amount of lemon juice and a sprinkle of salt, then serve.

Nutrition:

Calories: 167 Cal
Fat: 6 g
Fiber: 7 g
Carbs: 5 g
Protein: 3 g

288. Keto Vegan Cashew Cheese

Preparation Time: 5 Minutes
Cooking Time: 10 Minutes
Servings: 7

Ingredients

- A quarter teaspoon of dried thyme
- 1 clove of garlic (grated)

- Half a teaspoon of dried parsley
- 1 teaspoon of kosher salt
- 2 tablespoons of coconut oil
- A quarter teaspoon of dried dill
- A quarter teaspoon of dried pepper
- 2 tablespoons of lemon juice
- 1 teaspoon of dried basil leaves
- Almond crackers (for serving)
- 1 teaspoon of dried chives
- 1 cup of raw cashews

Directions:

2. Soak the cashews in water overnight or for eight hours, then drain.
3. Put the lemon juice, soaked cashews, coconut oil, garlic, pepper and salt right into a food processor, combination for 7-10 minutes the use of the S-blade attachment till a thick paste is formed.
4. Pour cashew cheese right into a medium-sized bowl, add the dried herbs and stir until nicely combined.
5. Line any small bowl with Saran wrap and pour the cashew cheese in it, fold the rims of the saran wrap and refrigerate for two hours.

Nutrition:

Calories: 197 Cal
Fat: 7 g
Fiber: 7.6 g
Carbs: 5.6 g
Protein: 4.2 g

289. Baba Ghanoush

Preparation Time: 10 Minutes
Cooking Time: 25 Minutes
Servings: 2

Ingredients:

- Half a teaspoon of fine sea salt
- A quarter cup of full-fat coconut milk
- 1 large eggplant
- 2 tablespoons of Thai green curry paste
- 2 limes
- A quarter cup of fresh cilantro (chopped)

Directions:

1. Set your broiler to high and location the racks as a minimum 6 inches from the heat source.
2. Cut the eggplant in half, area on a baking sheet with the reduce facet going through down, then poke holes within the eggplant the usage of a fork.
3. Broil the eggplant until soft, this is for about 25 minutes, then set

Desserts

apart to chill.

4. Grate two teaspoons of lime zest, then squeeze one tablespoon of juice from the lines.
5. Remove the flesh from the eggplants using a spoon, then positioned them in a meals processor and mixture until smooth.
6. Add the coconut milk, curry paste, lime juice and zest, cilantro and salt to taste, mixture again until smooth.
7. Serve heat or cold with a few crackers or vegetables.

Nutrition:

Calories: 57 Cal
Fat: 6 g
Fiber: 4 g
Carbs: 8 g
Protein: 4 g

290. Avocado Fries

Preparation Time: 10 Minutes
Cooking Time: 15 Minutes
Servings: 4

Ingredients:

- A quarter cup of almond milk
- Half a cup of almond flour
- 1 large avocado (not too ripe)
- 1 teaspoon of Cajun seasoning

Directions:

1. Preheat your oven to 450F.
2. Cut the avocado in half, pit and reduce into wedges. Put the Cajun Seasoning and almond flour, stir to combine. Pour the almond milk into a bowl and set aside.
3. Put the avocado slices into the milk, then put it inside the flour mixture, ensuring to coat the avocado completely. Line a baking sheet with parchment paper.
4. Place the covered avocados inside the baking sheet, area inside the oven and cook for 15 minutes.
5. Once the avocados are golden, dispose of them from the oven and set apart to chill for a couple of minutes before serving, but they may be higher when served hot.
6. Enjoy with some vegan mayo.

Nutrition:

Calories: 207
Cal Fat: 6 g
Fiber: 5 g
Carbs: 7.9 g
Protein: 4 g

291. Keto Vegan "Cheese" Sticks

Preparation Time: 5 Minutes
Cooking Time: 7 Minutes
Servings: 7

Ingredients:

- 1 tablespoon of olive oil
- 2 tablespoons of nutritional yeast
- 2 cans of hearts of palm
- A quarter teaspoon of garlic (minced)
- 2 tablespoons of soy flour
- 3 tablespoons of water
- 1 teaspoon of taco seasoning
- A quarter teaspoon of black pepper
- A pinch of salt

Directions:

1. Preheat your oven to 375F.
2. Line a baking sheet with parchment paper. Drain and rinse the hearts of palm, put in a bowl then set aside. In a huge bowl, blend the water, olive oil and dry substances collectively till fully mixed and smooth. Coat the hearts of palm in the combination then area them at the pre-lined baking sheet. Put in the oven and bake for 25 minutes or till the coating is absolutely organization to the touch. Serve with marinara sauce and enjoy!

Nutrition:

Calories: 57
Cal Fat: 3 g
Fiber: 4 g
Carbs: 3 g
Protein: 3 g

292. Keto Vegan Crack Bars

Preparation Time: 2 Minutes
Cooking Time: 10 Minutes
Servings: 20

Ingredients

- 1 cup of melted coconut oil
- 2 cups of shredded coconut flakes (unsweetened)
- A quarter cup of liquid stevia
- Half a cup of cranberries (unsweetened)

Directions:

1. Put the cranberries and coconut into a food processor, pulse on excessive till fully blended and a choppy paste is formed.
2. Put the cranberry mixture, stevia and coconut oil into a large blending bowl, blend till completely mixed.
3. Pour batter into a pre-coated 8 using an 8-inch baking tray.
4. Wet your palms and press the batter firmly into the tray.
5. Refrigerate for 8- 24 hours.
6. Cut into small squares and serve.

Nutrition:

Desserts

Calories: 97 Cal
Fat: 3 g Fiber: 7 g
Carbs: 4 g
Protein: 3 g

293. Vegetable Dip

Preparation Time: 10 Minutes
Cooking Time: 5 Minutes
Servings: 12

Ingredients:

- 2 tablespoons of dill leaves
- A quarter cup of walnut cheese
- 1 teaspoon of lemon juice
- 1 cup of sour cream
- 2 tablespoons of chives (roughly chopped)
- 1 clove of garlic
- A quarter cup of parsley leaves

Directions:

1. Put all the substances right into a food processor, blend until easy Pour into a bowl and serve with your favorite vegetables and enjoy.

Nutrition:

Calories: 56 Cal
Fat: 4 g
Fiber: 1 g
Carbs: 4 g
Protein: 3 g

294. Mongolian Stir Fry

Preparation Time: 5 Minutes
Cooking Time: 4 Minutes
Servings: 4

Ingredients:

- 1 tablespoon minced ginger
- 1 teaspoon minced garlic
- 1 tablespoon avocado oil
- 4 tablespoons soy sauce
- 1 teaspoon chili flakes
- 1 teaspoon cornstarch
- 1 tablespoon brown sugar 8 tablespoon water
- ½ teaspoon cayenne pepper
- 1-pound seitan, chopped

Directions:

2. In the combination, bowl whisk together minced ginger, minced garlic, avocado oil, soy sauce, chili flakes, cornstarch, brown sugar, cayenne pepper, and water. Preheat on the spot pot bowl on Sauté mode till hot. Transfer ginger combination in the instant pot and prepare dinner it for 1 minute. Then upload chopped seitan and stir well. Close the lid and set Manual mode (high stress) for 1 minute. Use quick strain release. Mix up the aspect dish well earlier than serving.

Nutrition:

Calories: 59
Cal Carbs: 5.6 g
Fat: 0.9 g
Protein: 6.6 g

295. Mushroom "Bacon"

Preparation Time: 5 Minutes
Cooking Time: 2 Minutes
Servings: 5

Ingredients:

- 6 oz. shiitake mushrooms
- 1 teaspoon salt
- ¼ teaspoon cayenne pepper
- 1 tablespoon olive oil

Directions:

1. Slice the mushrooms onto bacon form strips and sprinkle each strip with olive oil, cayenne pepper, and salt.
2. Then location mushroom "bacon" within the immediate pot and close the lid.
3. Set Manual mode (high strain) and cook dinner mushrooms for two minutes. Then use a short pressure release. The time of cooking depends on mushroom strips size.

Nutrition:

Calories: 43 Cal
Carbs: 4.7 g
Fat: 2.9 g
Protein: 0.5 g

SOUPS AND STEWS

296. Creamy Onion Soup

Preparation Time: 10minutes
Cooking Time: 65 Minutes
Servings: 4

Ingredients:

- 3 tbsp olive oil
- 3 cups thinly sliced white onions
- 2 garlic cloves, thinly sliced
- 2 tsp almond flour
- ½ cup dry white wine
- Salt and black pepper to taste
- 2 sprigs chopped thyme
- 2 cups hot vegetable broth
- 2 cups almond milk 1 cup grates Swiss cheese

Directions:

1. Heat the olive oil in a pot over medium warmness. Sauté the onions for 10 minutes or until softened, frequently stirring to avoid browning. Reduce the heat to low and cook similarly for 15 mins while once in a while, stirring.
2. Mix within the garlic, cook dinner also for 10 minutes, or until the onions caramelize.
3. Stir in the almond flour well, wine, and growth the heat. Season with salt, black pepper, thyme, and pour inside the hot vegetable broth. Cover the pot, convey to a boil, and then simmer for 30 minutes.
4. Pour within the almond milk and half of the Swiss cheese. Stir till the cheese melts, regulate the flavor with salt, black pepper, and dish the soup.
5. Top with the ultimate cheese and serve warm.

Nutrition:

Calories: 183 Cal
Fat: 14.7 g
Carbs: 8 g
Fiber: 2 g
Protein: 8 g

297. Lettuce and Cauliflower Soup

Preparation Time: 10 Minutes
Cooking Time: 30 Minutes
Servings: 4

Ingredients:

- 1 tbsp. olive oil
- 2 tbsp. butter
- 1 medium red onion, thinly sliced
- 3 garlic cloves, finely sliced
- 1 large head cauliflower, cut into florets

- 1 medium lettuce head, leaves extracted and chopped
- 4 cups vegetable stock
- 6 sprigs parsley, leaves extracted
- Salt and black pepper to taste
- 1 tbsp fresh dill leaves for garnishing 1 cup grated provolone cheese for topping

Directions:

1. Heat the oil and butter in a big saucepan over medium warmth and sauté the onion and garlic till softened and fragrant, 3 mins.
2. Stir inside the cauliflower, lettuce, and cook dinner until the lettuce wilts, 3 mins
3. Pour inside the vegetable stock, parsley and season with salt and black pepper. Close the lid, convey to a boil, and then simmer until the cauliflower softens.
4. Open the lid and the usage of an immersion blender, puree the soup until smooth. Adjust the taste with salt and black pepper.
5. Dish the soup, pinnacle with the provolone cheese, and serve warm.

Nutrition:

- Calories: 312 Cal
- Fat: 21 g
- Carbs: 15 g
- Fiber: 5 g
- Protein: 19 g

298. Spring Vegetable Soup

Preparation Time: 8 Minutes
Cooking Time: 13 Minutes
Servings: 4

Ingredients:

- 4 cups vegetable stock
- 3 cups green beans, chopped
- 2 cups asparagus, chopped
- 1 cup pearl onions, peeled and halved
- 2 cups baby spinach
- 1 tbsp. garlic powder
- Salt and white pepper to taste
- 2 cups grated cheddar cheese for topping

Directions:

1. In a big pot, upload the vegetable stock, green beans, asparagus, and pearl onions. Bring to a boil over medium warmth after which simmer till the veggies soften, 10 mins.
2. Stir inside the spinach, allow slight wilting, and regulate the taste with salt and white pepper.
3. Dish the soup, top with the cheddar cheese, and serve warm.

Desserts

Nutrition:

Calories: 405 Cal
Fat: 32.2 g
Carbs: 18 g
Fiber:4 g
Protein: 16 g

299. Creamy Garlicky Tofu Soup

Preparation Time: 10 Minutes
Cooking Time: 11 Minutes
Servings: 4

Ingredients:

- 1 tbsp olive oil
- 1 large white onion, finely chopped
- 3 tbsp minced garlic
- 1 tsp ginger puree
- 1 cup vegetable stock
- 2 parsnips, peeled and chopped
- Salt and black pepper to taste
- 2 (14 oz) silken tofu, drained and rinsed
- 2 cups almond milk
- 1 tbsp chopped fresh basil
- 1 tbsp chopped fresh parsley to garnish
- Chopped toasted pecans for topping

Directions:

1. Heat the olive oil in a saucepan and sauté the onion, garlic, and ginger puree until aromatic and soft, 3 mins
2. Mix within the vegetable stock, parsnips, salt, and black pepper. Cover and cook dinner till the parsnips soften, 6 minutes.
3. Add the silken tofu and right now puree the soup the usage of an immersion blender until very smooth.
4. Stir inside the almond milk, basil, and cook dinner also for two minutes with common stirring to prevent the tofu from curdling.
5. Dish the soup, garnish with the parsley, pecans, and serve warm.

Nutrition:

Calories:171 Cal
Fat: 13.9 g
Carbs: 12 g
Fiber: 6 g
Protein: 3 g

300. Kale Ginger Soup with Avocados

Preparation Time: 8 Minutes
Cooking Time: 8 Minutes
Servings: 4

Ingredients:

- 1 tbsp butter
- 1 tbsp sesame oil + extra for drizzling

- 1 small onion, finely sliced
- 3 garlic cloves, minced
- 2 tsp ginger paste
- 2 cups baby kale, chopped
- 2 cups chopped green beans
- 4 cups vegetable stock
- 3 tbsp chopped fresh cilantro + extra for garnish
- Salt and black pepper to taste
- 1 large avocado, pitted, peeled, and diced for topping

Directions:

1. Heat the butter and sesame oil in a huge pot over medium warmth.
2. Sauté the onions, garlic, and garlic until softened and fragrant, three minutes.
3. Mix within the kale, green beans, vegetable stock, and cilantro. Season with salt, black pepper, and prepare dinner covered till the vegetables soften, 5 minutes.
4. Open the lid, modify the flavor with salt, black pepper, and dish the soup.
5. Top with the avocado and serve warm.

Nutrition:

Calories: 212 Cal
Fat: 16.1 g
Carbs: 14 g
Fiber: 2 g
Protein: 5 g

301. Creamy Tomato & Turnip Soup

Preparation Time: 10 Minutes
Cooking Time: 18 Minutes
Servings: 4

Ingredients:

- 2 tbsp butter
- 1 large red onion, chopped
- 4 garlic cloves, minced
- 6 red bell peppers, deseeded and sliced
- 2 turnips, peeled and diced
- 3 cups chopped tomatoes
- 4 cups vegetable stock
- Salt and black pepper to taste
- 1 cup heavy cream
- ½ cup grated Swiss cheese 2 cups toasted chopped cashew nuts

Directions:

1. Melt the butter in a massive pot over medium warmness and sauté the onion and garlic till softened and fragrant, 3 mins.
2. Stir in the bell peppers, turnips, tomatoes, vegetable stock, and season with salt and black pepper.
3. Bring to a boil after which simmer

Desserts

until the turnips and very tender, 15 mins.

4. Insert an immersion blender and puree the soup till easy.
5. Mix inside the heavy cream and alter the taste with salt and black pepper.
6. Dish the soup, top with the Swiss cheese, cashew nuts, and serve warm.

Nutrition:

Calories: 486 Cal
Fat: 41.3 g
Carbs: 14 g
Fiber: 2 g
Protein: 17 g

302. Italian Cheese Soup

Preparation Time: 12 Minutes
Cooking Time: 20 Minutes
Servings: 4

Ingredients:

- 1 tbsp avocado oil
- 6 slices vegan bacon, chopped
- 4 tbsp butter
- 1 small white onion, roughly chopped
- 3 garlic cloves, minced
- 2 tbsp chopped fresh Italian mixed herbs
- 2 cups peeled and cubed rutabagas
- 3 ½ cups vegetable broth
- Salt and black pepper to taste
- 1 cup almond milk
- 1 cup grated provolone
- 2 tbsp. chopped scallions for garnishing

Directions:

1. Heat the olive oil in a medium pot over medium heat and cook dinner the vegan bacon till brown and crispy, 5 mins. Transfer to a plate and set aside.
2. Melt the butter in the pot and sauté the onion, garlic, and combined herbs till fragrant, three minutes.
3. Stir inside the rutabagas, season with salt, black pepper, and prepare dinner for 10 to 12 mins or until the rutabagas soften.
4. Open the lid, insert an immersion blender, and technique the soup until very smooth.
5. Stir within the almond milk and provolone cheese until the cheese melts.
6. Adjust the flavor with salt, black pepper, and dish the soup into serving bowls.
7. Garnish with the scallions and serve warm.

Nutrition:

Calories: 646 Cal
Fat: 63.7g
Carbs: 24 g
Fiber: 13 g
Protein: 8 g

303. Chilled Lemongrass and Avocado Soup

Preparation Time: 5 Minutes
Cooking Time: 5 Minutes
Servings: 4

Ingredients:

- 4 cups chopped avocado pulp
- 2 stalks lemongrass, chopped
- 4 cups vegetable broth
- 2 lemons, juiced
- 3 tbsp. chopped mint + extra to garnish
- Salt and black pepper to taste
- 2 cups coconut cream

Directions:

1. Over low warmness, bring the avocado, lemongrass, and vegetable broth to a gradual boil till the avocado warms through, three to five minutes.
2. Add the ultimate Ingredients and system till smooth the use of an immersion blender.
3. Adjust the flavor with salt, black pepper, and dish the soup.

Nutrition:

Calories: 391 Cal
Fat: 37.3 g
Carbs: 13 g
Fiber: 5 g
Protein: 7 g

304. Mixed Mushroom Soup

Preparation Time: 10minutes
Cooking Time: 29minutes
Servings: 4

Ingredients:

- 4 oz unsalted butter
- 1 small onion, finely chopped
- 1 clove garlic, minced
- 5 oz. white button mushrooms, chopped
- 5 oz. cremini mushrooms, chopped
- 5 oz. oyster mushrooms, chopped
- ½ lb. celery root, chopped
- ½ tsp dried rosemary
- 3 cups vegetable broth
- 1 tbsp plain vinegar
- 1 cup cashew cream
- 4 basil leaves, chopped
- 2 tbsp chopped blanched almonds

Directions:

1. Melt the butter in a medium pot and sauté the Ingredients up to the vegetable stock till softened, 5

Desserts

mins.

2. Mix in the vegetable broth, vinegar, and produce the meals to a boil. Reduce the warmth to low and simmer until the liquid reduces by one-third.

3. Mix in the cashew cream and puree the Ingredients the use of an immersion blender. Simmer for two mins.

4. Dish the soup, garnish with the basil, almonds, and serve warm.

Nutrition:

Calories: 325 Cal
Fat: 30.6 g
Carbs: 11 g
Fiber: 2 g
Protein: 8 g

305. Coconut Pumpkin Soup

Preparation Time: 8 Minutes
Cooking Time: 15 Minutes
Servings: 4

Ingredients:

- 2 tbsp + 2 tbsp butter
- 2 small red onions
- 2 garlic cloves
- 1 cup chopped pumpkins
- 2 cups vegetable broth
- Salt and black pepper to taste
- ½ cup coconut cream
- ½ lemon, juiced
- ¾ cup mayonnaise
- Pumpkin seeds for garnishing

Directions:

1. Melt 2 tbsp of butter in a medium pot and sauté the onion and garlic until softened and fragrant, three mins.

2. Stir in the pumpkins, vegetable broth, salt, and black pepper. Close the lid, permit boiling, after which simmer for 10 minutes

3. Open the lid, add the remaining butter, coconut cream, and puree the soup with an immersion blender until easy.

4. Mix inside the lemon juice, mayonnaise, and adjust the flavor with salt and black pepper.

5. Dish the soup, garnish with the pumpkin seeds and serve warm.

Nutrition:

- Calories: 566 Cal
- Fat: 57.7 g
- Carbs: 15 g
- Fiber: 7 g
- Protein: 6 g

306. Mushroom Bourguignon

Preparation Time: 10 Min
Cooking Time: 40 Min

Servings: 4

Ingredients:

- 2 tablespoons olive oil, isolated (see notes for without oil)
- 2 pounds' mushrooms, cut (darker, crimini)
- 1 cup pearl onions, stripped and closes cut (defrosted whenever solidified)
- 1 huge carrot, diced
- 1 yellow onion, diced
- 1 piling teaspoon crisp thyme leaves or 1/2 teaspoon dried mineral salt and broke pepper, to taste
- 2 or 3 cloves garlic, minced
- 1 cup full-bodied red wine
- 2 cups vegetable soup
- 2 tablespoons tomato glue
- 1 1/2 tablespoons flour

Directions

1. In a huge dutch broiler or full-size pot, warmth 1 tablespoon oil over medium-high warmth, consist of mushrooms and pearl onions burn till they start to take on a chunk of shading, around three to 4 minutes.
2. Decrease warmth to medium, consist of the carrots, onions, garlic, thyme, salt, and pepper, sauté for five to 7 minutes, blending once in a while, till onions are softly cooked.
3. Add the purple wine slowly to the pot and scrape any bits which can be adhered to the bottom or sides. Heat to medium-high and decrease wine significantly.
4. Mix in tomato glue and juices, warmness to the point of boiling, reduce the warmth to low and stew for 20 minutes, or until mushrooms are delicate. Let stew, secured or unfold aslant, blending at times, and recognize the great fragrance.
5. In a bit bowl, integrate the rest of the tablespoon oil, or water, with flour to make a glue, mix into the stew. Stew for 10 minutes. In the occasion that the sauce is excessively slight, come it down to the suitable consistency—season to taste.

Nutrition:

Calories:167 Cal
Fat:.4 g
Carbohydrate: 21.6 g
Fiber: 3.3 g
Protein: 7.1 g

SIDE DISHES

307. Basil Zucchinis and Eggplants

Preparation Time: 10 Minutes
Cooking Time: 20 Minutes
Servings: 4

Ingredients:
- 1 tablespoon olive oil
- 2 zucchinis, sliced
- 1 eggplant, roughly cubed
- 2 scallions, chopped
- 1 tablespoon sweet paprika
- Juice of 1 lime
- 1 teaspoon fennel seeds, crushed
- Salt and black pepper to the taste
- 1 tablespoon basil, chopped

Directions:
1. Heat up a pan with the oil over medium heat, upload the scallions and fennel seeds and sauté for 5 mins. Add zucchinis, eggplant and the alternative ingredients, toss, prepare dinner over medium heat for 15 mins more, divide between plates and serve as a facet dish.

Nutrition:
Calories: 97 Cal Fat: 4 g Fiber: 2 g Carbs: 6 g Protein: 2 g

308. Chard and Peppers Mix

Preparation time: 10 minutes
Cooking time: 20 minutes
Servings: 4

Ingredients:
- 2 tablespoons avocado oil
- 2 spring onions, chopped
- 2 tablespoons tomato passata
- 2 tablespoons capers, drained
- 2 green bell peppers, cut into strips
- 1 teaspoon turmeric powder
- A pinch of cayenne pepper Juice of 1 lime
- Salt and black pepper to the taste
- 1 bunch red chard, torn

Directions:
1. Heat up a pan with the oil over medium warmness, upload the spring onions, capers, turmeric and cayenne and sauté for 5 mins. Add the peppers, chard and the other ingredients, toss, cook over medium heat for 15 mins more, divide among plates and serve.

Nutrition:
Calories: 119 Cal Fat: 7 g Fiber: 3 g Carbs: 7 g Protein: 2 g

309. Balsamic Kale

Preparation time: 10 minutes
Cooking time: 20 minutes
Servings: 4

Ingredients:

- 1 tablespoon balsamic vinegar
- 2 tablespoons walnuts, chopped
- 1-pound kale, torn
- 1 tablespoon olive oil
- 1 teaspoon cumin, ground
- 1 teaspoon chili powder
- 3 garlic cloves, minced
- 2 tablespoons cilantro, chopped

Directions:

1. Heat up a pan with the oil over medium heat, upload the garlic and the walnuts and cook dinner for 2 mins.
2. Add the kale, vinegar and the other ingredients, toss, cook over medium warmness for 18 minutes more, divide between plates and function an aspect.

Nutrition:

Calories: 170
Cal Fat: 11 g
Fiber: 3 g
Carbs: 7 g
Protein: 7 g

310. Mustard Cabbage Salad

Preparation Time: 10 Minutes
Cooking Time: 0
Servings: 4

Ingredients:

- 1 green cabbage head, shredded
- 1 red cabbage head, shredded
- 2 tablespoons avocado oil
- 2 tablespoons mustard
- 1 tablespoon balsamic vinegar
- 1 teaspoon hot paprika
- Salt and black pepper to the taste
- 1 tablespoon dill, chopped

Directions:

1. In a bowl, mix the cabbage with the oil, mustard and the other ingredients, toss, divide among plates and function a facet salad.

Nutrition:

Calories: 150 Cal
Fat: 3 g
Fiber: 2 g
Carbs: 2 g
Protein: 7 g

311. Cabbage and Green Beans

Preparation Time: 10 Minutes
Cooking Time: 15 Minutes
Servings: 4

Ingredients:

- 1 green cabbage head, shredded
- 2 cups green beans, trimmed and

Desserts

- halved
- 2 tablespoons olive oil
- 1 teaspoon sweet paprika
- 1 teaspoon cumin, ground
- Salt and black pepper to the taste
- 1 tablespoon chives, chopped

Directions:

1. Heat up a pan with the oil over medium warmness, upload the cabbage and the paprika and sauté for 2 mins.
2. Add the green beans and the other ingredients, toss, prepare dinner over medium warmth for thirteen mins more, divide between plates and serve.

Nutrition:

Calories: 200 Cal
Fat: 4 g
Fiber: 2 g
Carbs: 3 g
Protein: 7 g

312. Green Beans, Avocado and Scallions

Preparation Time: 10 Minutes
Cooking Time: 20 Minutes
Servings: 4

Ingredients:

- 1-pound green beans, trimmed and halved
- 1 avocado, peeled, pitted and sliced
- 4 scallions, chopped
- 2 tablespoons olive oil
- 1 tablespoon lime juice
- Salt and black pepper to the taste
- Handful cilantro, chopped

Directions:

1. Heat up a pan with the oil over medium warmness, add the scallions and sauté for two mins.
2. Add the inexperienced beans, lime juice and the alternative ingredients, toss, prepare dinner over medium heat for 18 mins, divide between plates and serve.

Nutrition:

Calories: 200 Cal
Fat: 5 g
Fiber: 23 g
Carbs: 1 g
Protein: 3 g

313. Creamy Cajun Zucchinis

Preparation Time: 10 Minutes
Cooking Time: 20 Minutes
Servings: 4

Ingredients:

- 1-pound zucchinis, roughly cubed
- 2 tablespoons olive oil
- 4 scallions, chopped

- Salt and black pepper to the taste
- 1 teaspoon Cajun seasoning
- A pinch of cayenne pepper
- 1 cup coconut cream 1 tablespoon dill, chopped

Directions:

1. Heat up a pan with the oil over medium heat, upload the scallions, cayenne and Cajun seasoning, stir and sauté for 5 minutes.
2. Add the zucchinis and the opposite ingredients, toss, prepare dinner over medium warmness for 15 mins more, divide among plates and serve.

Nutrition:
Calories: 200 Cal
Fat: 2 g
Fiber: 1 g
Carbs: 5 g
Protein: 8 g

314. Herbed Zucchinis and Olives

Preparation Time: 10 Minutes
Cooking Time: 20 Minutes
Servings: 4

Ingredients:

- 1 cup kalamata olives, pitted
- 1 cup green olives, pitted
- 1-pound zucchinis, roughly cubed
- 1 tablespoon rosemary, chopped
- 1 tablespoon basil, chopped
- 1 tablespoon cilantro, chopped
- 2 tablespoons olive oil
- 3 garlic cloves, minced
- 1 tablespoon lemon juice
- 1 teaspoon lemon zest, grated
- 1 tablespoon sweet paprika
- A pinch of salt and black pepper

Directions:

1. Heat a pan with the oil over medium warmness, add the garlic, lemon zest and paprika and sauté for 2 minutes.
2. Add the olives, zucchinis and the other ingredients, toss, cook dinner over medium warmness for 18 mins more, divide between plates and serve.

Nutrition:
Calories: 200
Cal Fat: 20 g
Fiber: 4 g
Carbs: 3 g
Protein: 1 g

SALADS

315. Cherry Tomato Salad with Soy Chorizo

Preparation Time: 5 Minutes
Cooking Time: 5 Minutes
Servings: 4

Ingredients:

- 4 soy chorizos, chopped
- 2 ½ tbsp olive oil 2 tsp red wine vinegar
- 1 small red onion, finely chopped
- 2 ½ cups cherry tomatoes, halved
- 2 tbsp. chopped cilantro
- Salt and freshly ground black pepper to taste
- 3 tbsp. sliced black olives to garnish

Directions:

1. Over medium fire, heat half of tablespoon of olive oil in a skillet and fry soy chorizo till golden. Turn warmth off. In a salad bowl, whisk last olive oil and vinegar. Add onion, cilantro, tomatoes, and soy chorizo. Mix with dressing and season with salt and black pepper. Garnish with olives and serve.

Nutrition:

Calories: 138
Cal Fat: 8.95 g
Carbs: 5.63 g
Fiber: 0.4 g
Protein: 7.12 g

316. Roasted Bell Pepper Salad with Olives

Preparation Time: 10 Minutes
Cooking Time: 20 Minutes
Servings: 4

Ingredients:

- 8 large red bell peppers, deseeded and cut in wedges
- ½ tsp erythritol
- 2 ½ tbsp olive oil
- 1/3 cup arugula
- 1 tbsp mint leaves
- 1/3 cup pitted Kalamata olives
- 3 tbsp chopped almonds ½ tbsp balsamic vinegar
- Crumbled feta cheese for topping
- Toasted pine nuts for topping

Directions:

1. Preheat oven to 400o F.
2. Pour bell peppers on a roasting pan; season with erythritol and drizzle with 1/2 of olive oil. Roast in oven till barely charred, 20 mins. Remove from the oven and set

aside.

3. Arrange arugula in a salad bowl, scatter bell peppers on top, mint leaves, olives, almonds, and drizzle with balsamic vinegar and closing olive oil—season with salt and black pepper.

4. Toss; pinnacle with feta cheese and pine nuts and serve.

Nutrition:

Calories: 163 Cal
Fat: 13.3 g
Carbs: 6.53 g
Fiber: 2.2 g
Protein: 3.37 g

317. Tofu-Dulse-Walnut Salad

Preparation Time: 10 Minutes
Cooking Time: 15 Minutes
Servings: 4

Ingredients:

- 1 (7 oz.) block extra firm tofu
- 2 tbsp olive oil 2 tbsp butter
- 1 cup asparagus, trimmed and halved
- 1 cup green beans, trimmed
- 2 tbsp. chopped dulse
- Salt and freshly ground black pepper to taste
- ½ lemon, juiced
- 4 tbsp. chopped walnuts

Directions:

1. Place tofu in between two paper towels and permit soaking for 5 mins. After, get rid of towels and chop into small cubes.

2. Heat olive oil in a skillet and fry tofu till golden, 10 mins. Remove onto a paper towel-covered plate and set aside.

3. Melt butter in a skillet and sauté asparagus and green beans until softened, 5 minutes. Add dulse, season with salt and black pepper, and cook until softened. Mix in tofu and stir-fry for 5 mins. Plate, drizzle with lemon juice and scatter walnuts on top.

4. Serve warm.

Nutrition:

Calories 237
Fat 19.57g
Carbs 5.9g
Fiber 2.1g
Protein 12.75g

318. Almond-GojiBerry Cauliflower Salad

Preparation Time: 10 minutes
Cooking Time: 2 minutes
Servings: 4

Ingredients:

- 1 small head cauliflower, cut into florets

Desserts

- 8 sun-dried tomatoes in olive oil, drained
- 12 pitted green olives, roughly chopped
- 1 lemon, zested and juiced
- 3 tbsp chopped green onions
- A handful chopped almonds
- ¼ cup goji berries 1 tbsp sesame oil
- ½ cup watercress 3 tbsp chopped parsley
- Salt and freshly ground black pepper to taste
- Lemon wedges to garnish

Directions:

1. Pour cauliflower into a huge safe-microwave bowl, sprinkle with a few waters, and steam in microwave for 1 to 2 mins or until softened. In a massive salad bowl, combine cauliflower, tomatoes, olives, lemon zest and juice, green onions, almonds, goji berries, sesame oil, watercress, and parsley. Season with salt and black pepper, and blend well. Serve with lemon wedges.

Nutrition:

Calories 203
Cal Fat 15:.28 g
Carbs: 9.64 g
Fiber: 3.2 g
Protein: 6.67 g

319. Warm Mushroom and Orange Pepper Salad

Preparation Time: 10 Minutes
Cooking Time: 8 Minutes
Servings: 4

Ingredients:

- 2 tbsp. avocado oil
- 1 cup mixed mushrooms, chopped
- 2 orange bell peppers, deseeded and finely sliced
- 1 garlic clove, minced
- 2 tbsp. tamarind sauce
- 1 tsp maple (sugar-free) syrup
- ½ tsp hot sauce
- ½ tsp fresh ginger paste
- Sesame seeds to garnish

Directions:

1. Over medium fire, heat half of avocado oil in a huge skillet, sauté mushroom and bell peppers till slightly softened, 5 minutes.
2. In a small bowl, whisk garlic, tamarind sauce, maple syrup, hot sauce, and ginger paste. Add combination to greens and stir-fry for 2 to a few mins.
3. Turn warmth off and dish salad.

Drizzle with last avocado oil and garnish with sesame seeds. Serve with grilled tofu.

Nutrition:

Calories: 289
Cal Fat: 26.71 g
Carbs: 9 g
Fiber: 3.8 g
Protein: 4.23 g

320. Broccoli, Kelp, and Feta Salad

Preparation Time: 15 Minutes
Cooking Time: 0
Servings: 4

Ingredients:

- 2 tbsp. olive oil
- 1 tbsp. white wine vinegar
- 2 tbsp. chia seeds
- Salt and freshly ground black pepper to taste
- 2 cups broccoli slaw
- 1 cup chopped kelp, thoroughly washed and steamed
- 1/3 cup chopped pecans
- 1/3 cup pumpkin seeds
- 1/3 cup blueberries
- 2/3 cup ricotta cheese

Directions:

1. In a small bowl, whisk olive oil, white wine vinegar, chia seeds, salt, and black pepper. Set aside.
2. In a huge salad bowl, integrate the broccoli slaw, kelp, pecans, pumpkin seeds, blueberries, and ricotta cheese.
3. Drizzle dressing on the pinnacle, toss and serve.

Nutrition:

Calories 397
Fat 3.87g
Carbs 8.4g
Fiber 3.5g
Protein 8.93g

321. Roasted Asparagus with Feta Cheese Salad

Preparation Time: 10 minutes
Cooking Time: 20 minutes
Serving Size: 4

Ingredients:

- ½ tsp dried oregano
- 1 lb. asparagus, trimmed and halved
- 2 tbsp. olive oil
- ½ tsp dried basil
- Salt and freshly ground black pepper to taste
- ½ tsp hemp seeds
- 1 tbsp maple (sugar-free) syrup
- ½ cup arugula
- 4 tbsp crumbled feta cheese 2 tbsp hazelnuts

Desserts

- 1 lemon, cut into wedges

Directions:

1. Preheat oven to 350oF.
2. Pour asparagus on a baking tray, drizzle with olive oil, basil, oregano, salt, black pepper, and hemp seeds. Mix with your hands and roast in oven for 15 minutes.
3. Remove, drizzle with maple syrup, and hold cooking till slightly charred 5 minutes.
4. Spread arugula in a salad bowl and top with asparagus. Scatter with feta cheese, hazelnuts, and serve with lemon wedges.

Nutrition:

Calories: 146
Cal Fat: 12.87 g
Carbs: 5.07 g
Fiber: 1.6 g
Protein: 4.44 g

322. Fresh Veggie Salad

Preparation Time: 20 Minutes
Cooking Time: 0
Servings: 8

Ingredients:

For *Dressing*:

- 5 tablespoons olive oil
- 3 tablespoons fresh lemon juice
- 2 tablespoons fresh mint leaves, chopped finely
- 1 teaspoon Erythritol
- Salt and freshly ground black pepper, to taste

For *Salad*:

- 2 cups cucumbers, peeled and sliced
- 2 cups tomatoes, sliced
- 1 cup black olives 6 cups lettuce
- 1 cup mozzarella cheese, cubed

Directions:

1. For the dressing: in a bowl, upload all elements and beat till nicely combined.
2. Cover and refrigerate to sit back for approximately 1 hour.
3. For the salad: in a huge serving bowl, add all substances and mix. Pour dressing over salad and toss to coat properly. Serve immediately.

Nutrition:

Calories: 124
Cal Fat: 11.4 g
Carbs: 5.4 g
Protein: 2 g

323. Strawberry Salad

Preparation Time: 15 Minutes
Cooking Time: 0
Servings: 4

Ingredients:

- 6 cups fresh baby greens
- 2 cups fresh strawberries, hulled and sliced
- 1 tablespoon fresh mint leaves
- ¼ cup olive oil
- 2 tablespoons fresh lemon juice
- ¼ teaspoon liquid stevia
- 1/8 teaspoon paprika
- 1/8 teaspoon garlic powder
- Salt, to taste

Directions:

1. For the salad: in a large serving bowl, add greens, strawberries, and mint and blend.
2. For the dressing: in a bowl, upload closing substances and beat until properly combined.
3. Pour dressing over salad and toss to coat well.
4. Serve immediately.

Nutrition:

Calories: 141
Cal Fat: 14.7 g
Carbs: 1.8 g
Protein: 2 g

324. Tex Mex Black Bean and Avocado Salad

Preparation Time: 15 Minutes

Cooking Time: 0
Servings: 2

Ingredients

- 14 oz. black beans drained and rinsed
- 3 jars roasted red peppers, chopped
- 1 avocado, chopped ½ onion, chopped
- 1 red chili, chopped 1 lime, plus wedges to serve olive oil
- 1 teaspoon cumin seeds
- 2 handfuls rocket2 pitta bread, warmed

Directions:

1. Combine beans, peppers, avocado, onion and chili in a massive mixing bowl.
2. Add lime juice, cumin seeds and mix properly.
3. Serve the rocket on two plates with heat pittas and divide the bean mixture.

Nutrition:

Calories: 120
Cal Fat: 3 g
Fiber: 5 g Carbs: 3 g
Protein: 5 g

325. Lentil Fattoush Salad

Preparation Time: 10 Minutes

Desserts

Cooking Time: 42 Minutes
Servings: 2

Ingredients:

- ⅓ cup dry green lentils
- 1 whole wheat pita pocket, chopped into bite sized pieces
- 2 teaspoons olive oil
- 2 teaspoons zaatar
- 4 cups loosely packed arugula
- 2 stalks celery, chopped
- 1 carrot stick, chopped
- ¼ small hothouse cucumber, chopped
- 1 small radish, thinly sliced
- ¼ cup dates, chopped
- 2 tablespoons toasted sunflower seeds

For the *maple* Dijon vinaigrette:

- 2 tablespoons olive oil
- 2 tablespoons balsamic vinegar
- 1 tablespoon Dijon mustard
- 1 tablespoon maple syrup

Directions:

1. Place a small pot over medium heat. Add lentils and 2/3 cup water.
2. Bring it to a boil, decrease the warmth and convey it to a simmer for 35 minutes. Remove from the warmth and drain extra liquid.
3. Preheat the oven to 425F. Line a baking sheet with parchment paper.
4. Mix pita portions with olive oil and zaatar. Place on a baking sheet and bake for 7 minutes.
5. Mix arugula, lentils, veggies, dates, sunflower seeds and pita croutons.
6. Meanwhile in a separate bowl, blend the dressing components and set aside.
7. Add the dressing and toss properly before serving.

Nutrition:

Calories: 154 Cal
Fat: 8.4 g
Fiber: 4.4 g
Carbs: 4.3 g
Protein: 7.1 g

326. Sweet Potato Salad

Preparation: 10 Minutes
Cooking Time: 30 Minutes
Servings: 4

Ingredients:

- 2 sweet potatoes, peeled and cubed
- 1 tablespoon olive oil
- ½ teaspoon each of paprika, oregano and cayenne pepper

- 1 shallot, diced
- 2 spring onions, chopped
- 1 small bunch chives, chopped
- 3 tablespoons red wine vinegar
- 2 teaspoons olive oil
- 1 tablespoon pure maple syrup
- salt and pepper

Directions:

1. Preheat the oven to 300F and prepare a baking sheet by lining it with parchment paper.
2. Place candy potatoes inside the baking sheet.
3. Drizzle a few olive oil and spices, toss well and bake for 30 minutes.
4. In a separate bowl, mix shallots, scallions, chives, vinegar, olive oil and maple syrup.
5. Add baked candy potatoes to the dressing.

Nutrition:

Calories: 162 Cal
Fat: 8.0 g Fiber: 2.3 g
Carbs: 6.3 g
Protein: 8.1 g

SNACKS

327. Chipotle Tacos

Preparation Time: 10 Minutes
Cooking Time: 4 Hours
Servings: 4

Ingredients:

- 30 ounces canned pinto beans, drained
- ¾ cup chili sauce
- 3 ounces' chipotle pepper in adobo sauce, chopped
- 1 cup corn
- 6 ounces' tomato paste
- 1 tablespoon cocoa powder
- ½ teaspoon cinnamon, ground
- 1 teaspoon cumin, ground
- 8 vegan taco shells
- Chopped avocado, for serving

Directions:

1. Put the beans in your gradual cooker.
2. Add chili sauce, chipotle pepper, corn, tomato paste, cocoa powder, cinnamon and cumin.
3. Stir, cover and cook on Low for four hours. Divide beans and chopped avocado into taco shells and serve them.
4. Enjoy!

Nutrition:

Calories: 342
Fat: 3
Fiber: 6
Carbs: 12g
Protein: 10 g

328. Tasty Spinach Dip

Preparation Time: 10 Minutes
Cooking Time: 4 Hours
Servings: 12

Ingredients:

- 8 ounces' baby spinach
- 1 small yellow onion, chopped
- 8 ounces' vegan cashew mozzarella, shredded
- 8 ounces' tofu, cubed
- 1 cup vegan cashew parmesan cheese, grated
- 1 tablespoon garlic, minced
- A pinch of cayenne pepper
- A pinch of sea salts Black pepper to the taste

Directions:

1. Put spinach in your gradual cooker.
2. Add onion, cashew mozzarella, tofu, cashew parmesan, salt,

pepper, cayenne and garlic.

3. Stir, cover and cook on Low for 2 hours.
4. Stir your dip well, cover and cook dinner on Low for two extra hours.
5. Divide your spinach dip into bowls and serve.
6. Enjoy!

Nutrition:

Calories: 200 Cal
Fat: 3 g
Fiber: 4 g
Carbs: 6 g
Protein: 8 g

329. Candied Almonds

Preparation time: 10 minutes
Cooking time: 4 hours
Servings: 10

Ingredients:

- 3 tablespoons cinnamon powder
- 3 cups palm sugar
- 4 and ½ cups almonds, raw
- ¼ cup water
- 2 teaspoons vanilla extract

Directions:

1. In a bowl, mix water with vanilla extract and whisk.
2. In any other bowl, mix cinnamon with sugar and stir.
3. Dip almonds in water, then add them to the bowl with the cinnamon sugar.
4. Toss to coat in reality well, add almonds for your sluggish cooker, cover and prepare dinner on Low for 4 hours, stirring often.
5. Divide into bowls and function a snack.
6. Enjoy!

Nutrition:

Calories: 150 Fat: 3
Fiber: 4 Carbs: 6
Protein: 8

330. Eggplant Tapenade

Preparation Time: 10 Minutes
Cooking Time: 7 Hours
Servings: 6

Ingredients:

- 1 and ½ cups tomatoes, chopped
- 3 cups eggplant, chopped
- 2 teaspoons capers
- 4 garlic cloves, minced
- 1 tablespoon basil, chopped
- 2 teaspoons balsamic vinegar
- A pinch of sea salt
- Black pepper to the taste
- 6 ounces' green olives, pitted and sliced

Directions:

Desserts

1. Put tomatoes and eggplant pieces in your sluggish cooker.
2. Add garlic, capers, basil and olives, stir, cover and cook on Low for 7 hours.
3. Add salt, pepper, vinegar, stir gently, divide into small bowls and serve as an appetizer.
4. Enjoy!

Nutrition:

Calories: 140 Cal Fat: 3 g Fiber: 5 g Carbs: 7 g Protein: 5 g

331. Almond and Beans Fondue

Preparation Time: 10 Minutes
Cooking Time: 8 Hours
Servings: 4

Ingredients:

- ½ cup almonds
- 1 and ¼ cups water
- 1 teaspoon nutritional yeast flakes
- ¼ cup great northern beans
- A pinch of sea salt
- Black pepper to the taste
- Baby carrots, steamed for serving
- Tofu cubes for serving

Directions:

1. Put the water in your sluggish cooker.
2. Add almonds and beans, stir, cover and cook dinner on Low for 8 hours.
3. Transfer these to your blender, add yeast flakes, a pinch of salt and black pepper and pulse honestly well.
4. Transfer to bowls and serve with baby carrots and tofu cubes on the side.
5. Enjoy!

Nutrition:

Calories: 200
Cal Fat: 4 g
Fiber: 4 g
Carbs: 8 g
Protein: 10 g

332. Beans in Rich Tomato Sauce

Preparation Time: 10 Minutes
Cooking Time: 8 Hours And 10 Minutes
Servings: 6

Ingredients:

- 1-pound lima beans, soaked for 6 hours and drained
- 2 celery ribs, chopped
- 2 tablespoons olive oil
- 2 onions, chopped
- 2 carrots, chopped
- 4 tablespoons tomato paste
- 3 garlic cloves, minced

- A pinch of sea salt
- Black pepper to the taste
- 7 cups water
- 1 bay leaf
- 1 teaspoon oregano, dried
- ½ teaspoon thyme, dried
- A pinch of red pepper, crushed
- ¼ cup parsley, chopped
- 1 cup cashew cheese, shredded

Directions:
1. Heat up a pan with the oil over medium high heat, add onions, stir and prepare dinner for 4 minutes.
2. Add garlic, celery, carrots, salt and pepper, stir, cook dinner for 4-five minutes more and transfer to your sluggish cooker.
3. Add beans, tomato paste, water, bay leaf, oregano, thyme and red pepper, stir, cover and cook dinner on Low for eight hours.
4. Add parsley, stir, divide into bowls and serve bloodless with cashew cheese on the pinnacle.
5. Enjoy!

Nutrition:
Calories: 160 Cal
Fat: 3 g Fiber: 7 g Carbs: 9 g Protein: 12 g

333. Tasty Onion Dip

Preparation Time: 10 Minutes
Cooking Time: 8 Hours
Servings: 6

Ingredients:
- 3 cups yellow onions, chopped
- A pinch of sea salt
- 2 tablespoons olive oil
- 1 tablespoon coconut butter 1 cup coconut milk
- ½ cup avocado mayonnaise
- A pinch of cayenne pepper

Directions:
1. Put the onions in your sluggish cooker.
2. Add a pinch of salt, oil and coconut butter, stir nicely, cover and cook on High for 8 hours.
3. Drain extra liquid, switch onion to a bowl, add coconut milk, avocado mayo and cayenne, stir without a doubt nicely and serve with potato chips at the side.
4. Enjoy!

Nutrition:
calories 200
fat 4
fiber 4
carbs 9
protein 7

334. Special Beans Dip

Desserts

Preparation Time: 10 Minutes
Cooking Time: 2 Hours
Servings: 20

Ingredients:

- 16 ounces canned beans, drained
- 1 cup mild hot sauce
- 2 cups cashew cheese, shredded
- ¾ cup coconut milk
- ¼ teaspoon cumin, ground
- 1 tablespoon chili powder
- 3 ounces' tofu, cubed

Directions:

1. Put beans in your slow cooker.
2. Add hot sauce, cashew cheese, coconut milk, cumin, tofu and chili powder.
3. Stir, cover and cook for two hours.
4. Stir halfway.
5. Transfer to bowls and serve with corn chips on the side.
6. Enjoy!

Nutrition:

Calories 230
Fiber 6
Carbs 8
Protein 10
Fat 4

335. Sweet and Spicy Nuts

Preparation Time: 10 Minutes
Cooking Time: 2 Hours
Servings: 20

Ingredients:

- 1 cup almonds, toasted
- 1 cup cashews
- 1 cup pecans, halved and toasted
- 1 cup hazelnuts, toasted and peeled
- ½ cup palm sugar
- 1 teaspoon ginger, grated
- 1/3 cup coconut butter, melted
- ½ teaspoon cinnamon powder
- ¼ teaspoon cloves, ground
- A pinch of salt
- A pinch of cayenne pepper

Directions:

1. Put almonds, pecans, cashews and hazelnuts in your slow cooker.
2. Add palm sugar, coconut butter, ginger, salt, cayenne, cloves and cinnamon.
3. Stir nicely, cover and cook dinner on Low for 2 hours.
4. Divide into bowls and serve as a snack.
5. Enjoy!

Nutrition:

Calories: 110

Cal Fat: 3 g
Fiber: 2 g
Carbs: 5 g
Protein: 5g

336. Delicious Corn Dip

Preparation Time: 10 Minutes
Cooking Time: 2 Hours And 15 Minutes
Servings: 8

Ingredients:

- 2 jalapenos, chopped
- 45 ounces canned corn kernels, drained
- ½ cup of coconut milk
- 1 and ¼ cups cashew cheese, shredded
- A pinch of sea salt
- Black pepper to the taste
- 2 tablespoons chives, chopped
- 8 ounces' tofu, cubed

Directions:

1. In your gradual cooker, blend coconut milk with cashew cheese, corn, jalapenos, tofu, salt and pepper, stir, cowl and cook dinner on Low for two hours.
2. Stir your corn dip simply nicely, cover sluggish cooker again and prepare dinner on High for 15 minutes.
3. Divide into bowls, sprinkle chives on pinnacle and serve as a vegan snack!
4. Enjoy!

Nutrition:

Calories 150 Fat 3
Fiber 2Carbs 8Protein 10

Roasted Almonds

Preparation Time: 5 Minutes
Cooking Time: 10 Minutes
Servings: 16

Ingredients:

- 2 cups whole almonds
- 1 tablespoon chili powder
- ½ teaspoon ground cinnamon
- ½ teaspoon ground cumin
- ½ teaspoon ground coriander
- Salt and freshly ground black pepper, to taste
- 1 tablespoon olive oil

Directions:

1. Preheat the oven to 350 stages F. Line a baking dish with a parchment paper.
2. In a bowl, add all ingredients and toss to coat well.
3. Transfer the almond mixture into the organized baking dish in an unmarried layer.
4. Roast for about 10 minutes,

Desserts

flipping two times in a convenient way.

5. Remove from oven and hold apart to cool earlier than serving.
6. You can keep these roasted almonds in an airtight jar.

Nutrition:

Calories: 78 Cal
Fat: 6.9 g
Carbs: 2.9 g
Protein: 2.6 g

338. Cheese Biscuits

Preparation Time: 15 Minutes
Cooking Time: 15 Minutes
Servings: 8

Ingredients:

- 1/3 cup coconut flour, sifted
- ¼ teaspoon baking powder
- Salt, to taste
- 4 organic eggs
- ¼ cup butter, melted and cooled
- 1 cup cheddar cheese, shredded

Directions:

1. Preheat the oven to 400 tiers F. Line a large cookie sheet with a greased piece of foil.
2. In a big bowl, mix together flour, baking powder, garlic powder, and salt.
3. In every other bowl, add eggs and butter and beat properly.
4. Add egg combination into flour aggregate and beat till well combined. Fold in cheese.
5. With a tablespoon, location the mixture onto prepared cookie sheets in a single layer.
6. Bake for about 15 minutes or until top turns into golden brown.

Nutrition:

Calories: 142 Cal
Fat: 12.7 g Carbs: 0.8 g Protein: 8 g

339. Baked Veggie Balls

Preparation Time: 15 Minutes
Cooking Time: 25 Minutes
Servings: 8

Ingredients:

- 2 medium sweet potatoes, peeled and cubed into ½-inch size
- 2 tablespoons unsweetened coconut milk
- 1 cup fresh kale leaves, trimmed and chopped
- ½ small yellow onion, chopped finely
- 1 teaspoon ground cumin
- ½ teaspoon granulated garlic
- ¼ teaspoon ground turmeric

- Salt and freshly ground black pepper, to taste
- ¼ cup ground flax seeds

Directions:

1. Preheat the oven to 400 stages F. Line a baking sheet with parchment paper. In a pan of water, arrange a steamer basket.
2. Place the candy potato in a steamer basket and steam for approximately 10-15 mins.
3. In a massive bowl, location the sweet potato and coconut milk and mash well.
4. Add ultimate substances besides flax seeds and mix till well combined.
5. Make about 1½-2-inch balls from the aggregate.
6. Arrange the balls onto the prepared baking sheet in an unmarried layer and sprinkle with flax seeds.
7. Bake for about 20-25 mins.

Nutrition:
Calories: 61 Cal
Fat: 2.1 g
Carbs: 9 g
Protein: 1.5 g

340. Celery Crackers

Preparation Time: 15 Minutes
Cooking Time: 2 Hours
Serves: 15

Ingredients:
- 10 celery stalks
- 1 teaspoon fresh rosemary leaves
- 1 teaspoon fresh thyme leaves
- 2 tablespoons raw apple cider vinegar
- ¼ cup avocado oil
- Salt, to taste
- 3 cups flax seeds. Grounded roughly

Directions:

1. Preheat the oven to 225 stages F. Line 2 huge baking sheets with parchment paper.
2. In a meals processor, upload all ingredients except flax seeds and pulse until a puree forms.
3. Add flax seeds and pulse till nicely combined.
4. Transfer the dough right into a bowl and hold apart for about 2-3 minutes.
5. Divide the dough into 2 portions.
6. Place 1 portion in each organized baking sheet evenly.
7. With the again of a spatula, clean and press the dough to ¼-inch

Desserts

thickness.

8. With a knife, you are rating the squares in the dough.

9. Bake for approximately 2 hours, flipping once midway through.

10. Remove from the oven and keep apart to cool on the baking sheet for about 15 mins.

Nutrition:

Calories: 126 Cal
Fat: 7.6 g
Carbs: 7.1 g
Protein: 4.3 g

DESSERTS

Coconut Fat Bombs

Preparation Time: 1 Hr. 5 Minutes
Cooking Time: 0
Servings: 4

Ingredients:

- 20 drops liquid stevia
- 1 c. coconut flakes, unsweetened
- ¾ c. coconut oil
- 1 can coconut milk

Directions:

1. In a huge microwave-safe blending bowl, add coconut oil and heat on low energy for 20 seconds to melt.
2. Whisk in coconut milk and stevia into the oil.
3. Add coconut flakes; combine nicely.
4. Pour into candy molds or ice cube trays and freeze for 1 hour.
5. Serve and enjoy.

Nutrition:

Calories: 89.1
Cal Carbs: 0.87 g
Proteins: 0.33 g
Fats: 9.7 g

342. Coconut Cupcakes

Preparation Time: 1 Hour. 5 Minutes
Cooking Time: 0
Servings: 18

Ingredients:

- 1 tbsp. vanilla
- 1 t. baking soda
- 1 c. erythritol
- 4 t. baking powder
- 1 ¼ c. coconut milk
- ¾ c. coconut flour
- 14 tbsp. arrowroot powder
- 2 c. almond meal
- ½ c. coconut oil
- Whipped Cream:
- 1t. vanilla
- ¼ c. erythritol
- 2 13.5 oz. cans full-fat coconut milk, refrigerated overnight

Directions:

1. Prepare a muffin tin with muffin liners and convey the oven to 350 warmness setting.
2. In a huge mixing bowl, add all the substances and beat on medium-high speed till it turns to a batter-like consistency. If too dry, upload ¼ teaspoon of water at a time.
3. Fill the cupcake cups with the

Desserts

batter, three-quarters full. Bake for 20 mins or until the cupcakes are firm.

4. Place inside the refrigerator to cool.
5. While cupcakes are cooling, make the whipped cream.
6. Remove the coconut milk from the fridge and pour the clear coconut water from the milk.
7. In a big mixing bowl, upload the vanilla and erythritol; beat until fluffy. Ice the cupcakes and serve. Serve and enjoy.

Nutrition:

Calories: 202
Cal Carbs: 15.6 g
Proteins: 3.3 g
Fats: 15.8 g

343. Pumpkin Truffles

Preparation Time: 15 Minutes
Cooking Time: 0
Servings: 12

Ingredients:

- 1 t. cinnamon
- 2 tbsp. coconut sugar
- 3 tbsp. coconut flour
- ½ c. almond flour
- 1 t. pumpkin pie spice
- ¼ t. salt
- ½ t. vanilla extract
- ¼ c. maple syrup
- 1 c. pumpkin puree

Directions:

1. Bring a saucepan to medium warmness and add pumpkin puree, syrup, salt, and pumpkin pie spice, constantly stirring until thickened about five minutes.
2. Once thick, upload in vanilla and continue to stir for a further minute.
3. Remove from the heat and allow to cool.
4. Once cool, mix in the coconut and almond flour. Then put within the fridge to sit back for 10 minutes.
5. Remove from the fridge and mix again. If the dough is just too sticky, add in 1 tablespoon of almond flour until you can form a ball with the dough.
6. Form 12 balls using your fingers with the dough.
7. In a bit bowl, integrate coconut sugar and cinnamon.
8. Roll every ball into the cinnamon-sugar mixture.
9. Serve and enjoy.

Nutrition:

Calories: 66 Cal
Carbs: 10 g
Proteins: 1 g
Fats: 2 g

344. Raspberry Truffles

Preparation Time: 15 Minutes
Cooking Time: 0
Servings: 36

Ingredients:

- 2 tbsp. cocoa powder, unsweetened
- 6 oz. of the following: fresh raspberries, dry
- chocolate, bittersweet, finely chopped coconut milk, full-fat

Directions:

1. Prepare a cookie sheet with parchment paper and set to the side.
2. Warm a saucepan over medium warmness, and upload coconut milk.
3. Remove from the warmth and upload the chocolate with a rubber spatula, stirring to soften the chocolate
4. Once smooth, add the raspberries, five-8 at a time. Stir to coat.
5. Using forks, dispose of the raspberries from the chocolate sauce, allowing the excess sauce to drop again into the pan. Repeat this step until you have got coated all raspberries.
6. Place the raspberries inside the refrigerator for 1 hour or until firm.
7. In a shallow bowl with a lid, upload the cocoa powder.
8. Once truffles are firm, region 5 to eight cakes in the bowl and shake to coat with cocoa powder.
9. Return to the refrigerator till geared up to serve.

Nutrition:

Calories: 39
Cal Carbs: 3.8 g
Proteins: 0.6 g
Fats: 2.6 g

345. Pistachio Gelato

Preparation Time: 7 Hr. 60 Minutes
Cooking Time: -
Servings: 4

Ingredients:

- ½ t. almond extract
- 1 c. of the following: Medjool dates
- pistachios, unsalted, shells removed
- 1 big avocado
- 2 ½ c. cashew milk

Directions:

Desserts

1. In a blender, upload almond extract, dates, pistachios, avocado, and milk and blend till smooth.
2. Once smooth, pour right into a loaf pan, topping with chopped pistachios and freeze for eight hours or overnight.
3. Remove from the freezer and permit to fall for 15 minutes before serving.
4. Scoop and serve.

Nutrition:

Calories: 345 Cal
Carbs: 38.8 g
Proteins: 6.5 g
Fats: 19.8 g

346. Berry Bites

Preparation Time: 60 Minutes
Cooking Time: 0
Servings: 13

Ingredients:

- Dash Himalayan pink salt
- 1/16 t. stevia
- ½ t. vanilla
- ½ c. blackberries
- 2/3 c. coconut butter

Directions:

1. In a meals processor, add coconut butter, blackberries, vanilla, stevia, and salt; blend till well combined.
2. Using your hands, form them into 1 ½-inch ball, and area them on parchment a paper on a flat dish.
3. Place the dish within the freezer for 15 mins to set.
4. Store in refrigerator and serve cool.

Nutrition:

Calories: 75 Cal
Carbs: 2.8 g
Proteins: 0.8 g
Fats: 7.2 g

347. Espresso Cups

Preparation Time: 20 Minutes
Cooking Time: 0
Servings: 22

Ingredients:

- 15 drops vanilla stevia
- 1 ½ tbsp. instant espresso powder
- 1 tbsp. coconut milk
- 2 tbsp. cocoa powder
- 1/3 c. of the following: coconut oil almond butter

Directions:

1. In a saucepan over medium-low heat, soften the almond butter, coconut oil, coconut powder, coconut milk, coffee powder, and stevia. Stir frequently not to

scorch.

2. Pour into the candy molds or ice cube trays and freeze for 30 minutes.
3. Store within the fridge and serve cool.

Nutrition:

Calories: 77
Carbohydrates: 1 g
Proteins: 1 g
Fats: 8 g

348. Himalayan Raspberry Fat Bombs

Preparation Time: 55 Minutes
Cooking Time: 0
Servings: 4

Ingredients:

- 3 cups golden Himalayan raspberries
- 1 tsp vanilla extract
- 16 oz cream cheese, room temperature
- 4 tbsp unsalted butter
- 2 tbsp maple (sugar-free) syrup

Directions:

1. Line a 12-holed muffin tray with cake liners and set aside.
2. Pour raspberries, vanilla into a blender, and puree till smooth.
3. In a small saucepan, over medium heat, soften cream cheese and butter till nicely-combined.
4. In a medium bowl, evenly integrate a raspberry blend, cream cheese mix, and maple syrup. Pour the combination into muffin holes.
5. Refrigerate for 40 mins and serve after.

Nutrition:

Calories 227 Cal Fat 14.8g
Carbs 5.2g Fiber 2.1g
Protein 4.68g

349. Stewed Rhubarb

Preparation Time: 10 Minutes
Cooking Time: 7 Hours
Servings: 4

Ingredients:

- 5 cups rhubarb, chopped
- 2 tablespoons coconut butter
- 1/3 cup water
- 2/3 cup coconut sugar
- 1 teaspoon vanilla extract

Directions:

1. Put rhubarb in your slow cooker.
2. Add water and sugar, stir gently, cover and cook dinner on Low for 7 hours.
3. Add coconut butter and vanilla extract, stir and maintain inside the fridge until it's cold.

Desserts

4. Enjoy!

Nutrition:

Calories: 120 Cal
Fat: 2 g
Fiber: 3 g
Carbs: 6 g
Protein: 1 g

350. Peach Cobbler

Preparation Time: 10 Minutes
Cooking Time: 4 Hours
Servings: 4

Ingredients:

- ¼ cup coconut sugar
- 4 cups peaches, peeled and sliced
- ½ teaspoon cinnamon powder
- 1 and ½ cups vegan sweet crackers, crushed
- ¼ cup stevia
- ¼ teaspoon nutmeg, ground
- ½ cup almond milk
- 1 teaspoon vanilla extract
- Cooking spray

Directions:

1. In a bowl, blend peaches with coconut sugar and cinnamon and stir.
2. In a separate bowl, mix crackers with stevia, nutmeg, almond milk and vanilla extract and stir.
3. Spray your slow cooker with cooking spray and unfold peaches on the bottom.
4. Add crackers blend, unfold, cowl and cook on Low for four hours.
5. Divide cobbler between plates and serve.
6. Enjoy!

Nutrition:

Calories: 212
Cal Fat: 4 g
Fiber :4 g
Carbs: 7 g
Protein: 3 g

351. Apple Mix

Cooking Time: 4 Hours
Servings: 6

Ingredients:

- 6 apples, cored, peeled and sliced
- 1 and ½ cups almond flour
- Cooking spray
- 1 cup coconut sugar
- 1 tablespoon cinnamon powder
- ¾ cup cashew butter, melted

Directions:

1. Add apple slices to your gradual cooker after you've greased it with cooking spray
2. Add flour, sugar, cinnamon and

coconut butter, stir gently, cowl, cook dinner on High for 4 hours, divide into bowls and serve cold.

3. Enjoy!

Nutrition:

Calories: 200
Fat: 5
Fiber: 5
Carbs: 8
Protein: 4

352. Poached Plums

Preparation Time: 10 Minutes
Cooking Time: 3 Hours
Servings: 6

Ingredients:

- 14 plums, halved
- 1 and ¼ cups of coconut sugar
- 1 teaspoon cinnamon powder
- ¼ cup water

Directions:

1. Arrange plums on your slow cooker, upload sugar, cinnamon and water, stir, cowl, prepare dinner on Low for 3 hours, divide into cups and serve cold.
2. Enjoy!

Nutrition:

Calories: 150 Cal
Fat: 2 g
Fiber: 1 g
Carbs: 2 g

Protein: 3 g

353. Rice Pudding

Cooking Time: 5 Hours
Servings: 4

Ingredients:

- 6 and ½ cups of water
- 1 cup of coconut sugar
- 2 cups white rice, washed and rinsed
- 2 cinnamon sticks
- ½ cup coconut, shredded

Directions:

1. In your sluggish cooker, blend water with coconut sugar, rice, cinnamon and coconut, stir, cover and cook on High for five hours.
2. Divide pudding into cups and serve cold.
3. Enjoy!

Nutrition:

Calories: 213 Cal
Fat: 4 g
Fiber 6 g
Carbs: 9 g
Protein: 4 g

354. Cinnamon Rice

Preparation Time: 10 Minutes
Cooking Time: 35 Minutes
Servings: 4

Desserts

Ingredients:
- 3 and ½ cups water
- 1 cup coconut sugar
- 2 cups white rice, washed and rinsed
- 2 cinnamon sticks
- ½ cup coconut, shredded

Directions:
1. In your air fryer, blend water with coconut sugar, rice, cinnamon and coconut, stir, cowl and cook at 365 ranges F for 35 minutes.
2. Divide pudding into cups and serve cold.
3. Enjoy!

Nutrition:
Calories: 213
Cal Fat: 4 g
Fiber: 6 g
Carbs: 9 g
Protein: 4 g

355. Easy Buns

Cooking Time: 30 Minutes
Servings: 8

Ingredients:
- ½ cup coconut flour
- 1/3 cup psyllium husks
- 2 tablespoons stevia
- 1 teaspoon baking powder
- ½ teaspoon cinnamon powder
- ½ teaspoon cloves, ground
- 3 tablespoons flax meal combined with 3 tablespoons water
- Some chocolate chips, unsweetened

Directions:
1. In a bowl, mix flour with psyllium husks, swerve, baking powder, salt, cinnamon, cloves and chocolate chips and stir well.
2. Add water and flax meal, stir well till you obtain a dough, shape 8 buns and arrange them on a coated baking sheet.
3. Introduce inside the air fryer and prepare dinner at 350 degrees for 30 minutes.
4. Serve those buns warm.

Nutrition:
Calories: 140
Cal Fat: 3 g
Fiber: 3 g
Carbs: 7 g
Protein: 6 g

356. Zucchini Bread

Preparation Time: 10 Minutes
Cooking Time: 35 Minutes
Servings: 6

Ingredients:

- 1 cup natural applesauce
- 1 ½ banana, mashed
- 1 tablespoon vanilla extract
- 4 tablespoons coconut sugar
- 2 cups zucchini, grated
- 2 and ½ cups coconut flour
- ½ cup baking cocoa powder
- 1 teaspoon baking soda
- ¼ teaspoon baking powder
- 1 teaspoon cinnamon powder
- ½ cup walnuts, chopped
- Cooking spray

Directions:
1. Grease a loaf pan with cooking spray, upload zucchini, sugar, vanilla, banana, applesauce, flour, cocoa powder, baking soda, baking powder, cinnamon and walnuts, whisk well, introduce in the fryer and cook at 365 degrees F for 35 minutes. Leave the bread to cool down, slice and serve. Enjoy!

Nutrition:

Calories: 192
Fat: 3
Fiber: 6
Carbs: 8
Protein: 3

357. Pear Pudding

Preparation Time: 5 Minutes
Cooking Time: 30 Minutes
Servings: 4

Ingredients:
- 2 cups pears, chopped
- 2 cups coconut milk
- 1 tablespoon coconut butter, melted
- 3 tablespoons stevia
- ½ teaspoon cinnamon powder
- 1 cup coconut flakes ½ cup walnuts, chopped

Directions:
1. In a pudding pan, mix milk with stevia, butter, coconut, cinnamon, pears and walnuts, stir, introduce for your air fryer and cook dinner at 365 tiers F for 30 minutes
2. Divide into bowls and serve cold.
3. Enjoy!

Nutrition:

Calories: 202 Cal
Fat: 3 g
Fiber: 4 g
Carbs: 8 g
Protein: 7 g

358. Cauliflower Pudding

Preparation Time: 10 Minutes
Cooking Time: 30 Minutes
Servings: 4

Desserts

Ingredients:

- 2 and ½ cups water
- 1 cup coconut sugar
- 2 cups cauliflower rice
- 2 cinnamon sticks ½ cup coconut, shredded

Directions:

1. In a pan that suits your air fryer, mix water with coconut sugar, cauliflower rice, cinnamon and coconut, stir, introduce inside the fryer and cook at 365 degrees F for 30 minutes
2. Divide pudding into cups and serve cold.
3. Enjoy!

Nutrition:

Calories: 203 Cal
Fat: 4 g
Fiber: 6 g
Carbs: 9 g
Protein: 4 g

359. Exuberant Pumpkin Fudge

Preparation Time: 120 Minutes
Cooking Time: 0
Serving: 25

Ingredients:

- 1 and a ¾ cup of coconut butter
- 1 cup of pumpkin puree
- 1 teaspoon of ground cinnamon
- ¼ teaspoon of ground nutmeg
- 1 tablespoon of coconut oil

Directions:

1. Take an 8x8 inch square baking pan and line it with aluminum foil to start with
2. Take a spoon of the coconut butter and upload right into a heated pan; permit the butter melt over low heat. Toss inside the spices and pumpkin and preserve stirring it until a grainy texture has formed. Pour within the coconut oil and preserve stirring it vigorously so as to make certain that the whole thing is blended nicely. Scoop up the aggregate into the previously prepared baking pan and distribute lightly
3. Place a chunk of wax paper over the pinnacle of the mixture and press at the upper aspect to make flippantly straighten up the topsid. Remove the wax paper and throw it away. Place the mixture in your refrigerator and permit it cool for about 1-2 hours. Take it out and cut it into slices, then eat.

Nutrition:

Calories: 120 Cal
Protein: 1.2 g
Carbs: 4.2 g

Fats: 10.7 g

360. Bananas and Agave Sauce

Preparation Time: 10 Minutes
Cooking Time: 2 Hours
Servings: 4

Ingredients:

- Juice of ½ lemon
- 3 tablespoons agave nectar
- 1 tablespoon coconut oil
- 4 bananas, peeled and sliced diagonally
- ½ teaspoon cardamom seeds

Directions:

1. Arrange bananas in your slow cooker, upload agave nectar, lemon juice, oil and cardamom, cowl and prepare dinner on Low for 2 hours.
2. Divide bananas on plates, drizzle agave sauce all over and serve.
3. Enjoy!

Nutrition:

Calories: 120 Cal
Fat: 1 g
Fiber: 2 g
Carbs: 8 g
Protein: 3 g

LOW-CARB FRUITS AND BERRIES

Depending on your everyday carb target, you may be able to consist of a few other results as well, together with melons, cherries, apples, and summer fruits like plums:

What are the high-quality and the worst culmination and berries to consume on a low-carb diet? Here's the fast version: maximum berries are OK low-carb foods in moderate amounts, but the end result is candy from nature (and full of sugar). Others are blackberries, raspberries, strawberries, and blueberries.

BREAKFAST

361. Astonishing Hemp Seed Yogurt

Servings: 8
Preparation Time: 200 minutes Cooking Time: 0 minutes

Ingredients

- ¾ cup of hulled hemp seeds
- 3 cups of boiling water
- ¼ cup of lemon juice
- 2 teaspoon of xanthan gum
- Stevia as needed

Directions:

1. Take a pan and bring water to a boil
2. Take 1 cup of boiling water and mix them with hemp seeds in a blender
3. Process until the smooth lump-free mixture forms
4. While the blender is still processing, add xanthan gum and 2 cups of the remaining water
5. Process for 30 seconds more
6. Add lemon juice and blend for a little longer
7. Pour into a container and allow it to chill for 2-3 hours

Nutrition Values:

Calories: 166
Fat: 12G
Carbs: 4g
Protein: 10g

362. Sensual Portobello Mushrooms

Preparation Time: 10 minutes Cooking Time: 10 minutes Servings: 2

Ingredients:

- 2 Portobello mushrooms
- ½ cup of extra virgin olive oil
- 2 tablespoons of chopped

- onion
- 3 minced cloves of garlic
- 3 tablespoons of balsamic vinegar

Directions:
1. Carefully clear up mushrooms and remove stems
2. Keep the mushrooms for later use
3. Place the caps on a plate (gills upward)
4. Take a small sized bowl and add onion, vinegar, oil, and garlic
5. Mix everything well
6. Pour the mixture over the mushrooms caps and allow it to stand for about 60 minutes
7. Grill for about 10 minutes over your grill
8. Enjoy the grilled Portobello Mushrooms!

Nutrition Values:

Calories: 177
Fat: 14
Carbs: 7 Protein: 2.4g

363. Surprisingly Keto Tomato Tart

Servings: 8
Preparation Time: 10 minutes Cooking Time: 25 minutes

Ingredients

For Crust
- ½ a cup of coconut oil
- ¾ cup of coconut flour
- ½ a teaspoon of salt
- the mixture of 1 tablespoon of ground flaxseed + ¼ cup of water
- For Filling
- 4 ounce of heirloom tomatoes
- 3 ounce of cheese
- Black pepper and other herbs as needed

Directions:
1. Pre-heat your oven to 350 degrees Fahrenheit
2. Take a 9-inches pan and add all of the crust ingredients
3. Spread them out evenly and bake for 15-20 minutes until the crust starts to set
4. Remove the crust
5. Spread the cheese shredded over the crust
6. Slice up tomatoes into ¼ inch slices and arrange them on top of the Cheese
7. Sprinkle cracked pepper, oregano, basil and any other herbs of your choice
8. Cover and bake for 20-25 minutes until the cheese has

Desserts

9. melted, and the tomatoes are tender
10. Allow it to cool and enjoy!

Nutrition Values:

Calories: 212 Fat: 18g Carbs: 5g Protein: 2G

364. Kalamata Olive Tapenade

Preparation Time: 15 minutes Cooking Time: 0 minute Servings:4

Ingredients:

- 3 peeled garlic cloves
- 1 cup of pitted kalamata olives
- 2 tablespoons of capers
- 3 tablespoons of chopped fresh parsley
- 2 tablespoons of lemon juice
- 2 tablespoons of extra virgin olive oil
- Salt as needed
- Pepper as needed

Directions:

1. Take a food processor and add garlic cloves
2. Pulse them well until they are fully minced
3. Add olives, olive oil, capers, parsley, lemon juice to the food processor and blend them well until the whole mixture is finely chopped up
4. Season with some pepper and salt
5. Serve and enjoy!

Nutrition Values:

Calories: 81 Fat: 8g Carbs: 3g Protein: 0.5g

365. Silly Scallion Pancakes

Servings:4
Preparation Time: 5 minutes Cooking Time: 10 minutes

Ingredients

For Cakes

- ½ a cup of coconut flour
- 2 tablespoon of Psyllium Husk powder
- ½ a teaspoon of garlic powder
- ¼ teaspoon of salt
- 2-3 scallions sliced up into thin portions
- ¼ cup of sesame oil
- 1 cup of warm water

For Sauce

- 1 tablespoon of tamari sauce
- 1 teaspoon of rice wine vinegar
- 1 tablespoon of water
- 1 teaspoon of sesame oil
- 1 finely minced garlic clove

- Chili flakes as needed

Directions:
1. Take a frying pan and place it over medium-low heat
2. Add sesame oil and heat it up
3. Take a mixing bowl and add water, oil, garlic, salt, scallions, warm water and allow it to stand for 5 minutes to allow the flavors to mix up
4. Take another bowl and add coconut flour and the Psyllium Husk
5. Gently add the water to the dry ingredients, making sure to mix it well until the dough forms
6. Separate the dough into individual balls and flatten the balls into 4-inch rounds
7. Place the rounds in your skillet and fry for 5 minutes each side until they are golden
8. Keep repeating until the balls are used up
9. Enjoy!

Nutrition Values:
Calories: 206 Fat: 16g Carbs: 4g Protein: 4g

366. The Keto Crack Slaw

Servings: 2

Preparation Time: 5 minutes Cooking Time: 10 minutes

Ingredients
- 4 cups of shredded green cabbage
- ½ a cup of macadamia nuts chopped up
- 1 teaspoon of chili paste
- 1 teaspoon of vinegar
- 2 tablespoons of tamari
- 1 tablespoon of sesame oil
- 2 garlic cloves
- Sesame seeds as needed

Directions:
1. Take a pan and place it over medium-low heat and add tamari, sesame oil, vinegar, sesame oil, and chili paste
2. Add your green cabbage
3. Cover and allow it to cook for 5 minutes until the cabbage starts to tender
4. Stir everything and combine them well
5. Add the nuts
6. Cook for 5 minutes more until the nuts are tender
7. Serve and garnish

Nutrition Values:
Calories: 360 Fat: 33g Carbs: 7g Protein:

Desserts

7g

367. Feisty Grilled Artichokes

Preparation Time: 5 minutes Cooking Time: 30 minutes Servings:4

Ingredients:
- 2 large sized artichokes
- 1 quartered lemon
- ¾ cup of extra virgin olive oil
- 4 chopped up garlic cloves
- 1 teaspoon of salt
- ½ a teaspoon of ground black pepper

Directions:
1. Take a large sized bowl and fill it up with cold water
2. Squeeze a bit of lemon juice from the wedges
3. Trim the upper part of your chokes, making sure to trim any damaged leaves as well
4. Cut the chokes up in half lengthwise portions
5. Add the chokes to your bowl of lemon water
6. Bring the whole pot to a boil
7. Pre-heat your outdoor grill to about medium-high heat
8. Allow the chokes to cook in the boiling pot for 15 minutes
9. Drain the chokes and keep them on the side
10. Take another medium-sized bowl and squeeze the remaining lemon
11. Stir in garlic and olive to the lemon mix
12. Brush up the chokes with the garlic dip and place them on your pre-heated grill
13. Grill for about 10 minutes, making sure to keep basting them until the edges are just slightly charred
14. Serve with the dip and enjoy!

Nutrition Values:
Calories: 402 Fat: 40g Carbs: 10g Protein: 2.9g

368. The Thundering Cinnamon Chocolate Smoothie

Servings:1
Preparation Time: 5 minutes Cooking Time: 0 minutes

Ingredients
- ¾ cup of coconut milk
- ½ of a ripe avocado
- 2 teaspoons of unsweetened cocoa powder
- 1 teaspoon of cinnamon powder
- ¼ teaspoon of vanilla extract

- Stevia as needed
- ½ a teaspoon of coconut oil

Directions:
1. Add all of the ingredients to your blender and blend well until smooth
2. Allow them to chill and enjoy!

Nutrition Values:
Calories: 300 Fat: 30g Carbs: 14g Protein: 5g

369. Enchilada Macaroni

Servings: 4
Preparation Time: 20 minutes
Cooking Time: 45 minutes

Ingredients

For Sauce

- 1 cup of hemp seeds
- ½ a cup of nutritional yeast
- ¼ cup of sliced red, yellow or orange bell peppers
- ½ a teaspoon of salt
- ½ a teaspoon of onion powder
- ½ a cup of water
- For the Main Recipe
- 2 pack of Shirataki macaroni (Tofu)
- 1 can of young, green jackfruit in brine
- ¼ cup of enchilada sauce

Directions:
1. Pre-heat your oven to a temperature of 350 degrees
2. Fahrenheit
3. Drain and chop up your jackfruit with a knife and add 2 tablespoons of enchilada sauce, toss them well.
4. Keep it on the side
5. Blend the sauce ingredients in a blender and process them well
6. Drain and rinse the noodles thoroughly and transfer them to a baking dish
7. Add sauce, jackfruit to the baking dish and mix well
8. Bake for 45 minutes
9. Allow it to cool and enjoy!

Nutrition Values:
Calories: 192
Fat: 7.4g
Carbs: 4.1g
Protein: 9.6g

370. Squash Salad for the Green Lovers!

Preparation Time: 15 minutes Cooking Time: 30 minutes Servings: 4

Ingredients:

- 2 tablespoons of extra virgin olive

Desserts

- oil
- 1 small sized sliced onion
- 2 medium-sized coarsely chopped tomatoes
- 1 teaspoon of salt
- ¼ teaspoon of pepper
- 2 small zucchinis cut up into ½ inch slices
- 2 small sized yellow summer squash cut up into ½ inch slices
- 1 bay leaf
- ½ a teaspoon of dried basil

Directions:

1. Take a skillet and place it over medium heat
2. Add oil and allow it to heat up
3. Add onions and stir-fry them for about 5 minutes
4. Add tomatoes to the pan and mix well
5. Season the mixture with salt and pepper
6. Keep stirring for about 5 minutes until nicely cooked
7. Add bay leaf, zucchini, yellow squash, and basil
8. Lower down the heat and allow it to simmer for about 20 minutes, making sure to keep stirring it occasionally
9. Discard the bay leaf and enjoy!

Nutrition Values:

Calories: 65 Fat:5g Carbs: 5g Protein: 1.5g

371. Pumpkin Pecan Oatmeal

Preparation time: 10 minutes Cooking time: 8 hours Servings: 4

Ingredients:

- 1 and ½ cups water
- ½ cup pumpkin puree
- 1 teaspoon pumpkin pie spice
- 3 tablespoons stevia
- ½ cup steel cut oats
- ¼ cup pecans, chopped

Directions:

1. In your slow cooker mix water with oats, pumpkin puree, pumpkin spice, and stevia, stir, cover and cook on Low for 8 hours.
2. Sprinkle pecans on top, toss, divide into bowls and serve for breakfast.
3. Nutrition Value: calories 211, fat 4, fiber 7, carbs 8,
4. protein 3
5. Tasty Breakfast Burrito

Preparation time: 10 minutes Cooking time: 6 hours Servings: 8

Ingredients:

- 16 ounces tofu, crumbled
- 1 green bell pepper, chopped
- ¼ cup scallions, chopped
- 15 ounces canned black beans, drained
- 1 cup salsa
- ½ cup of water
- ¼ teaspoon cumin, ground
- ½ teaspoon turmeric powder
- ½ teaspoon smoked paprika
- A pinch of salt and black pepper
- ¼ teaspoon chili powder
- 3 cups spinach leaves, torn
- 8 tortillas for serving

Directions:

1. In your slow cooker, mix tofu with bell pepper, scallions, black beans, salsa, water, cumin, turmeric, paprika, salt, pepper, and chili powder, stir, cover and cook on Low for 6 hours.
2. Add spinach, toss well, divide this on your tortillas, roll, wrap them and serve for breakfast.
3. Enjoy!

Nutrition Value:

calories 211, fat 4, fiber 7, carbs 14, protein 4

372. Healthy Steel Cut Oats

Preparation time: 10 minutes Cooking time: 4 hours Servings: 6

Ingredients:

- 1 and ½ cups of water
- 1 and ½ cups of coconut milk
- 2 apples, cored, peeled and chopped
- 1 cup steel cut oats
- ½ teaspoon cinnamon powder
- ¼ teaspoon nutmeg, ground
- ¼ teaspoon allspice, ground
- ¼ teaspoon ginger powder
- ¼ teaspoon cardamom, ground
- 1 tablespoon flax seed, ground
- 2 teaspoons vanilla extract
- 2 teaspoons stevia
- Cooking spray

Directions:

1. Spray your slow cooker with cooking spray, add apple pieces, milk, water, cinnamon, oats, allspice, nutmeg, cardamom, ginger, vanilla, flax seeds, and stevia, stir, cover and cook on Low for 4 hours.
2. Stir oatmeal again divides into bowls and serve.

Desserts

Nutrition Value:
- calories 162, fat 3, fiber 7, carbs 8, protein 5
- Breakfast Tofu Casserole

Preparation time: 10 minutes Cooking time: 4 hours Servings: 4

Ingredients:
- 1 teaspoon lemon zest, grated
- 14 ounces tofu, cubed
- 1 tablespoon lemon juice
- 2 tablespoons nutritional yeast
- 1 tablespoon apple cider vinegar
- 1 tablespoon olive oil
- 2 garlic cloves, minced
- 10 ounces spinach, torn
- ½ cup yellow onion, chopped
- ½ teaspoon basil, dried
- 8 ounces mushrooms, sliced
- Salt and black pepper to the taste
- ¼ teaspoon red pepper flakes
- Cooking spray

Directions:
1. Spray your slow cooker with some cooking spray and arrange tofu cubes on the bottom.
2. Add lemon zest, lemon juice, yeast, vinegar, olive oil, garlic, spinach, onion, basil, mushrooms, salt, pepper, and pepper flakes, toss, cover and cook on Low for 4 hours.
3. Divide between plates and serve for breakfast.
4. Nutrition Value:
5. calories 216, fat 6, fiber 8, carbs 12, protein 4
6. Carrot Oatmeal

Preparation time: 10 minutes Cooking time: 7 hours Servings: 4

Ingredients:
- 2 cups of coconut milk
- ½ cup steel cut oats
- 1 cup carrots, shredded
- 1 teaspoon cardamom, ground
- ½ teaspoon agave nectar
- A pinch of saffron
- Cooking spray

Directions:
1. Spray your slow cooker with cooking spray, add milk, oats, carrots, cardamom, and agave nectar, stir, cover and cook on Low for 7 hours.
2. Stir oatmeal again, divide into bowls, sprinkle saffron on top and serve for breakfast.

Nutrition Value:

calories 182, fat 7, fiber 4, carbs 8,

protein 3

373. Delicious Scramble

Preparation time: 10 minutes Cooking time: 8 hours Servings: 4

Ingredients:

- 1-pound tofu, crumbled
- 1-pound white mushrooms, sliced
- 1 cup green onions, chopped
- 1 cup of corn
- 1 tablespoon olive oil
- A pinch of salt and black pepper
- 1 zucchini, chopped
- ¼ cup coconut aminos
- ½ cup nutritional yeast
- 3 pounds baby red potatoes, halved

Directions:

1. In your slow cooker, mix oil with tofu, mushrooms, green onions, corn, salt, pepper, zucchini, aminos, yeast and potatoes, toss, cover and cook on Low for 8 hours.
2. Divide between plates and serve for breakfast.

Nutrition Value: calories 222, fat 5, fiber 8, carbs 12,

protein 4

374. Blueberries Oatmeal

Preparation time: 10 minutes Cooking time: 8 hours Servings: 4

Ingredients:

- 1 cup blueberries
- 1 cup steel cut oats
- 1 cup of coconut milk
- 2 tablespoons agave nectar
- ½ teaspoon vanilla extract
- Coconut flakes for serving
- Cooking spray

Directions:

1. Spray your slow cooker with cooking spray, add oats, milk, agave nectar, vanilla and blueberries, toss, cover and cook on Low for 8 hours.
2. Stir your oatmeal one more time, divide into bowls, sprinkle coconut flakes all over and serve.
3. Nutrition Value: calories 182, fat 6, fiber 8, carbs 9,
4. protein 6
5. Sweet Apple and Pears Breakfast

Preparation time: 10 minutes Cooking time: 6 hours Servings: 6

Ingredients:

- 4 apples, cored, peeled and cut into medium chunks
- 1 teaspoon lemon juice

Desserts

- 4 pears, cored, peeled and cut into medium chunks
- 5 teaspoons stevia
- 1 teaspoon cinnamon powder
- 1 teaspoon vanilla extract
- ½ teaspoon ginger, ground
- ½ teaspoon cloves, ground
- ½ teaspoon cardamom, ground

Directions:

1. In your slow cooker, mix apples with pears, lemon juice, stevia, cinnamon, vanilla extract, ginger, cloves, and cardamom, stir, cover and cook on Low for 6 hours.
2. Divide into bowls and serve for breakfast.
3. Enjoy!

Nutrition Value: calories 201, fat 3, fiber 7, carbs 19,

protein 4

375. Almond Butter Oatmeal

Preparation time: 10 minutes Cooking time: 10 hours Servings: 2

Ingredients:

- ½ cup steel cut oats
- ½ cup almond milk
- Seeds from 1 vanilla bean
- 1 cup of water
- 4 tablespoons almond butter
- Stevia to the taste

Directions:

1. In 2 heatproof containers, divide oats, almond milk, vanilla seeds, water, stevia, and almond butter and stir.
2. Arrange containers in your slow cooker, fill slow cooker halfway with water, cover and cook on Low for 10 hours.
3. Serve warm for breakfast.

Nutrition Value:

calories 182, fat 3, fiber 7, carbs 18, protein 4

376. Banana Oatmeal

Preparation time: 10 minutes Cooking time: 8 hours Servings: 4

Ingredients:

- 1 banana, peeled and mashed
- 1 cup steel cut oats
- 2 cups almond milk
- 2 cups of water
- ¼ cup walnuts, chopped
- 2 tablespoons flax seed meal
- 2 teaspoons cinnamon powder
- 1 teaspoon vanilla extract

- ½ teaspoon nutmeg, ground

Directions:

1. In your slow cooker mix oats with almond milk, water, walnuts, flaxseed meal, cinnamon, vanilla, and nutmeg, stir, cover and cook on Low for 8 hours.
2. Stir oatmeal one more time, divide into bowls and serve for breakfast.

Nutrition Value:

calories 291, fat 7, fiber 6, carbs 42, protein 11

377. Delicious Frittata

Preparation time: 10 minutes Cooking time: 6 hours Servings: 4

Ingredients:

- 1-pound firm tofu, drained, pressed and crumbled
- 2 tablespoons olive oil
- ¼ cup nutritional yeast
- 1 yellow onion, chopped
- ¼ teaspoon turmeric powder
- 3 tablespoons garlic, minced
- 1 red bell pepper, chopped
- ½ cup kalamata olives pitted and halved
- 1 teaspoon basil, dried
- 1 teaspoon oregano, dried
- 1 tablespoon lemon juice
- Salt and black pepper to the taste

Directions:

1. Add the oil to your slow cooker and arrange crumbled tofu on the bottom.
2. Add yeast, onion, turmeric, garlic, bell pepper, olives, basil, oregano, lemon juice, salt, and pepper, toss a bit, cover and cook on Low for 6 hours.
3. Divide frittata between plates and serve for breakfast.
1. Nutrition Value:
2. calories 271, fat 4, fiber 7, carbs 20, protein 6

378. Apple Granola

Preparation time: 10 minutes Cooking time: 4 hours Servings: 3

Ingredients:

- ½ cup granola
- ½ cup bran flakes
- 2 green apples, cored, peeled and roughly chopped
- ¼ cup apple juice
- 1/8 cup maple syrup
- 2 tablespoons cashew butter
- 1 teaspoon cinnamon powder

Desserts

- ½ teaspoon nutmeg, ground

Directions:

1. In your slow cooker, mix granola with bran flakes, apples, apple juice, maple syrup, cashew butter, cinnamon, and nutmeg, toss, cover and cook on Low for 4 hours.
2. Divide apple granola into bowls and serve for breakfast.

Nutrition Value: calories 218, fat 6, fiber 9, carbs 17,

protein 6

379. Carrot and Zucchini Oatmeal

Preparation time: 10 minutes Cooking time: 8 hours Servings: 4

Ingredients:

- ½ cup steel cut oats
- 1 carrot, grated
- 1 and ½ cups of almond milk
- ¼ zucchini, grated
- A pinch of nutmeg, ground
- A pinch of cloves, ground
- ½ teaspoon cinnamon powder
- 2 tablespoons maple syrup
- ¼ cup pecans, chopped
- 1 teaspoon vanilla extract

Directions:

1. In your slow cooker, mix oats with carrot, zucchini, almond milk, cloves, nutmeg, cinnamon, maple syrup, pecans, and vanilla extract, stir, cover and cook on Low for 8 hours.
2. Stir your oatmeal one more time, divide into bowls and serve.

Nutrition Value:

calories 215,
fat 4,
fiber 7,
carbs 12,
protein 7

380. Cranberry Breakfast Quinoa

Preparation time: 10 minutes Cooking time: 2 hours Servings: 4

Ingredients:

- 1 cup quinoa
- 3 cups of coconut water
- 1 teaspoon vanilla extract
- 3 teaspoons stevia
- 1/8 cup coconut flakes
- ¼ cup cranberries, dried
- 1/8 cup almonds, chopped

Directions:

1. In your slow cooker, mix quinoa with coconut water, vanilla, stevia, coconut flakes, almonds

and cranberries, toss, cover and cook on High for 2 hours.

2. Stir quinoa mix one more time, divide into bowls and serve for breakfast.

Nutrition Value:

calories 246,
fat 5,
fiber 5,
carbs 30,
protein 7

381. Delicious Quinoa and Oats

Preparation time: 10 minutes Cooking time: 7 hours Servings: 6

Ingredients:

- ½ cup quinoa
- 1 and ½ cups steel cut oats
- 4 tablespoons stevia
- 4 and ½ cups of almond milk
- 2 tablespoons maple syrup
- 1 and ½ teaspoons vanilla extract
- Strawberries halved for serving
- Cooking spray

Directions:

1. Spray your slow cooker with cooking spray, add oats, quinoa, stevia, almond milk, maple syrup, and vanilla extract, toss, cover and cook on Low for 7 hours.
2. Divide into bowls, add strawberries on top, and serve for breakfast.

Nutrition Value:

calories 267,
fat 5,
fiber 8,
carbs 28,
protein 5

382. Breakfast Chia Pudding

Preparation time: 10 minutes Cooking time: 2 hours Servings: 4

Ingredients:

- ½ cup coconut chia granola
- ½ cup chia seeds
- 2 cups of coconut milk
- 2 tablespoons coconut, shredded and unsweetened
- ¼ cup maple syrup
- ½ teaspoon cinnamon powder
- 2 teaspoons cocoa powder
- ½ teaspoon vanilla extract

Directions:

1. In your slow cooker, mix chia granola with chia seeds, coconut milk, coconut, maple syrup, cinnamon, cocoa powder, and vanilla, toss, cover and cook on High for 2 hours.
2. Divide chia pudding into bowls and

Desserts

serve for breakfast.

Nutrition Value:

calories 261,
fat 4,
fiber 8,
carbs 10,
protein 4

MAINS

383. Stinky Roasted Garlic

Servings: 2
Preparation Time: 5 minutes Cooking Time: 20 minutes

Ingredients

- 2 medium garlic heads
- 2 tablespoon of olive oil

Directions

1. Pre-heat your oven to a temperature of 250 degrees Fahrenheit
2. Peel each of your garlic clove
3. Place the cloves in a single layer in a small sized baking dish and drizzle some olive oil
4. Bake for about 15 minutes until the garlic are tender

Nutrition Value:

Calories: 81 Fat: 7g Carbs: 5g Protein: 1g

384. The Crazy Tofu Bok Choy Salad

Servings: 5
Preparation Time: 30 minutes Cooking Time: 30 minutes

Ingredients

Oven Baked Tofu

- 15 ounces of extra firm tofu
- 1 tablespoon of Tamari
- 1 tablespoon of sesame oil
- 1 tablespoon of water
- 2 teaspoons of minced garlic
- 1 tablespoon of rice wine vinegar
- ½ a lemon juice

Bok Choy Salad

- 9 ounces of Bok Choy
- 1 green onion stalk
- 2 tablespoons of chopped cilantro
- 3 tablespoon of coconut oil
- 2 tablespoons of Tamari
- 1 tablespoon of Sambal Olek
- 1 tablespoon of peanut butter
- Juice of ½ a lime
- 7 drops of liquid Stevia

Directions

1. Press your tofu with heavy weight for 5 hours
2. Take a bowl and add all of the marinade ingredients -
1. Tamari, water, sesame oil, garlic, lemon juice, and vinegar
2. Chop up the tofu into square pieces and place them in a bag alongside the marinade

Desserts

3. Allow them to marinate for 30 minutes or overnight
4. Pre-heat your oven to 350 degrees Fahrenheit and place your tofu on a baking sheet lined up the parchment paper
5. Bake for 30-35 minutes
6. Add all of the salad dressing mixtures except Bok Choy in a bowl and mix well
7. Add chopped up Bok Choy
8. Toss well
9. Remove the tofu from your oven and assemble the salad by mixing the Bok Choy, Tofu, and Sauce

Nutrition Values:
Calories: 398
Fat: 30g
Carbs: 6g
Protein: 24g

385. A Spicy Red Coconut Curry for Keto Vegetarian

Servings: 4
Preparation Time: 10 minutes Cooking Time: 25 minutes

Ingredients

- 1 cup of broccoli florets
- 1 large sized handful of spinach
- 4 tablespoon of coconut oil
- ¼ medium onion
- 1 teaspoon of minced garlic
- 1 teaspoon of minced ginger
- 2 teaspoons of Tamari
- 1 tablespoon of red curry paste
- ½ a cup of coconut cream
- 2 teaspoons of special sauce

Special Sauce

- 1 and a ½ cup of shredded seaweed
- 6 cups of water
- 6 fat clove garlic crushed but not peeled
- 1 tablespoon of peppercorns
- 1 cup of mushroom Tamari
- 1 tablespoon of miso

Directions

1. Take a large saucepan and add garlic, peppercorns, water and bring to a boil
2. Lower down the heat and simmer for 20 minutes
3. Strain and return the liquid to the pot
4. Add Tamari and bring to a boil again and cook it is very salty
5. Remove the heat and stir in miso
6. This is your special sauce

7. Chop up your onion and mince garlic
8. Take a pan and place it over medium-high heat, add chopped up onions and minced garlic
9. Add two tablespoon of coconut oil and cook until translucent
10. Turn the heat down to medium-low and add broccoli to the pan, stir well
11. Once the broccoli is cooked, move the veggies on the side and add curry paste
12. Cook for 60 seconds
13. Add spinach and top and cook until wilt, add coconut cream alongside the remaining coconut oil
14. Stir and add Tamari, special sauce, ginger and allow it to simmer for 10 minutes more

Nutrition Values:

Calories: 310
Fat: 22G
Carbs: 5g
Protein: 25g

386. Quick and Easy Caesar Salad

Servings: 4
Preparation Time: 10 minutes Cooking Time: 0 minutes

Ingredients

- 1 piece of ripe avocado
- 3 tablespoon of lemon juice
- 2 tablespoons of water
- 3 minced garlic minced up
- 1 tablespoon of caper brine
- 1 tablespoon of capers
- 2 teaspoon of Dijon mustard
- Sea salt as needed
- Pepper as needed
- ¼ cup of hemp seeds
- 12 cups of chopped up romaine leaves

Directions

1. Take a bowl and add avocado, water, lemon juice, brine, garlic, capers, pepper and mustard salt
2. Add the contents to a blender and pulse until smooth
3. Add some water if your desired consistency is not reached
4. Spoon the dressing into a bowl
5. Add hemp seeds and mix
6. Add romaine lettuce to a large sized salad bowl and drop the dressing on top

Nutrition Values:

Calories: 281 Fat: 24g Carbs: 12G Protein: 6g

387. Creamy Roasted Pepper

Desserts

Soup

Servings: 4
Preparation Time: 0 minutes Cooking Time: 30 minutes

Ingredients

- 2 tablespoon of coconut butter
- ½ a cup of roasted red pepper chopped up
- 1 large sized finely chopped shallots
- 1 teaspoon of celery salt
- 1 tablespoon of seasoned salt
- 1 teaspoon of organic paprika
- 1 pinch of crushed red pepper flakes
- 4-5 cups of Cauliflower broken up into florets
- 4 cup of vegetable broth
- Just a splash of apple cider vinegar
- 1 pinch fresh thyme
- 1 cup of organic coconut milk

Directions

1. Take a heavy bottomed pot and add coconut oil over medium heat
2. Add chopped up shallots and Saute for 3 minutes
3. Add chopped up and roasted pepper alongside the seasonings
4. Stir well and cook for 2-3 minutes
5. Add cauliflower, fresh thyme, and stock
6. Bring it to a simmer and cover the pot, cook for 5-10 minutes
7. Work in small batches and puree the soup using an immersion blender
8. Bring back the whole blended soup back to your pot and stir in coconut milk

Nutrition Values:

Calories: 171
Fat: 16g
Carbs: 7g
Protein: 1g

388. Spiralized Asian Zucchini Salad

Servings: 10
Preparation Time: 10 minutes Cooking Time: 0 minutes

Ingredients

- 1 thinly spiralized medium zucchini
- 1 pound of shredded cabbage
- 1 cup of sunflower seeds
- 1 cup of sliced almonds
- ¾ cup of avocado oil
- 1/3 cup of white vinegar
- 1 teaspoon of Stevia

Directions

1. Cut up the spiralized zucchini into small portions using a kitchen knife
2. Take a large sized bowl and add sunflower seeds, cabbage, and almonds
3. Stir in zucchini
4. Take a small sized bowl and add oil, Stevia, and vinegar
5. Pour the dressing on top of the veggies and stir well
6. Chill for 2 hours and

Nutrition Values:

- Calories: 120
- Fat: 10g
- Carbs: 7g –
- Protein: 4g

389. Forever Together Courgette Salad

Preparation Time: 20 minutes Cooking Time: No cook required
Servings: 2

Ingredients

- Juice of 1 lemon
- 2 tablespoons of extra virgin olive oil
- ½ of a small pack of chopped up chives
- ½ of a small chopped up mint
- 300g of courgettes

Directions:

1. Take a large-sized bowl and pour lemon juice
2. Season with some salt and pepper
3. Whisk in olive oil and add the chopped-up herbs
4. Put Courgette through a Spiralizer using the noodle attachment
5. Tip the zoodles to your bowl
6. Add the prepped salad dressing
7. Toss everything well
8. Serve and enjoy!

Nutrition Values:

Calories: 144 Fat: 12G Carbs: 4g Protein: 4g

390. Roasted Cauliflower Soup

Servings: 6
Preparation Time: 15 minutes Cooking Time: 60 minutes

Ingredients

- 2 cauliflower head broken up into florets
- Olive oil cooking spray
- ¼ cup of olive oil
- 1 chopped up a large onion
- 4 cloves of chopped up garlic
- 6 cups of water

Desserts

- Salt as needed
- Pepper as needed

Directions

1. Add cauliflower florets to a large-sized bowl filled with salty water, wait for 20 minutes
2. Drain and arrange them on a sheet of aluminum foil on your baking sheet
3. Spray olive oil evenly over the cauliflower
4. Pre-heat your broiler to high and set the rack 6 inch away from the heat source
5. Broil for 20-30 minutes
6. Take a large soup pot and place it over medium heat
7. Add onion and cook for 5 minutes
8. Stir in garlic, roasted cauliflower and water and cook for 30 minutes
9. Blend the soup using an immersion blender and serve!

Nutrition Value:

Calories: 140
Fat: 10g
Carbs: 11g
Protein: 6g

391. Fine Pad Thai of Very Low Carb

Servings: 4
Preparation Time: 15 minutes Cooking Time: 20 minutes

Ingredients

- 1 bag of Kelp noodles
- ½ cup of peanut butter
- 1 medium-sized white onion
- ¼ cup of Tamari
- Juice of 1 lime
- 3 cloves of garlic
- 2 teaspoon of red pepper flakes
- Shredded up carrots, chopped scallions, sesame seeds, and cilantro

Directions

1. Soak your noodles under water and allow them to wilt
2. Take a food processor and add peanut butter, tamari, onion, lime juice, garlic, and pepper flakes
3. Process well
4. Drain the noodles and add ¼ of the sauce on top of the noodles
5. Give the whole mixture a toss
6. Serve with garnish and enjoy!

Nutrition Values:

Calories: 231
Fat: 16g

Carbs: 7g
Protein: 7g

392. Vegetarian White Pizza

Preparation Time: 15 MINUTES Servings: 2

Ingredients:

- 1 store-bought Pizza Crust
- ¼ cup Alfredo Sauce
- 1 tsp chopped Oregano
- ½ cup shredded Cheese
- 1 ½ cups Water

Directions:

1. Pour the water into your IP. Lower the trivet.
2. Line a baking dish that can fit into the IP with parchment paper.
3. Roll out the pizza crust and place inside the baking dish.
4. Spread the Alfredo sauce over the crust and sprinkle the cheese over.
5. Top with chopped oregano.
6. Place the dish on the lowered trivet and close the lid of the IP.
7. Set the IP to MANUAL and cook the pizza for 5 minutes on HIGH.
8. Do a quick pressure release. Serve and enjoy!

Nutrition Value:

Calories 390
Total Fats 20g
Carbs 30g
Protein 8g
Fiber: 2g

393. Mini Shephard's Pie

Preparation Time: 20 MINUTES Servings: 4

Ingredients:

- 1 cup diced Onion
- 2 cups steamed and Mashed Cauliflower
- 1 cup grated Potatoes
- 1 cup diced Tomatoes
- 1 ½ cup Water

Directions:

1. Add a splash of water to your IP and set it to SAUTE.
2. Add the onions and cook for 2 minutes.
3. Add the potatoes and cook on SAUTE for 5 minutes, stirring frequently.
4. Stir in the tomatoes and cook for 3 more minutes.
5. Divide the mixture between 4 greased ramekins.
6. Top with the mashed potatoes.
7. Pour the water into the IP and lower the trivet.
8. Place the ramekins on the trivet

Desserts

and close the lid.

9. Cook on HIGH for 5 minutes.
10. Serve and enjoy!

Nutrition Value:

Calories 225
Total Fats 14g
Carbs 5g
Protein 12g
Fiber: 0.3g

394. Mushroom Pasta

Preparation Time: 20 MINUTES Servings: 4

Ingredients:

- 1 ½ cups sliced Mushrooms
- 1 cup Coconut Milk
- 2 cups Water
- 1 tsp Arrowroot
- 2 cups Pasta, uncooked

Directions:

1. Add a splash of the coconut milk in the IP and set it to SAUTE.
2. Add mushrooms and cook for a few minutes.
3. Stir in the rest of the milk, water, and pasta.
4. Close the lid and set the IP to MANUAL.
5. Cook on HIGH for 7 minutes.
6. Do a quick pressure release and set the IP to SAUTE.
7. Whisk in the arrowroot and cook until the sauce thickens a bit.
8. Serve and enjoy!

Nutrition Value:

Calories 452
Total Fats 15g
Carbs 34g
Protein 15g
Fiber: 3g

395. Basil Risotto

Preparation Time: 30 MINUTES Servings: 6

Ingredients:

- 1 ½ tbsp Olive Oil
- 1 Onion, chopped
- 28 ounces Vegetable Broth
- 12 ounces Arborio Rice
- 1 ½ cups chopped Basil

Directions:

1. Heat the oil in the IP on SAUTE.
2. Add the onions and cook for 3 minutes.
3. Add the rice and cook for another minute.
4. Pour the broth over, give it a stir, and close the lid.
5. Cook on RICE for 15 minutes.
6. Do a quick pressure release.

7. Stir in the basil and cook on SAUTE for another minute.
8. Serve and enjoy!

Nutrition Value:

Calories 260
Total Fats 5g
Carbs 46g
Protein 7.8g
Fiber: 2g

396. Cheese and Asparagus Pasta

Preparation Time: 20 MINUTES Servings: 4

Ingredients:

- 1 cup shredded Cheese
- 2 cups Pasta
- 6 Asparagus Spears, chopped
- ½ cup Alfredo Sauce
- 3 ½ cups Veggie Broth

Directions:

1. Combine the pasta, asparagus, and broth, in the IP.
2. Close the lid and set it to MANUAL.
3. Cook on HIGH for 7 minutes.
4. Release the pressure quickly.
5. Drain the pasta and return it to the IP.
6. Stir in the sauce and cheese.
7. Cook on SAUTE for 2 minutes.
8. Serve and enjoy!

Nutrition Value:

Calories 480
Total Fats 12G
Carbs 39g
Protein 8g
Fiber: 2g

397. Carrot and Sweet Potato Medley

Preparation Time: 20 MINUTES Servings: 4

Ingredients:

- 2 tbsp Olive Oil
- 2 pounds Sweet Potatoes, cubed
- 1 Onion, chopped
- 2 pounds Baby Carrots, halved
- 1 cup Veggie Broth

Directions:

1. Heat the oil in your IP on SAUTE.
2. Add the onion and cook until soft, about 5 minutes.
3. Add the remaining ingredients, stir to combine, and close the lid.
4. Set the IP to MANUAL and cook on HIGH for 8 minutes.
5. Release the pressure quickly.
6. Serve and enjoy!

Nutrition Value:

Calories 413
Total Fats 7.5g
Carbs 76g

Desserts

Protein 7g
Fiber: 13g

398. Pesto Farfalle

Preparation Time: 10 MINUTES Servings: 4

Ingredients:
- 12 ounces Farfalle
- ¾ cup Pesto
- 4 cups Water
- 1 cup Cherry Tomatoes

Directions:
1. Combine the farfalle and water in your IP.
2. Close the lid and set the pot to MANUAL.
3. Cook on HIGH for 7 minutes.
4. Do a quick pressure release.
5. Drain the pasta and return to the pot.
6. Stir in the pesto sauce and cook on SAUTE for 1 more minute.
7. Quarter the cherry tomatoes and stir into the pasta.
8. Serve and enjoy!

Nutrition Value:
Calories 390
Total Fats 9g
Carbs 40g
Protein 8g
Fiber: 1g

399. Mexican Rice Casserole

Preparation Time: 35 MINUTES Servings: 4

Ingredients:
- 1 cup Black Beans, soaked overnight and drained
- 5 cups Water
- 2 cups Brown Rice
- 6 ounces Salsa Paste
- 2 tsp Cumin

Directions:
1. Combine all of the ingredients in your Instant Pot.
2. Close the lid and set the IP to MANUAL.
3. Cook on HIGH for 28 minutes.
4. Do a quick pressure release.
5. Serve garnished with lime and cilantro, if desired.

Nutrition Value:
Calories 322
Total Fats 2G
Carbs 60 g
Protein 6g
Fiber: 8g

400. Warm Collard Salad

Preparation Time: 5 minutes Cooking Time: 5 minutes Serving Size: 2

Ingredients

- ¾ cup coconut whipping cream
- 2 tbsp mayonnaise
- A pinch of mustard powder
- 2 tbsp coconut oil
- 1 garlic clove, minced
- Salt and freshly ground black pepper
- 2 oz. butter
- 1 cup collards, rinsed
- 4 oz. tofu

Directions

1. In a small bowl, whisk the coconut whipping cream,
1. mayonnaise, mustard powder, coconut oil, garlic, salt, and black pepper until well mixed; set aside.
2. Melt the butter in a large skillet over medium heat and sauté the collards until wilted and brownish. Season with salt and black pepper to taste.
3. Transfer the collards to a salad bowl and pour the creamy dressing over. Mix the salad well and crumble the tofu over.
4. Serve the salad immediately with cauli couscous.

Nutrition Value:
Calories: 495;
Total Fat: 46g;
Total Carbs: 8g;
Fiber: 3g;
Net Carbs: 5g;
Protein: 11g

401. Fried Broccoli Salad with Tempeh and Cranberries

Preparation Time: 5 minutes Cooking Time: 6 minutes Serving Size: 4

Ingredients

- 3 oz. butter
- ¾ lb tempeh slices, cut into 1-inch cubes
- 1 lb broccoli florets
- Salt and ground black pepper to taste
- 2 oz. almonds
- ½ cup frozen cranberries

Directions

1. In a deep skillet, melt the butter over medium heat until no longer foaming, and fry the tempeh cubes until brown on all sides.
2. Add the broccoli and stir-fry for 6 minutes. Season with salt and pepper. Turn the heat off. Stir in the almonds and cranberries to warm through. Share the salad

Desserts

into four bowls and serve.

Nutrition Value:

Calories: 740;
Total Fat: 72g;
Total Carbs: 12g;
Fiber: 5g;
Net Carbs: 7g;
Protein: 12g

402. Tangy Nutty Brussel Sprout Salad

Preparation Time: 13 minutes Cooking Time: 4 minutes Serving Size: 4

Ingredients

- 1 lb Brussels sprouts, trimmed
- 1 lemon, juice and zest
- ½ cup olive oil
- Salt and pepper to taste
- Spicy pecans and seed mix
- 1 tbsp butter
- 1 tsp chili paste
- 2 oz. pecans
- 1 oz. pumpkin seeds
- 1 oz. sunflower seeds
- ½ tsp cumin powder
- 1 pinch salt

Directions

1. Place the Brussels sprouts in a food processor and shred coarsely. Transfer to a salad bowl.
2. In a small bowl, mix the lemon juice, zest, olive oil, salt, and pepper, and drizzle the dressing over the Brussels sprouts. Toss and allow the vegetable to marinate for 10 minutes.
3. Meanwhile, melt the butter in a frying pan. Stir in the chili and then, toss the pecans, pumpkin seeds, sunflower seeds, cumin powder, and salt in the chili butter.
4. Sauté on low heat for 3 to 4 minutes just to heat the nuts but not exude the flavor. Turn the heat off and allow cooling. Pour the nuts and seeds mix in the salad bowl, toss, and enjoy the salad.

Nutrition Value:

Calories: 420;
Total Fat: 35g;
Total Carbs: 15g;
Fiber: 7g;
Net Carbs: 8g;
Protein: 12g

ENTREES

403. Tomato Cream Soup with Basil

Preparation Time: 20 minutes Servings: 2-4

Ingredients

- 1 carrot, chopped
- 2 tbsp olive oil
- 1 onion, diced
- 1 garlic clove, minced
- ¼ cup raw cashew nuts, diced
- 14 ounces canned tomatoes
- 1 tsp fresh basil leaves + extra to garnish
- 1 cup of water
- Salt and black pepper to taste
- 1 cup crème fraiche

Directions

1. Warm olive oil in a pot over medium heat and sauté the onion, carrot, and garlic for 4 minutes until softened. Stir in the tomatoes, basil, water, cashew nuts, and season with salt and black pepper.
2. Cover and bring to simmer for 10 minutes until thoroughly cooked. Puree the ingredients with an immersion blender. Adjust to taste and stir in the crème fraîche. Serve sprinkled with basil.

Nutrition Value:

Calories: 253,
Fat: 23.5g,
Net Carbs: 6.2g,
Protein: 4.1g

404. Coconut Green Soup

Preparation Time: 30 minutes Servings: 2-4

Ingredients

- 1 broccoli head, chopped
- 1 cup spinach
- 1 onion, chopped
- 1 garlic clove, minced
- ½ cup leeks
- 3 cups vegetable stock
- ½ cup of coconut milk
- 2 tbsp coconut oil
- 1 bay leaf
- Salt and black pepper, to taste

Directions

1. Warm coconut oil in a large pot over medium heat. Add onion, leeks, and garlic and cook for 5

Desserts

minutes. Add broccoli and cook for an additional 5 minutes. Pour in the stock over and add the bay leaf. Close the lid, bring to a boil, and reduce the heat. Simmer for about 10 minutes.

2. Add spinach and cook for 3 more minutes. Discard the bay leaf and blend the soup with a hand blender. Stir in the coconut cream, salt, and black pepper.

Nutrition Value:

Calories: 272, Fat: 24.5g, Net Carbs: 4.3g, Protein: 4.5g

405. Hearty Vegetable Soup

Preparation Time: 25 minutes Servings: 2-4

Ingredients

- 2 tsp olive oil
- 1 onion, chopped
- 1 garlic clove, minced
- ½ celery stalk, chopped
- 1 cup mushrooms, sliced
- ½ head broccoli, chopped
- ½ carrot, sliced
- 1 cup spinach, torn into pieces
- Salt and black pepper, to taste
- 2 thyme sprigs, chopped
- 3 cups vegetable stock
- 1 tomato, chopped
- ½ cup almond milk

Directions

1. Heat olive oil in a saucepan. Add onion, celery, garlic, and carrot; sauté until translucent, occasionally stirring, about 5 minutes.
2. Place in spinach, mushrooms, salt, rosemary, tomatoes, bay leaves, black pepper, thyme, and vegetable stock. Simmer the mixture for 15 minutes while the lid is slightly open.
3. Stir in almond milk and cook for 5 more minutes.

Nutrition Value:

Calories: 167; Fat: 6.2G, Net Carbs: 7.9g, Protein: 3.2g

406. Cream Soup with Avocado & Zucchini

Preparation Time: 35 minutes Servings: 2

Ingredients

- 3 tsp vegetable oil
- 1 leek, chopped

- 1 rutabaga, sliced
- 3 cups zucchinis, chopped
- 1 avocado, chopped
- Salt and black pepper to taste
- 4 cups vegetable broth
- 2 tbsp fresh mint, chopped

Directions

1. In a pot, sauté leek, zucchini, and rutabaga in warm oil for about 7-10 minutes. Season with black pepper and salt. Pour in broth and bring to a boil. Lower the heat and simmer for 20 minutes.
2. Lift from the heat. In batches, add the soup and avocado to a blender. Blend until creamy and smooth. Serve in bowls topped with fresh mint.

Nutrition Value: Calories: 378

Fat: 24.5g, Net Carbs: 9.3g, Protein: 8.2G

407. Mediterranean Artichoke & Red Onion Salad

Preparation Time: 30 minutes Servings: 2

Ingredients

- 6 baby artichoke hearts, halved
- ½ lemon, juiced
- ½ red onion, sliced
- ¼ cup cherry peppers halved
- ¼ cup pitted olives, sliced
- ¼ cup olive oil
- ¼ tsp lemon zest
- 2 tsp balsamic vinegar, sugar-free
- 1 tbsp chopped dill
- Salt and black pepper to taste
- 1 tbsp capers

Directions

1. Bring a pot of salted water to a boil. Add the artichokes to the pot. lower the heat and let simmer for 20 minutes until tender. Drain and place the artichokes in a bowl.
2. Add in the rest of the ingredients, except for the olives; toss to combine well. Transfer to a serving platter and top with the olives.

Nutrition Value:

Calories: 464,
Fat: 31.2g,
Net Carbs: 9.5g,
Protein: 13.4g

408. Fresh Avocado-Cucumber Soup

Preparation Time: 10 minutes + chilling time Servings: 2-4

Ingredients

Desserts

- 3 tbsp olive oil
- 1 small onion, chopped
- 4 large cucumbers, seeded, chopped
- 1 large avocado, peeled and pitted
- Salt and black pepper to taste
- 1 ½ cups water
- 1 tbsp cilantro, chopped
- 2 limes, juiced
- 1 garlic clove, minced
- 2 tomatoes, chopped
- 1 chopped avocado for garnish

Directions

1. Pour all the ingredient, except for the tomatoes and avocado in the food processor. Puree the ingredients for 2 minutes or until smooth. Pour the mixture in a bowl. Cover and refrigerate for 2 hours. Top with avocado and tomatoes.

Nutrition Value:

Calories: 343,
Fat: 26.4g
,Net Carbs: 5.3g,
Protein: 10g

409. Almond Parsnip Soup

Preparation Time: 25 minutes Servings: 2-4

Ingredients

- 1 tbsp olive oil
- 1 cup onion, chopped
- 1 celery, chopped
- 2 cloves garlic, minced
- 2 turnips, peeled and chopped
- 4 cups vegetable broth
- Salt and white pepper, to taste
- ¼ cup ground almonds
- 1 cup almond milk
- 1 tbsp fresh cilantro, chopped

Directions

1. Warm the oil in a pot over medium heat and sauté celery, garlic, and onion for 6 minutes. Stir in white pepper, broth, salt, and ground almonds. Boil the mixture.
2. Bring to the boil and simmer for 15 minutes. Transfer the soup to an immersion blender and puree. Serve garnished with sour cream and cilantro.

Nutrition Value:

Calories: 125;
Fat: 7.1g,
Net Carbs: 7.7g,
Protein: 4g

410. Sauteed Spinach with Spicy

Tofu

Preparation Time: 25 minutes Servings: 2-4

Ingredients

- 2 tbsp olive oil
- 14 ounces block tofu, pressed and cubed
- 1 celery stalk, chopped
- 1 bunch scallions, chopped
- 1 tsp cayenne pepper
- 1 tsp garlic powder
- 2 tbsp Worcestershire sauce
- Salt and black pepper, to taste
- 1-pound spinach, chopped
- ½ tsp turmeric powder
- ¼ tsp dried basil

Directions

1. In a large skillet over medium heat, warm 1 tablespoon of olive oil. Stir in tofu cubes and cook for 8 minutes. Place in scallions and celery; cook for 5 minutes until soft. Stir in cayenne, Worcestershire sauce, black pepper, salt, and garlic; cook for 3 more minutes; set aside.
2. In the same pan, warm the remaining 1 tablespoon of oil. Add in spinach and the remaining seasonings and cook for 4 minutes. Mix in tofu mixture and serve warm.

Nutrition Value:

Calories: 205;
Fat: 12.5g,
Net Carbs: 7.8g,
Protein: 7.7g

411. Cauliflower & Celery Bisque

Preparation Time: 30 minutes Servings: 2-4

Ingredients

- 2 tbsp olive oil
- 1 onion, finely chopped
- 1 garlic clove, minced
- 1 head cauliflower, cut into florets
- ½ cup celery, chopped
- 4 cups vegetable broth
- ½ cup heavy cream
- Salt and black pepper to taste
- 1 tbsp parsley, chopped

Directions

1. Set a large pot over medium heat and warm the olive oil. Add celery, garlic, and onion and sauté until translucent, about 5 minutes. Place in vegetable broth, and cauliflower.
2. Bring to a boil, reduce the heat and simmer for 15-20 minutes.

Desserts

Transfer the soup to an immersion blender and blend to achieve the required consistency; top with parsley to serve.

Nutrition Value:

Calories: 187;
Fat: 13.5g,
Net Carbs: 5.6g,
Protein: 4.1g

412. Crunchy Rosemary Almonds

Preparation Time: 10 minutes Servings: 4

Ingredients:

- 2 cups almonds
- 1 tsp smoked paprika
- 2 tbsp olive oil
- 2 tbsp rosemary, sliced
- 1 tsp salt

Directions:

1. Heat olive oil in a pan over medium-high heat.
2. Once the oil is hot, then add almonds and cook for 3 minutes.
3. Season almonds with paprika, rosemary, and salt.
4. Serve and enjoy.

Nutrition Value:

Calories 342
Fat 31 g
Carbs 11 g
Sugar 2 g
Protein 10 g
Cholesterol 0 mg

413. Simple Cauliflower Popcorn

Preparation Time: 50 minutes Servings: 4

Ingredients:

- 1 large cauliflower head, cut into florets
- 2 tbsp butter, melted
- 2 tbsp coconut oil, melted
- Salt

Directions:

1. Preheat the oven to 400 F.
2. Add cauliflower florets into the bowl.
3. Pour melted coconut oil and butter all over cauliflower florets.
4. Season with salt and toss well.
5. Place cauliflower florets on baking sheet and roast in preheated oven for 40 minutes. Stir after every 15 minutes.
6. Serve and enjoy.

Nutrition Value:

Calories 162
Fat 12 g
Carbs 11 g
Sugar 5 g

Protein 4 g
Cholesterol 15 mg

414. Easy Brussels sprouts Chips

Preparation Time: 15 minutes Servings: 2

Ingredients:

- 10 Brussels sprouts split leaves
- 1 tbsp extra virgin olive oil
- 1/4 tsp salt

Directions:

1. Preheat the oven to 350 F.
2. Add all ingredients to the bowl and toss well.
3. Place Brussels sprouts on baking sheet and roast in preheated oven for 10 minutes.
4. Serve and enjoy.

Nutrition Value:

- Calories 101
- Fat 7 g
- Carbs 8 g
- Sugar 2 g
- Protein 3 g
- Cholesterol 0 mg

415. Crispy Apple Chips

Preparation Time: 2 hours 5 minutes Servings: 6

Ingredients:

- 2 medium apples, cored and sliced
- 2 tbsp pumpkin pie spice
- Directions:
- Preheat the oven to 390 F.
- Arrange apple slices on a baking sheet.
- Sprinkle pumpkin pie spice on apple slices and bake in preheated oven for 2 hours. Serve and enjoy.

Nutrition Value:

Calories 45
Fat 0.4 g
Carbs 11 g
Sugar 7 g
Protein 0.3 g
Cholesterol 0 mg

416. Crisp Radish Chips

Preparation Time: 25 minutes Servings: 4

Ingredients:

- 16 oz fresh radishes
- 2 tbsp olive oil
- 1/2 tsp pepper
- 1/2 tsp sea salt

Directions:

1. Preheat the oven to 400 F.
2. Add all ingredients to the bowl and toss well.
3. Arrange sliced radishes on a baking sheet and bake in preheated oven for 15 minutes.

Desserts

4. Serve and enjoy.

Nutrition Value:

Calories 79
Fat 7 g
Carbs 4 g
Sugar 2 g
Protein 0.8 g
Cholesterol 0 mg

417. Fried Parsnip Chips

Preparation Time: 15 minutes Servings: 4

Ingredients:

- 2 medium parsnips, peeled and sliced
- Salt
- Oil for frying

Directions:

1. Heat oil in a large saucepan over medium-high heat.
2. Once the oil temperature reaches 350 F then add sliced parsnips into the batches in oil and fry for 30 seconds or until lightly golden brown.
3. Place fried parsnips chips on a paper towel to soak extra oil.
4. Sprinkle salt over fried parsnip chips and serve.

Nutrition Value:

Calories 50
Fat 2 g
Carbs 12 g
Sugar 3.2 g
Protein 0.8 g
Cholesterol 0 mg

418. Spicy Roasted Nuts

Preparation Time: 30 minutes Servings: 4

Ingredients:

- 1/2 cup almonds
- 1/2 cup walnuts
- 1/2 cup hazelnuts
- 1 tsp cinnamon
- 1 tsp ginger root
- 1 tsp fresh orange peel
- 1 tsp nutmeg
- 4 tbsp olive oil
- 1 tsp sea salt

Directions:

1. Preheat the oven to 375 F.
2. Add almonds, walnuts, and hazelnuts in a bowl and toss well.
3. Place nuts on a baking sheet and roast in preheated oven for 10 minutes.
4. Melt butter in a pan over medium heat.
5. Once butter is melted then add cinnamon, ginger root, orange peel, nutmeg, and salt in a pan and stir well.
6. Add roasted nuts in a pan and toss well.

7. Serve hot and enjoy.

Nutrition Value:

Calories 349
Fat 35 g
Carbs 6 g
Sugar 1 g
Protein 7 g
Cholesterol 0 mg

HIGH PROTEIN PLANT-BASED RECIPES

419. Tofu Scramble with Spinach

Ingredients (2 servings)

- 2 chopped tomatoes
- 2 minced cloves of garlic
- 2 tablespoons of olive oil
- 10 ounces of rinsed spinach
- ¾ cup of fresh sliced mushrooms
- 1 pound of firm tofu (crumbled, well-pressed)
- ½ teaspoon of soy sauce
- 1 teaspoon of fresh lemon juice (squeezed)
- ½ teaspoon of salt and pepper

How to make

1. Get a medium-size skillet, place on medium heat. Pour the olive oil in the skillet, add the garlic, mushrooms, and tomatoes to it. Sauté it for about 2 minutes.
2. Reduce the heat from medium to low heat then add the crumbled tofu, soy sauce, and spinach. Stir together
3. and pour in the lemon juice. Stir the mixture together and cover the skillet. Cook for 7 minutes, ensure you are stirring the mixture occasionally.
4. Sprinkle the salt and pepper to your desired taste. Stir together and cook for another 2 minutes.
5. Serve with toast or biscuit, and enjoy!

Note: You can add extra soy sauce to the scramble if you want more flavor. Also, you can replace the vegetables with zucchini, asparagus, bell peppers, chard or kale, or any green of your choice.

Nutritional value Calories: 527 Carbs: 43g

Protein: 36g Fat: 29g Fiber: 10g

420. Apple Pancakes

Ingredients (4 servings)

- 2 chopped apples
- ½ cup of soft/silken Tofu
- 1/3 cup of vegetable shortening
- 1 ½ cups of soy milk
- 2 ½ teaspoons of baking powder
- 1 ½ cups of flour
- ½ teaspoon of cinnamon
- ½ teaspoon of nutmeg
- 1/3 cup of chopped pecans
- 2 tablespoons of olive oil

How to make

1. Get a blender or food processor. Put the chopped apples, soft tofu, vegetable, flour, baking powder, and soy milk. Blend everything until it's well blended. Add the nutmeg, cinnamon to the mixture. Blend again until the apples are well minced, and all the ingredients are incorporated and blended.
2. Pick the pecans and gently fold the blended ingredients in the pecans.
3. Prepare a large skillet by oiling it.
4. Use a large spoon; take a spoonful of the pecans and drop in the skillet. Cook the pecans until bubbles appear; this usually takes a few minutes.
5. Flip the pecan to the other side and cook until both sides are lightly golden brown.
6. Serve and enjoy!

Nutritional value

Calories: 381
Carbs: 34g
Protein: 8g
Fat: 25g - Fiber: 5g

421. Chickpea Omelet

Ingredients (3 omelets)

- 1 cup of chickpea flour
- ½ teaspoon of powder onion
- ½ teaspoon of powder garlic
- ¼ teaspoon of white pepper
- ¼ teaspoon of black pepper
- 1/3 cup of yeast
- ½ teaspoon of baking soda
- 3 green chopped onions
- 4 ounces of mushrooms
- 1 cup of water

How to cook

1. Get a small bowl. Pour the chickpea in it. Add the garlic powder, onion powder, black pepper, white pepper, nutritional yeast, baking soda to the chickpea flour, and combine well.
2. Add the cup of water to it, stir everything together very well until a batter is formed. Make sure the batter is fine and smooth.
3. Place a frying pan over the medium heat. Use a spoon to scoop the batter from the bowl and place it in the pan. Make the pancakes 6-inches.
4. Sprinkle one tablespoon of green onions and mushroom to each of the batter scoops for the omelet.

Desserts

5. Flip each omelet when one side is browned. Flip to the other side and frying until it is also brown. This usually takes a minute. Do this for each of the omelets.
6. Serve the omelet and garnish with spinach, tomatoes, and hot sauce of your choice.
7. Serve and enjoy!

Nutritional value Calories: 297 Carbs: 26g

Protein: 20g Fat: 16g Fiber: 6g

422. Black Bean and Hummus Sandwich Wrap

Ingredients (2 servings)

- 1 roasted poblano pepper
- 8 ounce of roasted red bell pepper hummus
- ½ can of black beans
- ½ package of fresh spinach
- 1 chopped bell pepper
- 1 chopped onion
- 4 ounces of mushroom (sliced)
- ½ can of corn (drained and rinsed)
- 2 large wraps of whole grain

How to make

1. Preheat your over to 450 F and prepare a baking dish lined with baking sheet.
2. Get a medium-sized skillet or pot. Place over medium heat. Pour the onion into the pot and sauté it. Add bell pepper to it when the onion is transparent. Cook together for 2 minutes.
3. Pour the mushroom and corn into the pot and stir
4. together until it's well combined.
5. Prepare a clean countertop and spread the whole grain wraps on it. Use a spoon to spread the red bell pepper hummus on the wraps. Ensure its well spread. On each wrap, add the sautéed vegetables, poblano strips, beans, and spinach to it.
6. Roll the wraps with the ingredients in it into a burrito. Place each burrito in the baking dish and place it in the oven — Bake for 10 minutes.
7. Remove it and let it cool down a bit until it's warm. Top
8. with salsa and guacamole. Serve and enjoy!

Nutritional value Calories: 293 Carbs: 42.8g Protein: 13g

Fat: 8g - Fiber: 10g

423. Tempeh "Chicken" Salad

Ingredients (3 servings)

- 1 package of tempeh (cut the tempeh into ½ inch cubes)
- 2 tablespoons of olive oil
- 3 tablespoons of mayonnaise
- 2 teaspoons of lemon juice
- 2 tablespoons of minced onions
- 3 stalks of celery
- 1 tablespoon of dried parsley
- ¼ teaspoon of curry powder
- 2 cups of water to boil the tempeh

How to make

1. Get a large pot or skillet and pour the water. Place over high heat and let it boil.
2. Pour the tempeh in hot water. Leave it to simmer for 15 minutes then drain completely.
3. Put a frying pan on medium heat and add olive oil to heat. Add the boiled tempeh to it the pan. Fry for 5 minutes until all the sides are well cooked. Remove the frying pan from heat to cool down.
4. Get another large bowl, pour the cooled tempeh in it, add the mayonnaise, onion, celery, dried parsley, curry, and lemon juice. Keep stirring until the mayonnaise mixture is well combined with the tempeh, and evenly coats it.
5. Sprinkle salt and pepper to taste.
6. Serve the tempeh on a bed of lettuce, in between two toast pieces of bread. Serve and enjoy!

Nutritional value Calories: 250 Carbs: 5g

Protein: 7g
Fat: 23g
Fiber 1g

424. Black Bean and Sweet Potato Chili

Ingredients (6 servings)

- 2 minced cloves of garlic
- 1 diced small onion
- 2 tablespoons of olive oil
- 2 small sweet potatoes (chopped)
- 2 sliced carrots
- 1 can of black beans
- 1 can of diced tomatoes
- ½ cup of water
- 1 tablespoon of chili powder
- 1 teaspoon of cumin
- ½ teaspoon of cayenne
- ½ teaspoon of garlic powder
- ½ teaspoon of salt

Desserts

- ¼ teaspoon of black pepper

How to make

1. Place a Dutch oven over medium heat. Pour the olive oil, garlic, and onions, sauté for a few minutes.
2. Add the sliced carrots, chopped potatoes to the pot. Cook together with the onion until its soft. This usually takes 6 minutes.
3. Add the remaining ingredients to the veggies and reduce the heat from medium to low heat. Stir very well until it is well combined.
4. Partially cover the pot and let it simmer while stirring over low heat. Do this for 25 minutes. This should allow the flavors mingle, and also the sweet potatoes and carrots to be soft.
5. Remove from heat. Top with chopped cilantro, salsa, diced avocado, and green onions.
6. Serve and enjoy!

Nutritional value Calories: 384 Carbs: 67g

Protein: 19g
Fat: 6g - Fiber: 18g

425. Lentil Soup

Ingredients (4 servings)

- 1 teaspoon of vegetable oil
- 1 diced onion
- 1 sliced carrot
- 4 cups of vegetable broth
- 1 cup of dry lentils (brown lentils)
- ¼ teaspoon of dried thyme
- 2 bay leaves
- 2 teaspoons of lemon juice
- Salt and pepper to taste

How to make

1. Use a large pot placed over medium heat. Pour the vegetable oil, carrots, and onions, saute for 3 minutes.
2. Pour the vegetable broth to the mixture, add the thyme, bay leaves, lentils. Add salt and black pepper for taste.
3. Reduce the heat to low and let the mixture simmer together. Now cover the pot and cook the lentils until they are soft. This usually takes 40-45 minutes.
4. Remove the bay leaves from the soup. Pour the lemon
5. juice and stir it in until it's combined.
6. You can add more salt and pepper to your preference or not. Serve and enjoy!

Nutritional value Calories: 332 Carbs: 47g

Protein: 21g
Fat: 8g
Fiber: 7g

426. Indian Yellow Split Pea Dal

Ingredients (4 servings)

- 1 cup of uncooked yellow split peas
- 2 cups of vegetable broth
- 1 teaspoon of turmeric
- ¼ teaspoon of cayenne
- ½ teaspoon of salt
- 1 tablespoon of margarine
- 1 diced onion
- 1 ½ teaspoon of cumin (ground)
- 2 Whole cloves
- pepper for taste

How to make

1. Get a large pot and place it over medium heat. Pour the uncooked split peas and vegetable broth in it. Let it simmer.
2. When it is simmering, add the cayenne, turmeric, and salt. Cover the pot and let it cook until the yellow split peas are well cooked. This usually takes at least 20 minutes. Stir the mixture occasionally.
3. After 20 minutes and the split peas is not smooth and breaking up, you can cook for an additional 15 minutes until the dal as a smooth texture
4. Before the Dal is done, get another frying pan.
5. Place the frying pan on medium heat. Pour the margarine, onion, clove, and cumin. Let them heat together.
6. Cook the ingredients until they are soft. This usually takes 5 minutes.
7. Pour the onion mixture in the split pea, stir together until its well combined. Let it simmer for 5 minutes.
8. Add salt and pepper to your desired taste.
9. Serve hot and enjoy!

Nutritional value

Calories: 78
Carbs: 11g
Protein: 7g
Fat: 2G Fiber: 4g

427. Mexican Casserole with Black Beans

Ingredients (8 servings)

- 2 cups of minced garlic cloves
- 2 cups of Monterey Jack and cheddar

Desserts

- ¾ cup of salsa
- 1 ½ cups chopped red pepper
- 2 teaspoons ground cumin
- 2 cans black beans
- 12 corn tortillas
- 3 chopped tomatoes
- ½ cup of sliced black olives
- 2 cups of chopped onion

How to make

1. Preheat oven to 350 F and prepare a baking dish lined with baking sheets.
2. Place a large pot over medium heat. Pour the onion, garlic, pepper, cumin, salsa, and black beans in the pot — Cook the ingredients for 3 minutes stirring frequently.
3. Arrange the tortillas in the baking dish. Ensure they are well spaced and even overlapping the dish if necessary.
4. Spread half of the beans mixture on the tortillas. Sprinkle with the cheddar. Repeat the process across the tortillas until everything is well stuffed.
5. Cover the baking dish with foil paper and place in the oven. Bake it for 15 minutes. Remove from the oven to cool down a bit.
6. Garnish the casserole with olives and tomatoes
7. Serve and enjoy!

Nutritional value Calories: 595 Carbs: 72g

Protein: 33g
Fat: 21g
Fiber: 20g

428. Sweet-And-Sour Tempeh

Ingredients (3 servings)

- Tempeh
- 1 package of tempeh
- ¾ cup of vegetable broth
- 2 tablespoons of soy sauce
- 2 tablespoons olive oil
- Sauce
- 1 can of pineapple juice
- 2 tablespoons of brown sugar
- ¼ cup of white vinegar
- 1 tablespoon of cornstarch
- 1 red bell pepper
- 1 chopped white onion

How to make

1. Place a skillet on high heat. Pour in the vegetable broth and tempeh in it. Add the soy sauce to the tempeh. Let it cook until it softens. This

usually takes 10 minutes.

2. When it is well cooked, remove the tempeh and keep the liquid. We are going to use it for the sauce.

3. Put the tempeh in another skillet placed on medium heat. Saute it with olive oil and cook until the tempeh is browned. This should take 3 minutes.

4. Place a pot of the reserved liquid from the cooked tempeh on medium heat. Add the pineapple juice, vinegar, brown sugar, and cornstarch. Stir everything together until it's well combined. Let it simmer for 5 minutes.

5. Add the onion and pepper to the sauce. Stir in until the sauce is thick. Reduce the heat, add the cooked tempeh and pineapple chunks to the sauce. Leave it to simmer together.

6. Remove from heat and serve with any grain food of your choice.

7. Serve and enjoy!

Nutritional value Calories: 309 Carbs: 41g

Protein: 10g
Fat: 13g Fiber: 10g

429. Meatloaf Loaf

Ingredients (6 servings)

- 3 minced garlic cloves
- 1 diced onion
- 1 diced green bell pepper
- 3 tablespoons of vegetable oil
- 2 grounded packs of Gimme Lean beef substitute
- ¼ cup of uncooked oatmeal
- 2 slices of crumbled bread
- 3 tablespoons of ketchup
- 1 tablespoon of garlic salt
- ½ teaspoon of pepper
- ¼ cup of brown sugar
- ½ teaspoon of dry mustard

How to make

1. Preheat the oven to 375 F, prepare a baking dish by lightly greasing it.

2. Place a pan on medium heat, add oil, onion, garlic, and bell pepper. Let it saute for a few minutes.

3. In another large bowl, put the sautéed onions and pepper, beef substitute, crumbled bread, ketchup, oatmeal, salt, garlic. Combine the mixture very well.

4. Pour the mixture in the baking dish, cover the dish with a foil paper and place in the oven — Bake for 30 minutes.

5. In another bowl, put the ketchup,

Desserts

brown sugar, mustard. Whisk everything together until the mixture is smooth.

6. Drizzle the ketchup mixture on the baked loaf. Spread evenly across the length and breadth of the baking dish.

7. Place back in the oven and bake for another 15 minutes. Do not cover it this time.

8. Remove from the oven and allow it to cool before slicing.

9. Serve and enjoy!

Nutritional value

Calories: 212
Carbs: 33g
Protein: 7g
Fat: 8g
Fiber: 2g

SOUPS AND SALADS

430. White Bean Salad

Ingredients (4 servings)

- 2 cans of white beans
- 3 minced garlic cloves
- ½ cup of chopped parsley
- 2 tablespoons of olive oil
- 2 large diced tomatoes
- 1/3 cup of sliced black olives
- 2 tablespoons of red wine vinegar
- 1 tablespoon of lemon juice
- ½ teaspoon of salt
- ½ teaspoon of ground black pepper

How to make

1. Empty the canned white beans in a bowl and rinse well then drain.
2. Get a pot place over medium heat, pour the drained white beans, add onion, garlic, and parsley. Combine olive oil with the ingredients and heat until you perceive a pleasant smell.
3. This should happen within one minute. Make sure the
4. ingredients are not cooked until it's soft.
5. Remove the pot from heat and pour the contents in a large bowl.
6. Now, add the tomatoes, vinegar, black olives, and lemon juice. Stir gently until it's well combined, and all the ingredients are coated. Add the salt and black pepper to taste.
7. Serve warm or chill, enjoy!

Nutritional value

Calories: 586
Carbs: 100g
Protein: 33g
Fat: 7g Fiber: 29g

431. Gourmet Vegetarian Tabbouleh Salad with Edamame and Tofu Cheese

Ingredients (4 servings)

- 1 ¼ cups of bulgur wheat (uncooked)
- 2 cups of water
- ¼ cup pesto (cooked)
- 3 tablespoons of lemon juice
- 2 cups of chopped tomatoes
- ¾ cup of crumbled tofu cheese
- 1 can of chickpeas
- 1/3 cup of sliced green onions
- 2 tablespoons of minced parsley
- ¼ teaspoon of ground black

Desserts

pepper
- 2 cups of shelled edamame

How to make
1. Pour the bulgur wheat in a pot, add water, and place on heat. Cover the pot and cook for 30 minutes. Remove from heat and drain.
2. Get a small bowl, add the pesto and lemon juice together and whisk.
3. Get a large bowl, pour the pesto mixture to the drained bulgur, add the tofu, green onions, parsley, pepper, tomatoes, and edamame.
4. Stir everything together gently until it's well combined.
5. Serve the salad with pita halves and enjoy!

Nutritional value
Calories: 570
Carbs: 93g
Protein: 23g
Fat: 16g
Fiber: 14g

Quinoa Salad with Fresh Mint and Parsley

Ingredients (5 servings)
- 2 cups of quinoa
- ½ cup of almond nut
- 3 tablespoons of fresh parsley (chopped)
- ½ cup of chopped green onions
- 3 tablespoons of chopped fresh mint
- 3 tablespoons of olive oil
- 2 tablespoons of lemon juice
- 1 teaspoon of garlic salt
- ½ teaspoon of salt and pepper

How to make
1. Place a saucepan on high heat. Add the quinoa and water. Allow it to boil for about 15 minutes then reduce the heat and drain.
2. Pour the drained quinoa in a large bowl, add the parsley, almond nuts, and mint.
3. In another small bowl, add the olive oil, garlic salt, and lemon juice together. Whisk the mixture well until it's well combined and pour over the quinoa. Combine the mixture well until everything is well dispersed. Add the salt and black pepper to taste. Place the quinoa mixture bowl in the refrigerator. Leave it for 15 minutes for the flavors to blend in well. Toss together again. Serve and enjoy!

Nutritional value
Calories: 280
Carbs: 28g

Protein: 6g
Fat: 17g Fiber: 4g

433. Chickpea Spinach Salad

Ingredients (2 servings)

- 1 can of chickpea
- 1 handful of spinach
- ounces of tofu cheese
- 2 tablespoons of raisins
- ½ tablespoon of white vinegar
- 3 teaspoons of honey
- 4 tablespoon of olive oil
- ½ teaspoon of cumin
- ½ teaspoon of chili flakes
- ½ teaspoon of salt to taste

How to make

1. Empty the canned chickpeas in a bowl and rinse well then drain.
2. Add the chopped tofu cheese to it and spinach. Combine very well.
3. Drizzle the olive oil, honey, and lemon juice on the chickpea and spinach. Add the raisins to it and toss well.
4. Sprinkle the cumin powder and add salt and chili flakes to
5. taste. Toss together very well again until it's well combined.
6. Serve and enjoy!

Nutritional value

Calories: 658
Carbs: 52G
Protein: 23g
Fat: 40g
Fiber: 9g

434. Lentil Quinoa Salad with Spinach and Citrus

Ingredients (4 servings)

- ½ cup of dry lentils ½ cup of dry quinoa
- ¼ cup of diced red onion
- 2 segmented clementine
- 1 diced avocado
- ½ cup of halved grape tomatoes
- ¼ cup of parsley
- ¼ cup of pecans
- 4 big handfuls of spinach
- ¼ cup of unsweetened applesauce
- 2 tablespoons of balsamic vinegar
- 1 tablespoon of lemon juice
- 1 tablespoon of mustard
- ½ teaspoon of salt and pepper to taste

How to make

1. Rinse the dry lentils and pour it in a small pot, place over medium heat, and let it cook for 10 minutes. Drain the water, and keep covered.
2. Place a saucepan on high heat. Add the quinoa and water. Allow it to boil for about 15 minutes then reduce the heat and drain.

Desserts

3. Combine the cooked lentils and quinoa and
4. stir well until it's well combined.
5. Get another bowl, pour the applesauce in it, add the balsamic vinegar, mustard, and lemon juice. Whisk all the liquid ingredients together until it's smooth. Add desired salt and pepper to taste.
6. Combine the clementine, avocado, grape tomatoes, parsley, and pecans in a bowl.
7. Put the vegetables in each bowls and add a handful of spinach to the bowls.
8. Top each bowl with the lentil and quinoa mixture. Drizzle balsamic vinaigrette on each salad. Serve and enjoy!

Nutritional value

Calories: 338
Carbs: 50g
Protein: 12g
Fat: 13g
Fiber: 13g

435. Pasta Salad with Peanut Butter Dressing

Ingredients (2 servings)

- 5 ounces of pasta
- 1 chopped lettuce
- 1 chopped red cabbage
- 1 chopped purple kale
- 1 small chopped carrot
- 2 tablespoons peanut butter
- 2 tablespoons of soy sauce
- 2 tablespoons of maple syrup
- 2 tablespoons of malt vinegar
- ½ thumb of grated ginger
- 1 chopped garlic clove
- ½ cup of water
- 1 handful of roasted peanut

How to cook

1. Put the pasta in a medium-size pot, place on medium heat, add water, and cook until the pasta is tender.
2. Get a medium bowl, put the red cabbage, purple kale, lettuce and carrots in it.
3. In another bowl, put the peanut butter, maple syrup, malt vinegar, and soy sauce. Combine everything until it is smooth. Add the garlic and ginger to the mixture. Whisk together again.
4. Pour small water to the sauce to make it thin if it is thick.
5. If you are using a raw peanut, you can roast them on medium heat until the peanut is brown.
6. The pasta should be cooked and

tender, drain the water in it. Add the salad to it.

7. Scoop the sauce on the pasta and salad mixture
8. Garnish the salad with cilantro and lime.
9. Serve and enjoy!

Nutritional value

Calories: 660
Carbs: 104g
Protein: 26g
Fat: 17g Fiber: 15g

436. Red Lentil & Olive Salad with Tofu & Mint Yogurt Dressing

Ingredients (2 servings)

- 1 cup of red lentils
- 1 bay leaf
- 3 cups of water
- 1 cup of pitted Kalamata olives (chopped)
- 1½ cherry tomatoes
- 4-ounce tofu cheese
- ½ cup of blended cashew and coconut milk
- ¼ cup of olive oil
- ¼ cup of chopped mint
- ½ teaspoon of salt and pepper to taste

How to make

1. Get a pot, place over medium heat. Add the lentils and bay leaf to it. Pour the water in the pot and cover. Let it boil until the vegetables are soft and tender. This should take about 15 minutes. Ensure there is enough water in the pot.
2. When the vegetables are soft, drain the water out of the pot.
3. Add the tomato and chopped olives to the vegetable. Combine the vegetable mixture well and transfer to a bowl.
4. Place the vegetables in the refrigerator to cool off.
5. Pick another bowl to make the tofu yogurt dressing.
6. Pour the tofu cheese in the bowl, add the cashew and coconut milk, olive oil, and mint.
7. Use a blender or food processor, pour all the ingredients in it and blend until it is smooth and thick. Add salt and pepper to taste.
8. Remove the lentils from the refrigerator and serve in a bowl, drizzle the tofu yogurt on it. Serve and enjoy!

Nutritional value Calories: 310 Carbs: 38g

Protein: 10g Fat: 17g Fiber: 6g

Desserts

437. Kale Caesar Salad

Ingredients (4 servings)

- 1 bunch of dino kale (destemmed and chopped)
- 1 bunch of romaine lettuce (destemmed and chopped)
- ¼ cup of roasted chickpeas
- 2/3 cup of lemon juice
- ¼ cup of olive oil
- 1 tablespoon of water
- ¼ teaspoon of salt
- 1 ½ tablespoon of mustard
- 2 tablespoon of flaxseed (grounded)
- ½ cup of raw walnuts
- 2 teaspoons of garlic cloves

How to make

1. Put the walnut in a bowl, add water and soak for 10 minutes and drain.
2. Use a medium-sized bowl, put the kale and lettuce in it, toss together to combine.
3. Use a food processor or blender, add the mustard, lemon juice, flaxseed, drained walnuts, and garlic. Blend everything until it is smooth. Transfer the kale and lettuce to the plate, drizzle the blended ingredients on it. Ensure it is spread evenly. Sprinkle little grounded flaxseed, pepper, and salt to taste. Toss everything together again. Serve with the roasted chickpeas. Serve and enjoy!

Nutritional value

Calories: 260
Carbs: 10g
Protein: 13g
Fat: 7g - Fiber: 6g

438. High Protein Kidney Bean Salad

Ingredients (2 servings)

- 1 can of kidney beans
- ½ can of sweet corn
- ½ diced cucumber (chopped)
- ¾ cup of crumbled tofu cheese
- ½ cup of cilantro (chopped)
- 1 spring onions (chopped)
- 1 tablespoon of lime juice
- 2 tablespoon of olive oil
- 1 teaspoon of mustard
- 1 teaspoon of cumin
- ½ teaspoon of dried oregano
- 1 teaspoon of honey
- ½ teaspoon of salt and pepper to taste

How to make

1. Empty the cans in a bowl and rinse. Drain the kidney beans and corn.
2. Get another bowl, add the drained kidney beans and corn, add the chopped cucumber, cilantro, onions and crumble tofu. Toss everything together until it's well combined. Get a small bowl, add the mustard, cumin,
3. oregano, honey, and lime juice. Whisk together until it's combined and smooth. Add desired salt and pepper to taste. Whisk together again.
4. Transfer the salad into plates, drizzle the dressing mixture on it and mix.
5. Serve and enjoy!

Nutritional value

Calories: 539
Carbs: 54g
Protein: 23g
Fat: 28g
Fiber: 13g

439. Sweet Potato Salad

Ingredients (4 servings)

- 2 large sweet potatoes (peeled and sliced)
- 1 tablespoon of olive oil
- ½ teaspoon of paprika
- ½ teaspoon of oregano
- ½ teaspoon of cayenne pepper
- 1 diced shallot
- 2 diced spring onions
- Small chopped chives
- 3 tablespoons of red wine vinegar
- 2 tablespoons of olive oil
- 1 tablespoon of maple syrup
- ½ teaspoon of salt and pepper to taste

How to make

1. Preheat oven to 390F (200C) and prepare a baking sheet lined with parchment paper
2. Get a bowl, add the sweet potatoes, and add the paprika, cayenne pepper, and oregano to it. Mix with olive oil.
3. Spread the mixture in the baking sheet and place in the oven. Bake until it is roasted. This should take 30-35 minutes.
4. Remove and let it cool.
5. In another bowl, mix the shallot, spring onions, chives, vinegar, maple syrup, and olive oil. Mix everything until it's well combined.
6. Transfer the baked sweet potatoes to a bowl, dress it with the shallot mixture. Place in a refrigerator for

Desserts

1 hour for the flavors to blend. (You can serve it without refrigerating).

7. Remove from refrigerator and serve.
8. Serve and enjoy!

Nutritional value

Calories: 257
Carbs: 48g
Protein: 4g
Fat: 6g
Fiber: 7g

440. Greek-Style Salad

Preparation Time: 3 hours 15 minutes
Servings 4

Nutrition Value:

208 Calories;
15.6g Fat;
6.2G Carbs;
7.6g Protein;
5.1g Fiber

Ingredients

For Sunflower Seed Dressing:
- 1 cup sunflower seeds, raw and hulled
- 2 cups of water
- 2 tablespoons scallions, chopped
- 1 garlic clove, chopped
- 1 lime, freshly squeezed
- Salt and black pepper, to taste
- 1/2 teaspoon red pepper flakes crushed
- 1/4 teaspoon rosemary, minced
- 2 tablespoons coconut milk

For the salad:
- 1 fresh head lettuce, separated into leaves
- 3 tomatoes, diced
- 3 cucumbers, sliced
- 2 tablespoons Kalamata olives, pitted

Directions

1. Soak the sunflower seeds in water at least 3 hours. Drain the sunflower seeds; transfer them to your blender and add the remaining ingredients for the dressing.
2. Puree until creamy, smooth and uniform.
3. Put all the salad ingredients into four serving bowls. Toss with the dressing and serve immediately. Bon appétit!
4. 64.   Moroccan Carrot Salad with Harissa

Preparation Time: 10 minutes Servings 4

Nutrition Value:

196 Calories;
17.2G Fat;
6g Carbs;

1.2g Protein;
3.5g Fiber

Ingredients

- 1-pound carrots, coarsely shredded
- 1/4 cup fresh cilantro, chopped
- For the Vinaigrette:
- 3 garlic cloves, smashed
- Sea salt and ground black pepper, to taste
- 1/3 cup extra-virgin olive oil
- 1 lime, freshly squeezed
- 2 tablespoons balsamic vinegar
- 1/2 teaspoon ground cumin
- 1/2 teaspoon harissa

Directions

1. Place the shredded carrots and fresh, chopped cilantro in a salad bowl.
2. Combine all ingredients for the vinaigrette; mix until everything is well incorporated.
3. Add the vinaigrette to the carrot salad and toss to coat well. Bon appétit!

441. Warm Savoy Cabbage Slaw

Preparation Time: 25 minutes Servings 4
Nutrition Value: 118 Calories; 7g Fat; 6.7g Carbs; 2.9g Protein; 5g Fiber

Ingredients

- 2 pounds Savoy cabbage, torn into pieces
- 2 tablespoons almond oil
- 1 teaspoon garlic, minced
- 1/2 teaspoon dried basil
- 1/2 teaspoon red pepper flakes, crushed
- Salt and ground black pepper, to the taste

Directions

1. Cook the Savoy cabbage in a pot of a lightly salted water
2. approximately 20 minutes over moderate heat. Drain and reserve.
3. Now, heat the oil in a sauté pan over medium-high heat. Now, cook the garlic until just aromatic.
4. Add the reserved Savoy cabbage, basil, red pepper, salt, and black pepper; stir until everything is heated through.
5. Taste adjust the seasonings and serve warm over cauliflower rice.

442. Taco Salad Boats

Preparation Time: 25 minutes Servings 4

Nutrition Value:

140 Calories;
10.8g Fat;

Desserts

7.2G Carbs;
4.3g Protein;
5g Fiber

Ingredients

- 1 head romaine lettuce, stems removed
- 1/2 cup canned black beans
- 1 cup tomatoes, chopped
- 1 medium bunch of scallions, sliced
- 2 peppers, shredded
- 1 cup red cabbage, shredded
- 1 ripe avocado, peeled, pitted and diced
- 1/2 cup sesame butter
- 1 tablespoon apple cider vinegar
- 1 tablespoon fresh lime juice
- 1 teaspoon chili powder
- Sea salt and ground black pepper, to taste
- 1/2 red pepper flakes

Directions

- Pull the leaves off of the romaine hearts and arrange them on a tray.
- In a mixing bowl, combine the black beans with the tomatoes, scallions, peppers, red cabbage, and avocado. Fill the romaine "boats" with the bean mixture.
- Then, mix the sesame butter with the apple cider vinegar, lime juice, chili powder, salt, and black pepper.
- Drizzle the sauce over the filling.
- Garnish with red pepper flakes and serve immediately. Bon appétit!

443. Cauliflower Salad with Pecans

Preparation Time: 15 minutes + chilling time Servings 4

Nutrition Value:

281 Calories; 26.8g Fat; 5.6g Carbs; 4.2g Protein; 3.8g Fiber

Ingredients

- 1 head fresh cauliflower, cut into florets
- 1 cup spring onions, chopped
- 4 ounces bottled roasted peppers, chopped
- 1/4 cup extra-virgin olive oil
- 1 tablespoon wine vinegar
- 1 teaspoon yellow mustard
- Coarse salt and black pepper, to your liking
- 1/2 cup green olives, pitted and chopped
- 1/2 cup pecans, coarsely chopped

Directions

1. Steam the cauliflower florets for 4 to 6 minutes; set aside to cool.
2. In a salad bowl, place the spring onions and roasted peppers.
3. In a mixing dish, whisk the olive oil, vinegar, mustard, salt, and pepper. Drizzle over the veggies in the salad bowl.
4. Now, add the reserved cauliflower and toss to combine well. Scatter the green olives and pecans over the top and serve.

444. Crunchy Broccoli Salad

Preparation Time: 5 minutes + chilling time Servings 4

Nutrition Value:

245 Calories;
22.8g Fat;
6g Carbs;
4.2g Protein;
4.3g Fiber

Ingredients

- 1-pound frozen broccoli, thawed and broken into small florets
- 1 cup green onions, chopped
- 1 bell pepper, sliced
- 1/4 cup pecan, slivered
- 1/3 cup extra-virgin olive oil
- 2 tablespoons balsamic vinegar
- 1/2 teaspoon basil
- 1/2 teaspoon oregano
- Sea salt and freshly ground black pepper

Directions

1. Thoroughly combine all ingredients in a salad bowl.
2. Cover and let it sit in your refrigerator until ready to serve. Bon appétit!

445. Kale Salad with Crispy Tofu Cubes

Preparation Time: 15 minutes Servings 4
Nutrition Value: 327 Calories; 29.1g Fat; 7.2G Carbs; 13.2g Protein; 3.7g Fiber

Ingredients

- 2 tablespoons coconut oil
- 1 (14-ounce) block extra-firm tofu, pressed and cubed
- 1 bunch kale, torn into small pieces
- 1 shallot, sliced
- 1 garlic clove, pressed
- 1/4 cup cilantro leaves, divided
- 1 jalapeno pepper, seeded and minced
- 1/4 cup olive oil
- 1 lemon, juices
- Sea salt and ground black pepper, to taste

Desserts

- 1 (1-inch) piece fresh ginger, peeled and grated
- 1 tablespoon coconut aminos
- 1 tablespoon sunflower seeds, lightly toasted
- 1 tablespoon pumpkin seeds, lightly toasted

Directions

1. Heat the coconut oil in a saucepan over medium heat; now, cook the tofu cubes until they are golden brown on all sides. Reserve.
2. Mix the kale, shallot, garlic, cilantro, and jalapeno pepper in a salad bowl; then, drizzle the salad with olive oil and lemon juice.
3. Add the salt, pepper, ginger, and coconut aminos; toss to combine well. Top with the reserved tofu cubes. Scatter lightly toasted seeds over your salad and serve.

446. Cucumber and Zucchini Ribbon Salad

Preparation Time: 15 minutes Servings 4

Nutrition Value:
252 Calories;
23.1g Fat;
6.1g Carbs;
3.5g Protein;
2.7g Fiber

Ingredients

- 2 medium cucumbers, julienned
- 2 medium zucchinis, julienned
- 1 teaspoon of sea salt
- 2 tomatoes, sliced
- 1 WHIte onion, chopped
- 1 cup rocket lettuce, torn into pieces
- 1/3 cup extra-virgin olive oil
- 1 teaspoon fresh garlic, pressed
- 2 tablespoons balsamic vinegar
- 1 tablespoon Dijon mustard
- Sea salt and ground black pepper, to taste
- 2 tablespoons sesame seeds, lightly toasted
- 2 tablespoons sunflower seeds, lightly toasted

Directions

1. Toss the cucumber and zucchini with 1 teaspoon of sea salt in a fine-mesh sieve; place the sieve over the bowl.
2. Let it sit for about 20 minutes; then, squeeze the cucumber and zucchini gently to remove any excess liquid. Transfer them to a large bowl.
3. Add in the tomatoes, onion, and rocket lettuce. Make the vinaigrette by whisking the olive oil, garlic, balsamic vinegar,

mustard, salt, and black pepper to taste.
4. Dress your salad and serve garnished with lightly toasted seeds. Eat immediately or place in your refrigerator until ready to serve!

447. Crazy Asian Zucchini Salad:

Servings: 10
Preparation Time: 10 to 15minutes

Nutrition Value:

Calories: 120
Protein: 4g
Fat: 1g
Carbs: 7.3g

Ingredients:

- 1 lb. Cabbage (shredded
- 1/3 cup White vinegar
- 1 cup Sunflower seeds (shelled)
- 1 cup Almonds (sliced)
- 1 ½ teaspoon Stevia drops – about
- ¾ cup Avocado oil
- 1 Zucchini (thinly spiralized)

Direction:

1. First of all, please check that you've all the ingredients on the market. Toss together the cabbage, zucchini, almonds & sunflower seeds in a bowl.
2. Now whisk together the vinegar, oil & stevia in a bowl.
3. One thing remains to be done. Add the dressing to the salad & toss.
4. Finally, refrigerate for about 2 hours.

448. Iconic Creamy Kale Salad:

Servings: 3
Preparation Time: 20 to 30 minutes

Nutrition Value:

- Calories: 78
- Protein: 1.1 g
- Fat: 6.4 g - Carbs: 3.2 g

Ingredients:

- 1 bunch spinach
- 1 ½ tablespoon lemon juice
- 1 cup sour cream
- 1 cup roasted macadamia
- 2 tablespoons sesame seeds oil
- 1 ½ garlic clove, minced
- ½ teaspoon black pepper
- ¼ teaspoon salt
- 2 tablespoons lime juice
- 1 bunch kale

Toppings:

- 1 ½ Avocado, diced
- 1/4 cup Pecans, chopped

Direction:

1. First of all, please confirm you've all the ingredients out there.

Desserts

1. Chop kale and wash kale then remove the ribs.
2. Now transfer kale to a large bowl.
3. One thing remains to be done. Add sour cream, lime juice, macadamia, sesame seeds oil, pepper, salt, garlic.
4. Finally, mix thoroughly. Top with your avocado and pecans. Serve & enjoy.

449. Tasty Corn & Avocado Salad

Servings: 4
Preparation Time: 4 to 5 minutes

Nutrition Value:
- Calories: 144
- Protein: 3.2 g
- Fat: 13 g
- Carbs: 8 g

Ingredients:

450. Salad:

- 1 Corn on the cob (cooked, cut off husk)
- 4 ½ Grape tomatoes(quartered)
- ¼ cup Red onions (sliced)
- 1 Romaine head (chopped)
- ½ Avocado(sliced)

Dressing:
- Just a pinch Black pepper
- 1 ½ tablespoon Shallots(minced)
- 2 tablespoons White wine vinegar
- ½ teaspoon Kosher salt
- 6 tablespoons buttermilk
- 2 tablespoons Dijon mustard
- ¼ teaspoon Garlic powder
- 2 tablespoons virgin olive oil

Direction:
1. First of all, active and assemble all the ingredients in one place. Now for the dressing, whisk together all the dressing, whisk together all the dressing ingredients.
2. Finally, combine all the salad ingredients in a bowl along with the dressing & toss together. Finally, we've completed the recipe. Enjoy.

451. Coolest Arugula & Blueberry Salad:

Servings: 6 to 7
Preparation Time: 5 to 10minutes

Nutrition Value:
- Calories: 121
- Protein: 6 g
- Fat: 13 g
- Carbs: 5 g

Ingredients:
- 2 cups Blueberries

- 2 ½ tablespoons Balsamic vinegar
- 1 tablespoon Dijon mustard
- 10 oz. Arugula
- 2 ½ tablespoons Fresh orange juice
- ¼ cup Avocado oil

Direction:
1. First of all, ahead and assemble all the ingredients in one place. Now toss together the blueberries & arugula in a bowl.
2. Only one thing remains to be done now. Whisk along the remainder of the ingredients in another bowl.
3. Finally, pour the dressing over the dish and toss.
4. Finally, we've completed the recipe. Enjoy.

452. Fantastic Clean Avocado Saladwith Cilantro:

Servings: 4 to 6
Preparation Time: 10 to 15minutes
Nutrition Value:
Calories: 126 Protein: 2.1g Fat: 10g Carbs: 10g

Ingredients:
- 1 chopped up a sweet
- Pepper as needed
- green bell pepper (chopped up)
- 1 large sized chopped up red tomato
- Salt as needed
- ¼ cup of chopped up fresh cilantro
- avocados peeled, pitted and diced
- ½ of a juiced

Direction:
1. First of all, please confirm you've all the ingredients obtainable. Take a medium-sized bowl and add onions, bell pepper, tomato, avocados, cilantro& lime juice
2. Then mix well & coat everything well
3. One thing remains to be done. Season with some salt & pepper
4. Finally, serve chilled!

453. Curious Courgette Salad with Herbed Vinaigrette:

Servings: 4 to 5
Preparation Time: 20 to 25 minutes

Nutrition Value:
- Calories: 76
- Protein: 2.1 g
- Fat: 4.1 g
- Carbs: 3.1 g

Ingredients:
- 2 ½ tablespoons Olive oil
- Salt and pepper to taste

Desserts

- ½ pack Chopped chives
- 1 lemon juice
- 1 pack Chopped mint
- 10 ½ oz. Courgettes

(spiralized using the large noodle attachment of the spiralizer)

Direction:

1. First of all, go ahead and assemble all the ingredients in one place. Combine the salt, lemon juice, pepper and olive oil in a bowl and whisk together.
2. Mix in the herbs.
3. Combine the courgette noodles & the dressing in a bowl and toss together. Finally, we've completed the recipe. Enjoy.

454. Keto Red Curry

Servings: 6-8
Preparation Time: About 40 minutes

Ingredients:

- 1 cup broccoli florets
- 1 large handful of fresh spinach
- 4 Tbsp. coconut oil
- ¼ medium onion
- 1 tsp. garlic, minced
- 1 tsp. fresh ginger, peeled and minced
- 2 tsp. soy sauce
- 1 Tbsp. red curry paste
- ½ cup coconut cream

Directions:

1. Add half the coconut oil to a saucepan and heat over medium-high heat.
2. When the oil is hot, add the onion to the pan and saute for 3-4 minutes, until it is semi-translucent.
3. Add the garlic to the pan and saute, stirring, just until fragrant, about 30 seconds.
4. Lower the heat to medium-low and add broccoli florets. Saute, stirring, for about 1-2 minutes.
5. Push the vegetables to the side of the pan and add the red curry paste. Saute until the paste is fragrant, then mix everything together.
6. Add the spinach on top of the vegetable mixture. When the spinach begins to wilt, add the coconut cream and stir.
7. Add the rest of the coconut oil, the soy sauce, and the minced ginger. Bring to a simmer for 5-10 minutes.
8. Serve hot.

Nutrition Value:

Total Fat: 41 g
Carbs: 8 g
Protein: 4 g

455. Kale Soup

Servings: 6-8
Preparation Time: About 40 minutes

Ingredients:

- 4 cups fresh kale, chopped
- ½ cup canned white beans
- 2 cloves garlic, minced
- ½ onion, diced
- ½ cup celery, diced
- ¼ tsp. freshly ground black pepper
- Salt to taste
- 1 cup of water

Directions:

1. Place all ingredients into a heavy stockpot.
2. Bring to a low simmer and cook until fragrant, about 30 minutes. Add water if necessary, during cooking.
3. Transfer the soup to serving bowls and serve hot.

Nutrition Value:

- Total Fat: 15 g Carbs: 15 g
- Protein: 9 g

456. Creamy Jalapeno Soup

Servings: 8-10
Preparation Time: About 45 minutes

Ingredients:

- 3 Tbsp. butter
- 2 cloves garlic, minced
- ½ onion, chopped
- ½ bell pepper, chopped
- 2 jalapeno peppers, seeded and chopped
- 3 cups vegetable stock
- ½ cup heavy cream
- ¼ tsp. paprika
- 1 tsp. cumin
- 1 tsp. salt
- ½ tsp. freshly ground black pepper

Directions:

1. Heat the oil in a heavy stockpot over medium-high heat. When the butter is melted, add onion, bell pepper, and jalapenos and sauté until the onion is soft about 5 minutes.
2. Bring to a low simmer and cook until the chicken is thoroughly cooked and the vegetables are tender about 30 minutes. Add water if necessary, during cooking.
3. Stir in the cream, stirring to

Desserts

combine.

4. Transfer to serving bowls and serve hot.

Nutrition Value:

Total Fat: 40 g
Carbs: 4 g
Protein: 41 g

457. Chinese Chili Soup

Servings: 8-10
Preparation Time: About 40 minutes

Ingredients:

- ¼ cup sesame oil
- 6 dried red Thai chilis
- 5 cloves garlic, crushed
- 2 Tbsp. fresh ginger, peeled and sliced
- 3 cups vegetable stock
- ¼ cup of soy sauce
- ¼ cup dry sherry
- Salt to taste
- ¼ cup fresh Thai basil, chopped

Directions:

1. Heat the oil in a heavy stockpot over medium-high heat. Add the garlic, chilis, and ginger to the pot and sauté just until fragrant, about a minute.
2. Lower the heat and add all the other ingredients, excluding the basil, to the pot.
3. Bring to a low simmer and cook until the soup is fragrant about 30 minutes. Add water if necessary, during cooking.
4. Bring the soup to a boil again and stir in the basil, stirring until the basil is fragrant and wilted.
5. Transfer to serving bowls and serve hot.

Nutrition Value:

Total Fat: 15 g
Carbs: 7 g
Protein: 31 g

458. Mushroom Soup

Servings: 8-10
Preparation Time: About 40 minutes

Ingredients:

- 1 onion, chopped
- 3 cloves garlic, minced
- 2 cups fresh button mushrooms, chopped
- 1 medium yellow summer squash, chopped
- 3 cups vegetable stock
- Salt and pepper to taste
- 1 tsp. poultry seasoning

Directions:

1. Add all ingredients to a heavy stockpot.
2. Bring to a low simmer and cook until the soup is fragrant about 30 minutes. Add water if necessary, during cooking.
3. Transfer soup to serving bowls and serve hot.

Nutrition Value:
Total Fat: 15 g
Carbs: 9 g
Protein: 30 g

459. Vietnamese-Style Vegetable Soup

Servings: 6-8
Preparation Time: About 40 minutes

Ingredients:

- 1 onion, diced
- 2 Tbsp. tomato paste
- 2 Whole star anise
- 1 Tbsp. fresh ginger, peeled and minced
- 3 cloves garlic, minced
- 6 cups of water
- 1 tsp. ground pepper
- ½ tsp. Chinese five-spice
- ½ tsp. curry powder
- 2 carrots, peeled and sliced

Directions:

1. Place all ingredients in a heavy stockpot.
2. Bring to a low simmer and cook until the soup is fragrant about 30 minutes. Add water if necessary, during cooking.
3. Serve the stew hot.

Nutrition Value:
Total Fat: 9 g
Carbs: 8 g
Protein: 15 g

460. Green Chili Soup

Servings: 6-8
Preparation Time: About 2 hours

Ingredients:

- ½ cup dry navy beans, soaked for an hour in hot water
- 1 onion diced
- 3 New Mexico green chili peppers, chopped
- 5 cloves garlic, minced
- 1 cup cauliflower, diced
- 4 cups vegetable stock
- ¼ cup fresh cilantro, chopped
- 1 tsp. ground coriander
- 1 tsp. ground cumin
- 1 tsp. salt

Directions:

1. Put all the ingredients, into a large,

Desserts

heavy stockpot.

2. Bring to a low simmer and cook until the beans are tender about 60 minutes. Add water if necessary, during cooking.
3. Using an immersion blender, blend the soup until it is smooth.
4. Return the soup to a simmer.
5. Transfer the soup to serving bowls and serve hot.

Nutrition Value:

Total Fat: 5 g
Carbs: 13 g
Protein: 22 g

461. Vegetarian Red Chili

Servings: 6-8
Preparation Time: About 35 minutes

Ingredients:

- 3 tsp. chili powder
- 2 tsp. ground cumin
- 2 tsp. salt
- 1 tsp. dried oregano
- 1 Tbsp. olive oil
- 1 onion, chopped
- 2 cloves garlic, minced
- 1 cup canned diced tomatoes
- 1 Tbsp. canned chipotle chilis, chopped
- 2 corn tortillas, torn into small pieces
- ½ cup of water

Directions:

1. In a small bowl, mix chili powder, cumin, salt, and oregano.
2. In a blender or food processor, blend tomatoes, chilis, and tortilla pieces until smooth.
3. Heat the oil in a heavy stockpot over medium-high heat. When the oil is hot, sauté the onions until they're softened, about 3 minutes. Add the garlic and sauté for
4. about a minute more.
5. Stir in the spice mixture and sauté until fragrant, about 30 seconds.
6. Add the tomato/tortilla mixture to the pot, along with 2 cups water.
7. Bring to a low simmer and cook until fragrant about 20 minutes. Add water if necessary, during cooking.
8. Transfer the chili to serving bowls and serve hot.

Nutrition Value:

Total Fat: 24 g
Carbs: 12 g
Protein: 30 g

462. Vegetarian Green Chili

Servings: 6-8
Preparation Time: About 30 minutes

Ingredients:

- 3 tomatillos, sliced
- 3 jalapeno peppers, seeded and chopped
- 2 New Mexico green chili peppers, seeded and chopped
- 6 cloves garlic, minced
- 1 tomato, chopped
- 3 cups vegetable stock
- 2 tsp. cumin
- Salt and pepper to taste

Directions:

1. Put the tomatillos, jalapenos, New Mexico chilis, garlic, chicken stock, and tomato into a heavy stockpot.
2. Add the cumin, salt, and pepper on top of the meat.
3. Bring to a low simmer and cook until fragrant, about 20 minutes. Add water if necessary, during cooking.
4. Using an immersion blender, blend the sauce in the pot
5. until it's smooth.
6. Transfer the chili to serving bowls and serve hot,
7. garnished with chopped fresh cilantro.

Nutrition Value:
Total Fat: 4 g
Carbs: 4 g
Protein: 26 g

463. Tortilla Soup

Servings: 6-8
Preparation Time: About 30 minutes

Ingredients:

- 2 corn tortillas, torn into pieces
- ½ onion, chopped
- 1 cup tomatoes, chopped
- 2 cloves garlic
- 1 Tbsp. canned chipotle chili in adobo sauce, chopped
- ½ jalapeno pepper
- ¼ cup fresh cilantro, chopped
- 1 tsp. salt
- 1 Tbsp. olive oil
- 4 cups of water

Directions:

1. In a blender or food processor, combine onion, tomatoes, garlic, chipotle, jalapeno, and cilantro. Blend until the mixture is smooth.
2. Heat the oil in a heavy stockpot over medium-high heat. When the oil is hot, add the blended mixture to the pot. Cook, stirring, until fragrant, about a minute or two.

Desserts

3. Add the tortillas, chicken, and water to the pot.
4. Bring to a low simmer and cook until fragrant, about 20 minutes. Add water if necessary, during cooking.
5. Transfer to serving bowls and serve hot.

Nutrition Value:

Total Fat: 5 g
Carbs: 5 g
Protein: 12 g

464. Keto Vegetable Soup

Servings: 6-8
Preparation Time: About 45 minutes

Ingredients:

- 1 turnip, cut into bite-size pieces
- 1 onion, chopped
- 6 stalks celery, diced
- 1 carrot, sliced
- 15 oz. pumpkin puree
- 1 lb. green beans frozen or fresh
- 8 cups chicken stock
- 2 cups of water
- 1 Tbsp. fresh basil, chopped
- ¼ tsp. thyme leaves
- 1/8 tsp. rubbed sage
- Salt to taste
- 1 lb. fresh spinach, chopped

Directions:

1. Put all the ingredients, excluding the spinach, into a heavy stockpot.
2. Bring to a low simmer and cook until the vegetables are tender about 30 minutes. Add water if necessary, during cooking.
3. Add the spinach and stir until it's wilted about 5 minutes.
4. Transfer to serving bowls and serve hot.

Nutrition Value:

- Total Fat: 0 gram
- Carbs: 10 g
- Protein: 3 g

465. Keto Cabbage Soup

Servings: 6-8
Preparation Time: About 45 minutes

Ingredients:

- ¼ cup onion, diced
- 1 clove garlic, minced
- 1 tsp. cumin
- 1 head cabbage, chopped
- 1 ¼ cup canned diced tomatoes
- 5 oz. canned green chilis
- 4 cups vegetable stock
- Salt and pepper to taste

Directions:

1. Heat a heavy stockpot over medium-high heat. When the oil is hot, add the onions and sauté for 5-7 minutes more. Add the garlic and sauté for one more minute.

2. Bring to a low simmer and cook until the vegetables are tender about 30 minutes. Add water if necessary, during cooking.

3. Transfer to serving bowls and serve hot.

Nutrition Value:

- Total Fat: 18 g
- Carbs: 6 g
- Protein: 17 g

Sauces and Dips

466. Vegetarian Black Soup

Ingredients (4 servings)

- 2 15-ounce cans of black beans (undrained)
- 16-ounce of vegetable broth
- ½ cup of salsa
- Shredded cheese (optional)
- Sour cream (optional)
- Chopped onion (optional)
- Fresh chopped cilantro (optional)

How to make

1. Mash a can of black beans with a potato masher or make use of the food processor as a substitute. If using a food processor, add more water until they are mostly smooth
2. Pour the two cans of beans into a medium-sized saucepan
3. Add salsa, vegetable broth and chilli powder to the saucepan
4. Boil all the ingredients
5. As soon as all the ingredients are boiled, it is ready to serve
6. Depending on your preference, the vegetarian black soup can go with shredded cheese, sour cream, onion, and cilantro. Instead of this, you can make use of cheese and sour cream as an alternative. Serve and enjoy!

Nutritional Value

- Calories: 157 Carbs: 30g. Protein: 7g Fat: 1g Fiber: 9g
- Vegetarian Bean and Barley Vegetable Soup

Ingredients (6 servings)

- ½ of a large onion (diced)
- 2 to 3 cloves of garlic (minced)
- 2 tablespoons of oil/margarine
- 2 ribs of celery (diced)
- 2 medium of sized carrots (diced)
- Any other vegetables of your choice (about ½ cup each)
- 8 cups of water
- 1 cup of pearled barley (uncooked)
- 1 cup of pinto beans
- 1/3 cup of tomato paste
- ¼ teaspoon of salt
- ½ teaspoon of barley
- ¼ teaspoon of celery (optional)
- ½ teaspoon of pepper
- ½ teaspoon of thyme
- ½ teaspoon of oregano
- 1 teaspoon of onion powder
- 2 large bay of leaves
- Salt and pepper

How to make

1. Saute the onions and garlic in the oil or margarine, in a large soup or stockpot for two minutes
2. Add celery, carrots and other vegetables of your choice and allow to cook between 3 and 5 minutes
3. Add vegetable broth and other vegetables. Let it simmer. Mix the remaining ingredients. Once it is simmering, bring the heat to medium-low and cover pot
4. Let it simmer for up to 30 minutes or an hour. Stir occasionally until barley is soft and fluffy
5. Remove bay leaves before serving food
6. Before serving the soup, taste and add more spices, pepper and salt if necessary
7. Serve soup and enjoy!

Nutritional Value

Calories: 116
Carbs: 19g.
Protein: 5g.
Fat: 3g Fiber: 6g

467. Vegetarian Curried Corn Soup

Ingredients (3 servings)

- 2 tablespoon of vegetable oil
- ½ cup of green bell pepper (well chopped)
- ½ cup of red bell pepper (well chopped)
- ¼ cup of shallots (minced)
- 2 tablespoon of curry powder
- ½ tablespoon of salt
- 3 cups of fresh corn or as alternative 16-ounce bag frozen corn (3 cups)
- ½ tablespoon of freshly ground pepper
- 3 cups plain of soymilk or any non-diary milk
- 1 cup of vegetable stock
- ½ cup of shredded cheddar cheese

How to make

1. Heat the oil in a large saucepan with medium-high heat. After heating oil, add ball peppers and cook for about four minutes. While cooking stir occasionally until the bell peppers are tender
2. Add shallots in the last one minute and stir until it is browned. Add curry powder and stir and stair for another minute
3. Add the corn, pepper, pepper, vegetable stock and boil. Reduce heat and cook until vegetable is

Desserts

tender in 5 minutes

4. Add 2 cups of corn mixture to a food processor or a blender. Add a cup of soymilk. Blend until the mixture is almost smooth
5. After boiling, pour the mixture into the saucepan. Add and stir the remaining soymilk under medium heat. Cook for about 5 minutes
6. Sprinkle each serving with two tablespoon cheese. Serve and enjoy!

Nutritional Value

Calories: 100
Carbs: 20g
Protein: 3g
Fat: 3g
Fiber: 7g

468. Vegetarian Thai Coconut Vegetable Soup

Ingredients (4 servings)

- 1 onion (diced)
- 2 bell peppers (red, diced)
- ¼ teaspoon of cayenne
- ½ tablespoon of coriander
- ½ tablespoon of cumin
- 4 tablespoons of olive oil
- 1 can of chickpeas
- 1 carrot (sliced)
- 3 cloves of garlic
- ½ cup of basil or cilantro (fresh chopped)
- 1 teaspoon of salt
- 3 limes (freshly squeezed juice)
- ½ cup of vegetable broth
- 1 cup of coconut milk
- 1 cup of peanut butter
- 2½ cups of tomatoes (finely diced)

How to make

1. Saute onions, garlic and pepper in olive oil in a large pot. Make ingredients to be soft for at least 3 to 5 minutes
2. Leaving out basil, add the rest of the ingredients and allow it to simmer. Cook over low heat for an hour
3. Add half of it to the food processor, allow it to be very smooth and return to the pot
4. Add either of basil or cilantro, and your coconut food is ready. Before serving the soup, taste and add more seasoning if necessary. Serve, and enjoy!

Nutritional Value

Calories: 120 Carbs: 44g Protein: 10g Fat: 10g Fiber: 2g

469. Vegetarian Minestrone Soup

Ingredients (6 servings)

- Pepper (to taste)
- 1 bay leaf
- Salt (to taste)
- 3 cloves of garlic (minced)
- Optional: 1 cup green of beans (chopped)
- ½ onions (chopped)
- 2 stalks of celery (chopped)
- 2 carrots (chopped)
- 1 tablespoon of oregano
- 1 tablespoon of basil (chopped)
- 4 cups of tomatoes (diced)
- 4 cups of vegetable broth
- 3 Zucchini (chopped)
- 1½ cups of macaroni pasta

How to make

1. In a large pot, put vegetable broth then add diced tomatoes, basils, oregano, carrots, celery, onion, zucchini, green beans, garlic and bay leaves.
2. Slowly cook the soup to a low simmer and allow the soup to cook over very low heat for a minimum of 45 minutes, which could also extend to one hour. Cook
3. until the vegetables are tender. Note that you should stir the soup occasionally while it is cooking
4. Add salt and pepper and the macaroni pasta to the soup. Then bring the heat up a little to a medium-low level. Once this is done, allow the soup to simmer for another 10 or 20 minutes, or allow soup to simmer up until the pasta is done cooking
5. Before serving the soup, taste and add more spices, pepper, and salt if necessary
6. Remove the bay leaf from the soup.
7. Serve and enjoy!

Nutritional Value

Calories: 120
Carbs: 44g.
Protein: 10g
Fat: 10g
Fiber: 2g

470. Fat-Free Cabbage Soup Recipe

Ingredients (4 servings)

- 1 pound of cabbage (chopped)
- 2 cups of vegetable broth
- Dash salt (to taste)
- Dash pepper (to taste)
- 2 onions (chopped)
- Dash Tabasco or hot sauce (to taste)

Desserts

- ¼ cup of cilantro (chopped)
- 2 cloves of garlic (minced)

How to make

1. In a large saucepan, add chopped onions, minced garlic, vegetable broth, Tabasco or hot sauce together with a bit of salt with pepper. Once all these ingredients are combined, cover saucepan and allow it to simmer in medium-low heat for 20 minutes or more. Note that you should stir the soup occasionally while it is cooking. After about 20 minutes of cooking, carefully pour half of the soup into a blender or food processor. Process or blend the soup together until it is smooth.
2. As a substitute to this, note that you can make use of an immersion blender to process the soup until it is blended halfway. You can decide to process the soup a
3. bit more or less, depending on your preference and how you like the soup
4. If you used the non-emersion blender method, return the blended portion of the soup to the saucepan and reheat it when needed
5. Add fresh chopped cilantro, add more pepper, and hot sauce how you want it. Serve and enjoy!

Nutritional Value

Calories: 72
Carbs: 12G
Protein: 3g.
Fat: 3g
Fiber: 4g

471. Easy Vegetarian Pumpkin Soup

Ingredients (4 servings)

- 1 tablespoon of margarine
- 1 onion (diced)
- 1 16-ounce can of pumpkin puree
- 1 1/3 cups of vegetable broth
- ½ tablespoon of nutmeg
- ½ tablespoon of sugar
- Salt (to taste)
- Pepper (to taste)
- 3 cups of soymilk or any milk as a substitute

How to make

1. Using a large saucepan, add onion to margarine and cook it between 3 and 5 minutes until the onion is clear
2. Add pumpkin puree, vegetable broth, sugar, pepper, and other ingredients and stir to combine.

3. Cook in medium heat for between 10 and fifteen minutes
4. Before serving the soup, taste and add more spices, pepper, and salt if necessary
5. Serve soup and enjoy!

Nutritional Value

Calories: 118 Carbs: 16g Protein: 2G Fat: 6g Fiber: 3g

472. Gazpacho Soup

Ingredients (3 servings)

- 1 large cucumber (to be sliced into chunks)
- 4 big ripe tomatoes (coarsely chopped)
- ½ bell pepper (any color)
- 2 cloves of garlic (minced)
- 1 celery rib (chopped)
- 1 tablespoon of lemon juice
- ¼ tablespoon of celery pepper
- 1 tablespoon of fresh basil (chopped)
- 1 tablespoon of fresh parsley (chopped)
- Dash black pepper
- ½ tablespoon salt
- 3 tablespoons of red wine (vinegar/balsamic vinegar)
- ½ sweet onions (quartered)

How to make

1. To make the gazpacho place the cucumber chunks, chopped tomatoes, bell pepper, garlic, celery, lemon juice, and onion in the food processor or blender. You may choose to blend or process in batches if needed
2. Add the vinegar (red/balsamic), salt, pepper to the blender or food processor and blend or process together until it is smooth or nearly smooth (the texture depends on you)
3. The next step is to pour soup into a serving bowl and stir in the fresh chopped parsley and basil
4. Cover the serving bowl with plastic wrap or foil or cover it with a plastic wrap and put the bowl inside the refrigerator for about 30 minutes or until when you are set to serve the gazpacho soup.
5. You can decide to add some extra fresh herbs to the soup for presentation as well as some avocado slices or crusty croutons
6. Serve gazpacho soup with the following: green salad some artisanal or homemade bread as a substitute, balsamic vinegar, and

Desserts

olive oil for dipping for a light but complete meal.

7. Serve and enjoy!

Nutritional Value

- Calories: 87 Carbs: 18g Protein: 3g Fat: 1g Fiber: 2g
- Crockpot Vegetarian Split Pea Soup

Ingredients (8 servings)

- 2 cups of split pea soup (uncooked)
- 8 cups of vegetable broth (or water)
- 2 potatoes (chopped)
- 2 cubes of bouillon (vegetarian)
- Optional: 2 ribs of celery (chopped)
- 1 onion (diced)
- 2 cloves of garlic (minced)
- 2 carrots (sliced)
- 1 teaspoon of dry mustard
- 1 teaspoon of sage
- 1 teaspoon of thyme
- 1 teaspoon of cumin

How to make

1. Add peas, vegetable broth, and bouillon cubes in crock-pot or slow cooker. Stir it and break up the bouillon cubes a bit
2. Add chopped potatoes, onions, celery, carrot and garlic
3. Add mustard, cumin, sage, thyme, and bay leaves, and stir
4. Season soup lightly with salt and pepper
5. Cook for about 4 hours/till peas split
6. Taste and check seasoning
7. Serve, and enjoy!

Nutritional Value

Calories: 198
Fat: 5g
Carbs: 21g
Fiber: 7g
Protein: 18g

Desserts and Snacks

473. Crockpot Lasagna with Spinach Tofu

Ingredients (6 servings)

- 1 container of soft (silken) tofu
- 1 container firm or extra firm tofu
- ¼ cup of soy milk
- ½ teaspoon of garlic powder
- 2 teaspoon of lemon juice
- 3 teaspoons of fresh basil (chopped)
- 1 teaspoon of salt
- 2 (10-ounce) packages of frozen spinach (thawed and patted dry)
- 4 cups of tomato sauce
- 1 (10-ounce) box of lasagna noodles

How to make

1. Get a blender. Put silken tofu, firm or extra-firm tofu, soymilk, garlic powder, lemon juice, basil, and salt in the food processor or blender. Grind it together until it is very smooth. After grinding, add thawed spinach to the mixture.
2. Get a crockpot or slower cooker. Get a cup of tomato sauce. Put the tomato sauce in the bottom of the crockpot or slower cooker. Mix the spinach. Put 1/3 of the lasagna noodles on top of the sauce and 1/3 of the tofu and spinach mixture on top of the noodles. Now repeat the layers. Ensure that the sauce is on top.
3. In the crockpot, cook the noodles on very low heat between 6 and 8 hours. Or cook the noodles on very low heat till they are soft.
4. After cooking, put some nutritional yeast on top of the noodles. Serve, and enjoy.

474. Black Bean Veggie Burger

Ingredients (1 serving)

- ½ onion (chopped small)
- 1 (14-ounce) can of black beans (well-drained)
- 2 slices of bread (crumbled)
- ½ teaspoon of seasoned salt
- 1 teaspoon of garlic powder
- 1 teaspoon of onion powder
- ½ cup of flour
- Dash salt (to taste)
- Dash pepper (to taste)
- Oil for frying (divide)

How to make:

Desserts

1. Grease the bottom of a small frying pan and place it over medium-high heat. Combine onions and sauté and pour it in the small frying pan. Fry them until they are soft. This process usually takes between 3 and 5 minutes.

2. Get a large bowl. Mash the black beans inside it. Ensure that the beans are almost smooth.

3. Saute your onions and crumble the bread. In the bowl, add the sautéed onions, mashed black beans, crumbled bread, seasoned salt, garlic powder, and onion powder. Ensure you mix to combine well.

4. Add some flour to the ingredients by adding a teaspoon per time. Stir everything together until it is well combined. While mixing, make sure that it is very thick. To achieve this, you may want to use your hand to work your flour well.

5. Make the mixed black beans into patties. Ensure that each of the patties is approximately ½ inch thick. The best way to do this is to make a ball with the black beans. After doing this, flatten the ball gently. Place your frying pan on medium-low heat. Add some oil. Fry your black bean patties in the frying pan until it is slightly firm and lightly browned on each side. This usually takes about 3 minutes. Ensure you adjust the

6. head well because if the pan is too hot, the bean burgers will be brown in the middle and will not be well cooked in the middle.

7. To serve, assemble your veggie burgers and enjoy it with all the fixings. You can also serve also get a plate, serve them with a little ketchup or hot sauce or no bunds. To increase the nutrition of the meal, you can add a nice green salad.

8. Serve and enjoy!

Nutritional Value

Calories: 353
Fat: 10g
Carbs: 50g
Fiber: 15g
Protein: 16g

475. Blueberry Tofu Smoothie

Ingredients (1 serving)

- 6 ounces of silken tofu
- 1 medium banana
- 2/3 cups of soy milk
- 1 cup of frozen or fresh blueberries (divided)
- 1 tablespoon of honey

- 2-3 ice cubes (optional)

How to make

1. Drain the silken tofu in order to remove the excess water (silken tofu as a high water content)
2. Peele and slice the banana. Place the sliced banana on a baking sheet and freeze them. This process usually takes up to 15 minutes. This helps to make the smoothie thicker.
3. Get a blender. Blend the banana, tofu, and soy milk. This usually takes up to 30 seconds.
4. Add ½ cup of the blueberries to the banana, tofu, and soymilk. Then blend it until it is very smooth.
5. Put the remaining blueberries. Add honey and ice cubes. Blend it until it is well combined.
6. Serve and enjoy.

Nutritional Value

Calories: 365
Fat: 11g
Carbs: 43g
Fiber: 4g
Protein: 28g

476. Fluffy 1-Bowl Sugar Cookies

Ingredients (24 servings)

- ½ cup of softened butter
- ½ cup of organic cane sugar
- 1 tablespoon of vanilla extract
- 3 tablespoons of aquafupuaba
- ¾ tablespoon of baking powder
- ¼ tablespoon of sea salt
- 1 2/3 tablespoon of gluten-free flour blend
- 2/3 cups of almond flour
- 1/3 cup of cornstarch or arrowroot
- 1 tablespoon of unsweetened almond milk Frosting (optional)
- ½ cup of powder
- 1 ½ cup of sifted organic powdered sugar
- ¼ tablespoon of vanilla extract
- 1-3 tablespoon of unsweetened almond milk
- Natural food dye

How to make

1. Get an oven, preheat the oven to 350 degrees F (176 C). Put two baking sheets inside the oven
2. Soften your butter in a large mixing bowl. Beat or whisk the butter until it is creamy and smooth. Do this for about a minutes. Be careful so that the better is not melted or cold.
3. Add some sugar to the butter. Mix it over medium speed until it

Desserts

becomes and light. This usually takes 1 minute. Add chickpeas brine and vanilla. Mix again until it is very smooth

4. Add sea salt and baking powder. Blend or whisk to so the ingredients will mix very well. Ass gluten-free flour blend, almond flour, and corn starch and blend. Ensure that the ingredients are well mixed. If desired, you can use a wooden spoon to mix. Add almond milk and stir again.

5. Now, the dough should be very thick, moldable, and a bit difficult to mix. If it is too soft, add a mixture of the gluten-free flour blend, almond flour, and cornstarch

6. until it is thick. If it is too thick, mix with extra almond milk.

7. Put the dough in the refrigerator and let it chill. This usually takes 25 minutes. Then use a scooper or a tablespoon to measure out 1 ½ tablespoon of the dough. Roll it carefully to make balls. Be careful because the dough will still be soft. Arrange these balls on the parchment-lined baking sheets. Leave the space of an inch between them. Use your palm to press each of the balls and slightly smash the balls.

8. As an alternative. Make a well-floured surface. Roll the dough on this surface until it is about ¼ inch thick. Press the cookie cutters into the dough. Ensure that the cutters dipped into gluten-free flour. Use the floured spatula to scoop on the baking sheets. This procedure works whether you are using the cut-out method or traditional circles.

9. Bake the cookies. This should take 10 minutes. Make sure they are fluffy and that their edges are starting to become dried out. Leave it on the baking sheet for about 10 minutes for it to cool then transfer it to a plate for it to be completely cool.

10. To make frosting (optional). Get a mixing bowl. Add softened butter. Whisk or beat it until it is soft and fluffy. This should take about 1 minute. Pour some powdered sugar into the bowl and whip. Add the vanilla

11. extract and whisk. Keep adding sugar and whisking until the frosting can be separated. If you want a thinner frosting, add some almond milk to it. When it is too thick, add more almond milk. If you

want, add some food coloring now.

12. Frost the cookies or leave it to be plain.

Nutritional value

Calories: 122
Carbs: 17g
Protein: 2G
Fat: 5g
Fiber: 1g

477. Banana Cream Pie

Ingredients (8 servings) Crust

- ¾ cup of gluten-free rolled oats
- ¾ cup of raw almond
- ¼ teaspoon full of salt (optional)
- 2 tablespoon of organic sugar cane or coconut sugar
- ¼ cups of melted coconut oil
Filling
- 2 tablespoons of cornstarch
- 1/3 cups of organic sugar cane or sub coconut sugar
- 1 pinch of sea salt (optional)
- 1 ½ cups of unsweetened plain almond milk
- 1 tablespoon of pure vanilla extract
- 1 medium just-ripe banana (sliced)
Coconut Whip
- 1 14-ounce can of coconut cream (or two cans full of full-fat Coconut milk per one can of coconut cream, refrigerated overnight)
- ½ tablespoon of vanilla extract
- 3-5 tablespoon of organic powdered sugar

For Toppings
- Coconut Whipped Cream
- 1-2 more just ripe bananas (sliced)

How to make

1. Preheat oven to 350 degrees F (176 C). Then put parchment paper on an 8-by-8-inch baking dish or as an alternation, grease a standard pie dish and set it aside.
2. Get a high-speed blender. Add oats, almonds, sea salts (optional) and sugar. Blend these ingredients on high speed until it is very smooth.
3. Add melted coconut oil. Blend until the ingredient forms a loose dough. Scrape down the sides if you want. You should be able to form a dough by squeezing the mixture with two fingers instead of crumbling it. Add extra melted coconut if the dough is too dry.
4. Get a pie can or baking dish. Pour the mixture and spread it evenly. Find an object with a flat bottom such as a drinking glass. Use it to

Desserts

press the parchment paper on top. Make sure that it is uniform and well pack in the up and bottom sides.

5. Bake dough for 15 minutes. Increase the heat to 375 F (190 C). Bake for an additional 10 minutes till the edges are golden brown and there is some browning on the

6. surface. Remove the dough from the oven and allow it to cool.

7. Add cornstarch, sugar, and salt together in a small saucepan. Add some almond milk to it to prevent clumps

8. Place the pudding on medium heat. When it is bubbling and whisking frequently, reduce the heat and keep cooking for 4 minutes. Ensure that you use a rubber spatula to scrape the sides and bottom of the pan from time to time.

9. Remove from heat when visible ribbon forms when you drizzle some over the top with your spatula. Add some vanilla and let it cool for 10 minutes. Get a glass or ceramic bowl. Transfer it into this glass and cover with a plastic wrap. Ensure the wrap is touching the surface. Refrigerate until it is cool. This should take between 2 and 3 hours.

10. Get a medium-large glass mixing bowl and put it in the freezer. Remove the coconut cream can from the fridge. Make sure you don't remove the top by shaking or turning it. Scoop the hardened surface into the chilled bowl. Ensure that you leave out the watery liquid potion. This is useful for smoothies or baking.

11. Get a hand-held mixer. Use the mixer to whip the coconut cream till it starts looking like whipped cream. Do this for a minute. Add vanilla extract and some

12. powdered sugar. Beat the cream until it is airy and light. Do this for 3 minutes then put in the refrigerator.

13. When the pudding is very cool, add some coconut whipped cream and mix it together until it is well combined. Put it in the refrigerator.

14. Get sliced bananas, add it to the bottom of the baked crust. Add crusted-coconut whip mixture. Smooth the top with a spoon, cover with plastic wrap and put it in the refrigerator. Let it cool for 4 hours.

15. Serve with whipped coconut cream and sliced bananas.

16. Serve and enjoy!

Nutritional Value

Calories: 230
Fat: 12G
Carbs: 29g
Fiber: 2g
Protein: 3g

478. Gluten-Free Black Beans Brownies

Ingredients (12 servings)

- 1 15-oz can of black beans
- 2 large flax eggs
- 3 tablespoon of coconut oil
- ¾ cup cocoa powder
- ¼ tablespoon of salt
- 1 tablespoon pure vanilla extract
- ½ cup of organic cane sugar
- 1 ½ tablespoon of baking powder
  Toppings
- Crushed walnuts
- Pecans
- Daily-free semisweet chocolate chips

How to make

1. Preheat the oven to 350 degrees F, prepare a baking dish lined with parchment paper.
2. Get a 12-slot standard size muffin pot and grease. Rinse your black beans well and drain.
3. Get the bowl of a food processor and prepare flax egg
4. Leave out walnuts and other toppings and add the remaining ingredients and purre
5. If the batter is too thick, add 1 or 2 tablespoons of water.
6. Get the muffin tin and pour the batter in it. Ensure that the top is smooth
7. Bake the batter until the tops are dry, and the edges start to pull away from the sides. This takes 25 minutes.
8. Remove the pan and let it cool
9. Serve and enjoy!

Nutritional Value

Calories: 113
Fat: 5g
Carbs: 18g
Fiber: 3g
Protein: 3g

479. Tahini Chocolate Banana Soft Serve

Ingredients (2 servings)

- 2 cups of ripe sliced frozen bananas
- 2 tablespoons of tahini
- 3 tablespoons cacao

Desserts

- 1-2 tablespoons of maple syrup
- 1-2 pitted dates (optional)
- 1 tablespoon vanilla extract (optional)
- 1 pinch of salt (optional) For Toppings (optional)
- 1-2 tablespoon of magic shell

How to make

1. Get a high-speed blender. Add sliced frozen bananas. Blend until it is creamy.
2. Add tahini, cacao powder, and maple syrup and blend. You can also add vanilla extract or a pinch of sea salt for more flavor. Ensure they are well mixed
3. Transfer it into serving bowls. Serve and enjoy!

Nutritional Value

Calories: 304
Fat: 19g
Carbs: 34g -
Fiber: 8g -
Protein: 3g

480. Raw Oreos

Ingredients (35 servings) FILLING

- 1 cup of coconut butter
- ¼ teaspoon of vanilla extract
- Organic powdered sweetener (to taste) COOKIE
- 1 ½ cups of raw almond or walnuts
- 6-7 whole Medjool or deglet nour dates
- 3 tablespoon of melted coconut oil
- 1 tablespoon of syrup
- 1/3 cup of cocoa powder
- 1 pinch of sea salt

How to make

1. Add coconut butter and vanilla and sweetener to taste. Set it aside
2. Add nuts and pulse. Add dates, coconut oil, maple syrup, cocoa powder, salt, and blend it well.
3. Add more cocoa powder for chocolate flavor and dates for sweetness and salt
4. Get a cutting board, line it with parchment or wax paper. Place dough in the center. Form in a 1-inch disc and top with a piece of wax paper
5. Roll dough into a ¼-inch-thick rectangle. Remove top wax paper. Use a cookie cutter to cut the dough
6. Use a spatula to transfer cookie on a flat plate. Put the plate in the freezer for 10-15 minutes
7. Add coconut butter with half of the

cookies. Put it back in the freezer for about some time and add coconut butter to the other half

Nutritional Value

Calories: 140
Fat: 7g
Carbs: 20g
Fiber: 1g
Protein: 0g

481. Peanut Butter Cup Cookies

Ingredients (18 servings)

- ½ cup of softened butter
- 2/3 cup of organic cane sugar
- 1 tablespoon of vanilla extract
- 3 tablespoons of aquafaba
- ¼ cup of salted creamy peanut butter
- ¾ tablespoon of baking powder
- 1 pinch of sea salt
- 2/3 cup of almond flour
- ¼ cup of cornstarch or arrowroot
- 1 1/3 cup of gluten-free flour blend
- 15-18 mini peanut butter cups

How to make

1. Pre-heat oven to 375 degrees F (190 C). Put parchment paper on two baking sheets
2. Get a mixing bowl and add softened butter
3. Add sugar and mix until it is fluffy. Add vanilla and chickpea, peanut butter, and mix very well. Add baking powder
4. The dough should be thick by now. Put it in the refrigerator for 5 minutes.
5. Use a scooper to measure out 1 ½ tablespoon of dough. Roll it into balls and place them on baking sheets. Smash them slightly with your palm
6. Bake until the edges are starting to dry out. Remove from oven and press an unwrapped peanuts butter in the middle of the cookie. Don't crack too much. Transfer them to a wire rack

Nutritional Value

Calories: 115
Fat: 6g
Carbs: 14g
Fiber: 0.6 g -
Protein: 3g

482. Gluten-Free Cinnamon Rolls

Ingredients (7 servings) WET

- ¾ scant cup of unsweetened almond milk
- 2 tablespoon of organic cane sugar
- 1 tablespoon of butter
- 1 packet of active dry yeast DRY

Desserts

- 2 cups of DIY gluten-free flour blend
- ¾ cup of almond flour
- 2 tablespoon of sea salt
- 4 tablespoons of butter FILLING
- 3 tablespoons of melted butter
- 2/3 of organic brown sugar
- 1 tablespoon of ground cinnamon FROSTING
- cream cheese frosting
- Simple powdered sugar glaze

How to make

1. Preheat oven to 350 degrees F (176 C). Use butter oil to coat baking dish
2. Heat the dairy-free milk. Ensure you do not overheat as this may kill the yeast
3. Add butter and sugar to the dairy milk. Add yeast and stir. Leave it for some time until the surface is puffy
4. Whisk together gluten-free flour blend, almond flour, cane sugar, baking powder, and sea salt. Use a fork to mix the ingredients
5. To dry the ingredients, add the almond milk mixture and stir. A dough that looks like moist will be formed. Set it aside
6. Get a large cutting board and wrap it with a plastic wrap. Clean the surface and add gluten-free flour to it.
7. Put the dough in the center of the surface and cover it with another plastic wrap. Roll the dough to a large rectangle shape with the rolling pin.
8. Remove the top plastic wrap and brush on the butter. Sprinkle brown sugar and cinnamon on it with your finger. Make sure it is uniform. Remove the bottom wrap from the cutting board. Use it to roll the dough into a cylinder.
9. Use the serrated knife to cut the dough into equal rolls. Carefully transfer it inside the pie dish or cake pan
10. Cover it with a plastic wrap and towel. Put it in a warm oven and let it rise till the rolls are almost touching.
11. Remove the wrap and towel. Put the rolls on the center rack of the oven. Bake. This usually takes 30-35 minutes.
12. Let the rolls cool for like 20 minutes before frosting.

Nutritional Value

Calories: 429
Fat: 17g
Carbs: 69g
Fiber: 5g
Protein: 6g

Made in the USA
Middletown, DE
22 August 2020